Sarcoma

Editor

ANDREW J. WAGNER

HEMATOLOGY/ONCOLOGY CLINICS OF NORTH AMERICA

www.hemonc.theclinics.com

Consulting Editors
GEORGE P. CANELLOS
H. FRANKLIN BUNN

October 2013 • Volume 27 • Number 5

ELSEVIER

1600 John F. Kennedy Boulevard • Suite 1800 • Philadelphia, Pennsylvania, 19103-2899

http://www.theclinics.com

HEMATOLOGY/ONCOLOGY CLINICS OF NORTH AMERICA Volume 27, Number 5
October 2013 ISSN 0889-8588, ISBN 13: 978-0-323-26100-5

Editor: Patrick Manley
Developmental Editor: Donald Mumford

Hematology/Oncology Clinics (ISSN 0889-8588) is published bimonthly by Elsevier Inc., 360 Park Avenue South, NewYork, NY10010-1710. Months of issue are February, April, June, August, October, and December. Business and Editorial Offices: 1600 John F. Kennedy Blvd., Ste. 1800, Philadelphia, PA 19103–2899. Customer Service Office: 3251 Riverport Lane, Maryland Heights, MO63043. Periodicals postage paid at New York, NY and at additional mailing offices. Subscription prices are $367.00 per year (domestic individuals), $599.00 per year (domestic institutions), $179.00 per year (domestic students/residents), $417.00 per year (Canadian individuals), $732.00 per year (Canadian institutions) $496.00 per year (international individuals), $732.00 per year (international institutions), and $241.00 per year (international and Canadian students/residents). International air speed delivery is included in all *Clinics* subscription prices. All prices are subject to change without notice. **POSTMASTER:** Send address changes to *Hematology/Oncology Clinics of North America*, Elsevier Health Sciences Division, Subscription Customer Service, 3251 Riverport Lane, Maryland Heights, MO 63043. Customer Service (orders, claims, online, change of address): Elsevier Health Sciences Division, Subscription Customer Service, 3251 Riverport Lane, Maryland Heights, MO 63043. Tel: 1-800-654-2452 (U.S. and Canada); 314-447-8871 (outside U.S. and Canada). Fax: 314-447-8029. E-mail: journalscustomerservice-usa@elsevier.com (for print support); journalsonlinesupport-usa@elsevier.com (for online support).

Reprints. For copies of 100 or more, of articles in this publication, please contact the Commercial Reprints Department, Elsevier Inc., 360 Park Avenue South, New York, New York 10010-1710; Tel.: 212-633-3874, Fax: 212-633-3820, E-mail: reprints@elsevier.com.

Hematology/Oncology Clinics of North America is covered in *MEDLINE/PubMed (Index Medicus), EMBASE/ Excerpta Medica, and BIOSIS.*

Printed and bound by CPI Group (UK) Ltd, Croydon, CR0 4YY

Transferred to digital print 2012

Contributors

CONSULTING EDITORS

GEORGE P. CANELLOS, MD
William Rosenberg Professor of Medicine, Department of Medical Oncology, Dana-Farber Cancer Institute, Boston, Massachusetts

H. FRANKLIN BUNN, MD
Professor of Medicine, Division of Hematology, Brigham and Women's Hospital, Harvard Medical School, Boston, Massachusetts

EDITOR

ANDREW J. WAGNER, MD, PhD
Assistant Professor of Medicine, Harvard Medical School, Dana-Farber Cancer Institute, Boston, Massachusetts

AUTHORS

JAKOB K. ANNINGA, MD, PhD
Department of Clinical Oncology, Leiden University Medical Center, Leiden, The Netherlands

CRISTINA R. ANTONESCU, MD
Professor, Department of Pathology, Memorial Sloan-Kettering Cancer Center, New York, New York

CHRISTINE M. BARNETT, MD
Fellow, Hematology and Medical Oncology, Division of Hematology/Oncology, Portland VA Medical Center, OHSU Knight Cancer Institute, Oregon Health and Science University, Portland, Oregon

SEBASTIAN BAUER, MD
Associate Professor, Department of Medical Oncology, Director, Sarcoma Center, West German Cancer Center, University Hospital Essen, University of Duisburg-Essen, Essen, Germany

JUDITH V.M.G. BOVÉE, MD, PhD
Professor, Department of Pathology, Leiden University Medical Center, Leiden, The Netherlands

PAOLO G. CASALI, MD
Adult Sarcoma Medical Oncology Unit, Department of Cancer Medicine, Fondazione IRCCS Istituto Nazionale Tumori, Milan, Italy

PHILIPPE A. CASSIER, MD
Department of Medical Oncology, Léon Bérard Cancer Center, Lyon, France

EDWIN CHOY, MD, PhD
Assistant Professor in Medicine, Division of Hematology Oncology, Yawkey Center for Outpatient Care, Massachusetts General Hospital, Harvard Medical School, Boston, Massachusetts

RASHMI CHUGH, MD
Assistant Professor, Division of Hematology/Oncology, Department of Internal Medicine, University of Michigan, Ann Arbor, Michigan

ANGELA CIOFFI, MD
Research Clinical Oncologist, Departments of Medicine and Pediatrics, Mount Sinai School of Medicine, New York, New York

ANNE-MARIE CLETON-JANSEN, PhD
Department of Pathology, Leiden University Medical Center, Leiden, The Netherlands

CHRISTOPHER L. CORLESS, MD, PhD
Professor, Department of Pathology, OHSU Knight Cancer Institute, Oregon Health and Science University, Portland, Oregon

GREGORY M. COTE, MD, PhD
Instructor in Medicine, Division of Hematology Oncology, Yawkey Center for Outpatient Care, Massachusetts General Hospital, Harvard Medical School, Boston, Massachusetts

ANGELO P. DEI TOS, MD
Anatomic Pathology, Department of Oncology, General Hospital of Treviso, Treviso, Italy

SUMANA DEVATA, MD
Hematology/Oncology Fellow, Division of Hematology/Oncology, Department of Internal Medicine, University of Michigan, Ann Arbor, Michigan

HANS GELDERBLOM, MD, PhD
Professor, Department of Clinical Oncology, Leiden University Medical Center, Leiden, The Netherlands

SUZANNE GEORGE, MD
Clinical Director, Senior Physician, Center for Sarcoma and Bone Oncology, Dana-Farber Cancer Institute, Assistant Professor of Medicine, Harvard Medical School, Boston, Massachusetts

ALESSANDRO GRONCHI, MD
Department of Surgery, Sarcoma Service, Fondazione IRCCS Istituto Nazionale dei Tumori, Milan, Italy

MICHAEL C. HEINRICH, MD
Professor, Division of Hematology/Oncology, Departments of Medicine and Cell and Developmental Biology, Portland VA Medical Center, OHSU Knight Cancer Institute, Oregon Health and Science University, Portland, Oregon

JOERN HENZE, MD
Department of Medical Oncology, Sarcoma Center, West German Cancer Center, University Hospital Essen, University of Duisburg-Essen, Essen, Germany

HEIKKI JOENSUU, PhD, MD
Professor of Oncology, Physician-in-Chief, Department of Oncology, Helsinki University Central Hospital, Helsinki University, Helsinki, Finland

ALICE LEVARD, MD
Department of Medical Oncology, Léon Bérard Cancer Center, Lyon, France

ROBERT G. MAKI, MD, PhD, FACP
Professor of Medicine, Pediatrics, and Orthopaedics, Tisch Cancer Institute, Mount Sinai School of Medicine, New York, New York

ANDREA MARRARI, MD
Adult Sarcoma Medical Oncology Unit, Department of Cancer Medicine, Fondazione IRCCS Istituto Nazionale Tumori, Milan, Italy

CHANDRAJIT P. RAUT, MD, MSc
Department of Surgery, Brigham and Women's Hospital; Center for Sarcoma and Bone Oncology, Dana-Farber Cancer Institute; Associate Professor of Surgery, Harvard Medical School, Boston, Massachusetts

SONIA REICHERT, MD
Medical Oncology Fellow, Department of Medicine, Mount Sinai School of Medicine, New York, New York

CÉSAR SERRANO, MD
Fletcher Laboratory, Postdoctoral Research Fellow, Department of Pathology, Brigham and Women's Hospital, Harvard Medical School; Clinical Research Fellow, Center for Sarcoma and Bone Oncology, Dana-Farber Cancer Institute, Harvard Medical School, Boston, Massachusetts

SILVIA STACCHIOTTI, MD
Adult Sarcoma Medical Oncology Unit, Department of Cancer Medicine, Fondazione IRCCS Istituto Nazionale Tumori, Milan, Italy

LOUIS TASSY, MD
Department of Medical Oncology, Léon Bérard Cancer Center, Lyon, France

JOSEPH VADAKARA, MD
Fellow, Department of Medical Oncology, Fox Chase Cancer Center, Philadelphia, Pennsylvania

JOLIEKE G. VAN OOSTERWIJK, MSc
Department of Pathology, Leiden University Medical Center, Leiden, The Netherlands

MARGARET VON MEHREN, MD
Professor, Department of Medical Oncology, Fox Chase Cancer Center, Philadelphia, Pennsylvania

Contents

> Mutation-activated signaling from the KIT and PDGFRA kinases has been
> successfully targeted in gastrointestinal stromal tumors (GISTs), with sub-
> tle differences between the mutations serving to refine prognosis and more
> precisely tailor therapy. There is a growing understanding of the molecular
> drivers of GISTs lacking mutations in KIT or PDGFRA, so called wild-type
> GISTs, further aiding in management decisions. This article provides an
> overview of all the known molecular subtypes of GIST and provides infor-
> mation about clinical correlates, treatment, and prognosis depending on
> the subtype.

> Adjuvant imatinib prolongs recurrence-free survival and probably overall
> survival of patients who have undergone surgery for gastrointestinal stromal
> tumor (GIST). Estimation of the risk of recurrence with a prognostication tool
> and tumor mutation analysis is essential before imatinib initiation, because
> approximately 60% of patients with GIST with operable tumor are cured by
> surgery alone and some mutated tyrosine kinases are insensitive to imati-
> nib. Adjuvant imatinib is usually administered for 3 years at the dose of
> 400 mg once daily. Early detection of tumors that recur despite adjuvant
> therapy with longitudinal imaging of the abdomen is likely beneficial.

> Gastrointestinal stromal tumors (GIST) are the most common mesenchy-
> mal tumors of the gastrointestinal tract. Before the advent of tyrosine kinase
> inhibitors (TKIs) there were few treatment options available to patients with
> metastatic GIST. Surgery was the mainstay of treatment and the prognosis
> was dismal. With the advent of imatinib and second-line TKIs the prognosis
> of metastatic GIST has improved dramatically; however, there is still a need
> for therapies for patients with disease refractory to TKI therapy. Newer
> agents are under investigation and may have promise. This article dis-
> cusses the current standard of care in terms of standard and investigational
> pharmacotherapy in the management of metastatic GIST.

> Surgery remains the only potentially curative therapy in the management of
> localized adult soft tissue sarcomas and gastrointestinal stromal tumors.

There are over 50 different unique histologic types of soft tissue sarcomas, with different patterns of recurrence and prognosis. Surgical principles and sensitivity to locoregional and systemic treatments vary considerably based on the histologic type and anatomic location, as discussed in detail in this review.

Liposarcoma is one of the most common sarcoma subtypes with a heterogeneous biology and clinical behavior. This article gives a comprehensive overview on clinically relevant aspects of pathology and imaging. Prognostic factors and treatment strategies are discussed for different clinical situations and histologic subtypes. This information will be of value to clinicians and interdisciplinary sarcoma teams.

This article presents an overview of the current literature about the biology, pathology, and the clinical management of leiomyosarcoma. In addition, the article emphasizes and discusses the current systemic treatment options available for patients with leiomyosarcoma, which range from cytotoxic chemotherapy to target therapies. Particular leiomyosarcoma subtypes, such as uterine leiomyosarcoma and inferior vena cava leiomyosarcoma, are discussed separately.

Although benign hemangiomas are among the most common diagnoses among connective tissue tumors, angiosarcomas and other sarcomas arising from blood vessels are rare, even among sarcomas. Because endothelial tumors have unique embryonal derivation compared with other sarcomas, it is not surprising they have unique characteristics. Herein are reviewed some of these unique characteristics and therapeutic options for patients with some of these diagnoses, highlighting the potential of new agents for these tumors, which will in all likelihood also impact treatment on more common cancers.

Desmoid tumors are rare, clonal collections of benign fibrous tissue that exhibit a highly variable clinical course. This article presents a comprehensive review of desmoid tumors and summarizes the current literature pertaining to clinical presentation, diagnostic modalities, pathogenesis, prognostic factors, and management options.

The improvement in outcome for patients with localized and metastatic Ewing sarcoma since the development of cytotoxic chemotherapy remains one of the most profound advances in oncology and one of the proudest achievements of sarcoma researchers. Identification of molecular targets for new treatments has become an intense area within Ewing sarcoma research. The development of improved preclinical Ewing sarcoma models and advanced molecular techniques will build on knowledge of EWS/FLI1 function, EWS/FLI1 transcription targets, and the other critical driver events in these tumors.

HEMATOLOGY/ONCOLOGY CLINICS OF NORTH AMERICA

Preface

Sarcoma

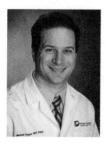

Andrew J. Wagner, MD, PhD
Editor

Our understanding of the biology and treatment of sarcomas has blossomed over the last few decades, led by the evolution of improved diagnostic techniques, classification of tumors, understanding of their behavior, and the molecular identification of translocations, mutations, and other genetic drivers. Whereas most past sarcoma clinical studies tended to lump sarcomas into one malignant entity, often because of the rarity of the subtypes, the establishment and collaboration of international centers that focus on sarcoma have permitted the rapid study of smaller and better defined subsets of disease.

The markedly improved treatment of advanced gastrointestinal stromal tumor (GIST) that quickly followed the identification of KIT mutations serves as a paradigm-changing approach to the management of nearly all solid tumors. Subsequent studies provided prognostic information for the risk of tumor recurrence and predictive information for the treatment response of tumors, led the way for the development of other lines of systemic therapy, and helped to guide surgical management of disease. On the basis of these approaches to GIST treatment and in parallel with these discoveries, key diagnostic, pathogenic, and therapeutic advances have been made in other sarcoma subtypes with continued promise for new findings and improved outcomes.

These topics are reviewed in this issue of *Hematology/Oncology Clinics of North America*, with articles contributed by a collection of international authors expert in the diagnosis and management of sarcomas. I am grateful for their contributions as well as for the editorial assistance of Patrick Manley and his staff at Elsevier for their support in putting together this issue. With further work in this field, I look forward to

Hematol Oncol Clin N Am 27 (2013) xi–xii
http://dx.doi.org/10.1016/j.hoc.2013.08.001
0889-8588/13/$ – see front matter

a future edition that recapitulates and extends the success seen to date in GIST in other sarcoma subtypes.

Andrew J. Wagner, MD, PhD
Harvard Medical School
Dana-Farber Cancer Institute
450 Brookline Avenue
Boston, MA 02215, USA

E-mail address:
andrew_wagner@dfci.harvard.edu

Gastrointestinal Stromal Tumors
Molecular Markers and Genetic Subtypes

Christine M. Barnett, MD[a], Christopher L. Corless, MD, PhD[b],
Michael C. Heinrich, MD[c,d],*

KEYWORDS

- GIST • KIT • PDGFRA • RTK-wild-type • SDH

KEY POINTS

- Recent advances in the knowledge of gastrointestinal stromal tumors (GISTs) have been translated into improved diagnosis and treatment.
- The current understanding is that GISTs represent a heterogeneous collection of molecular entities linked by a common histology and presumed cell of origin.
- Most GISTs are driven by a pathogenic mutant kinase, but other disease-initiating molecular abnormalities have been identified.
- The type of underlying molecular defect in a given patient's GIST has a significant impact on treatment response and potential mechanisms of primary and secondary resistance.

Gastrointestinal stromal tumors (GISTs) were not widely recognized before 1998. They are now regarded as the most common mesenchymal tumor of the gastrointestinal (GI) tract, with an incidence of more than 5000 cases per year in the United States. These tumors have become a paradigm for the expanding use of gene-based

Disclosures: None (C.M. Barnett); honoraria from Novartis; consulting fees from Novartis and Pfizer; research support from Novartis, Pfizer, and Bayer (C.L. Corless); honoraria from Onyx; consulting fees from Novartis, Pfizer, Ariad, MolecularMD; research support from Novartis, Pfizer, AROG, Ariad, Imclone; equity interest: MolecularMD (M.C. Heinrich).
^a Hematology and Medical Oncology, Division of Hematology/Oncology, Portland VA Medical Center, OHSU Knight Cancer Institute, Oregon Health & Science University, Mail Code L586, 3181 Southwest Sam Jackson Park Road, Portland, OR 97239, USA; ^b Department of Pathology, OHSU Knight Cancer Institute, Oregon Health & Science University, 3181 Southwest Sam Jackson Park Road, Mail Code L-471, Portland, OR 97239, USA; ^c Division of Hematology/Oncology, Department of Medicine, Portland VA Medical Center, OHSU Knight Cancer Institute, Oregon Health & Science University, R&D-19 3710, U.S. Veterans Hospital Road, Portland, OR 97239, USA; ^d Division of Hematology/Oncology, Department of Cell and Developmental Biology, Portland VA Medical Center, OHSU Knight Cancer Institute, Oregon Health & Science University, R&D-19 3710, U.S. Veterans Hospital Road, Portland, OR 97239, USA
* Corresponding author. Division of Hematology/Oncology, Department of Cell and Developmental Biology, Portland VA Medical Center, OHSU Knight Cancer Institute, Oregon Health & Science University, R&D-19 3710, U.S. Veterans Hospital Road, Portland, OR 97239.
E-mail address: heinrich@ohsu.edu

Hematol Oncol Clin N Am 27 (2013) 871–888
http://dx.doi.org/10.1016/j.hoc.2013.07.003
0889-8588/13/$ – see front matter Published by Elsevier Inc.

diagnostics and molecularly targeted therapies. This review focuses on recent advances in our understanding of GIST biology and how this knowledge has been translated into improved diagnosis and treatment. In addition, the evolving molecular classification of GIST is updated, with particular emphasis on those 10% to 15% of GISTs that lack gain-of-function KIT or platelet-derived growth factor receptor α (PDGFRA) receptor tyrosine kinase (RTK) mutations. These GISTs were previously classified as wild-type (WT) GIST, but we now propose the use of the term RTK-WT as a more accurate subclassification of this group of GISTs.

PATHOLOGY AND DIAGNOSIS

GISTs most commonly arise in the stomach (60%) but also present in the small intestine (25%), rectum (5%), and other sites along the GI tract, including the esophagus, colon, appendix, and gallbladder. Rarely, the tumors appear unattached from the GI tract. These so-called extraintestinal GISTs may occupy the mesentery or omentum. GISTs are rare outside the abdominal cavity, but there is a well-documented report of a primary GIST of the pleura.[1]

Historically, GISTs were considered to be sarcomas of smooth muscle origin, because of their predominantly spindle cell morphology and their association with the muscularis propria. However, studies using electron microscopy and immunohistochemistry suggested that these tumors differ from classic leiomyosarcoma, and in 1983, Mazur and Clark[2] proposed the term stromal tumor. The subsequent discovery that most stromal tumors arising in the GI tract were CD34-positive provided further support for their distinction from leiomyosarcoma.

During the 1990s, several investigators noted similarities between GISTs and a little known population of cells in the gut wall designated as the interstitial cells of Cajal (ICCs). ICCs are now known to serve as pacemakers for peristaltic gut contractions. Studies during this period showed that ICCs express KIT tyrosine kinase (CD117) and are developmentally dependent on stem cell factor (SCF) signaling through this kinase.[3] This finding led to the observation by 2 different groups in 1998 that GISTs commonly express CD117.[4,5] It is now well established that 95% of GISTs are immunohistochemically positive for CD117.

In 2004, DOG-1 (also known as anoctamin 1) was described as another high-specific marker for GISTs.[6] DOG-1 is a calcium-activated chloride channel that is highly expressed in ICCs and is detectable in 98% of GISTs, regardless of CD117 expression.[7] Only a small percentage of other sarcomas stain positively for DOG-1. The combination of CD117 and DOG-1 expression is essentially diagnostic for GIST.[6,7]

The use of CD117 and DOG-1 has helped define the range of morphologies associated with GIST. Although most GISTs are composed of a uniform population of spindled cells, some have an epithelioid appearance and others comprise a mixture of spindled and epithelioid cells. Tumor cellularity varies widely among GISTs. Low-grade lesions may show areas of central calcification, or show a bandlike alignment of nuclei that mimics a schwannoma. High-grade tumors often ulcerate the overlying mucosa and may undergo significant hemorrhagic necrosis. The variety in GIST histology dictates a broad morphologic differential (**Table 1**). Spindle cell GISTs should be distinguished from nerve sheath tumors and smooth muscle neoplasms, whereas epithelioid GISTs may resemble malignant melanoma, paraganglioma, or carcinoid tumor. Judicious use of immunohistochemistry is key to establishing an accurate diagnosis.

Table 1
GIST pathologic mimics

Tumor	Primary Morphology	Distinguishing Features	Immunomarkers	Other Information
Schwannomas	Spindle cells	Wavy fascicles; peripheral cuff of lymphocytes	Strong S-100 positivity	—
Desmoid fibromatosis	Spindle cells	Collagenous matrix	Nuclear β-catenin positivity in 75%	
Inflammatory myofibroblastic	Fascicular	Plasma cell-rich inflammatory infiltrate	ALK expression in 50%	Children and young adults
Smooth muscle tumors	Spindle cells	Bright eosinophilic cytoplasm; well-defined cell borders	Desmin positive	—
Dedifferentiated liposarcoma	Spindle cells	Pleomorphic nuclei	MDM2; CDK4	—
Malignant melanoma	Variable	Intranuclear inclusions	Melan-A, HMB45, S-100	50% are CD117 positive
Angiosarcoma	Spindle cells	Highly vascular	CD31	Commonly CD117 positive
Sarcomatoid carcinoma	Spindle cells	Prominent nucleoli; chromatin clearing	Cytokeratins	—
Carcinoid tumors	Epithelioid cells	Nested; stippled chromatin pattern	Synaptophysin, chromogranin	—
Paraganglioma	Epithelioid cells	Nested	Synaptophysin; S-100	—
PECOMA	Epithelioid cells	—	HMB45	—

In 2008, a subset of GISTs was found to be immunohistochemically negative for the expression of succinate dehydrogenase subunit B (SDHB).[8] Further studies have shown that some tumors also lack succinate dehydrogenase subunit A (SDHA) staining. The implications of these findings are discussed later.

Once a diagnosis of primary GIST has been established, the prognosis of the tumor can be assessed by taking into account 3 pathologic features: tumor size, site of origin, and mitotic index. In general, tumors arising in the stomach are less likely to recur than those arising in the small intestine or rectum. Tumors larger than 5 cm are more prone to recur or metastasize, as are tumors with more than 5 mitoses in 5 mm². Tumor rupture before or during surgery is associated with a high rate of recurrence. Several risk assessment tools that incorporate these factors have been developed.[9–11]

MOLECULAR TYPES OF GIST

In 1998, Hirota and colleagues[4] published the first report of gain-of-function mutations of KIT in GIST. KIT is the most commonly mutated oncogene in GIST, with 75% to 80% of GISTs harboring such mutations. Subsequently, it was discovered that approximately 10% of GISTs have homologous gain-of-function mutations in the PDGFRA RTK, which is a member of the same RTK family as KIT. The remaining 10% to 15% of GISTs lack mutations in either PDGFRA or KIT, and have commonly been designated as WT GIST. Recently, several other oncogenic mutations have been found in these tumors, leading us to propose that such tumors be designated as RTK-WT GIST. The molecular subtypes of GIST serve as a classification system that is useful for diagnostic, prognostic, and treatment planning purposes (**Table 2**).

KIT-mutant GIST

KIT is a type III RTK, belonging to a family that includes PDGFRA and B, CSF1R, and FLT3. Binding of dimeric SCF to the extracellular domain of KIT results in receptor

Table 2
Molecular classification of GISTs

Genetic Type	Relative Frequency (%)	Anatomic Distribution	Notable Features
KIT mutation	77	—	—
Exon 8	Rare	Small bowel	
Exon 9	8	Small bowel, colon	Better responses higher-dose imatinib
Exon 11	67	All sites	Respond well to imatinib
Exon 13	1	All sites	Imatinib responsive
Exon 17	1	All sites	Many are imatinib sensitive
PDGFRA mutation	10	—	—
Exon 12	1	All sites	Sensitive to imatinib
Exon 14	<1	Stomach	Sensitive to imatinib
Exon 18 D842V	5	Stomach, mesentery, omentum	Imatinib resistant
Exon 18 other	1	All sites	Some but not all are imatinib sensitive
RTK-WT	13	All sites	—
RTK-WT/SDHB negative	—	—	—
SDH mutation (A/B/C/D)	~2	Stomach, small bowel	Carney-Stratakis syndrome
Carney triad	Rare	Stomach	Not heritable
Other (SDHA/B/C/D WT)	50–70 of pediatric GIST but <2 GIST	Stomach only	Most pediatric and adults <age 30–40 y
RTK-WT/SDHB positive	—	—	—
BRAF V600E mutation	~2	All sites	—
RAS mutations	<1	Stomach	—
NF1-related	~1	Small bowel	Multiple lesions, rarely malignant
Other	5–10	All sites	Most RTK-WT GIST in adults >30 y old

homodimerization, leading to KIT tyrosine kinase activity, and subsequent activation of multiple pathways, including those involved with the PI3K/AKT and RAS signaling networks.[12]

Normally, KIT is autoinhibited, favoring an inactive state unless bound by SCF.[13] Mutations in the KIT receptor act to release this autoinhibition, allowing the receptor to shift into a more constitutively active state without binding SCF and thereby sustaining increased growth signaling.[13]

The functional importance of KIT mutations in GIST pathogenesis is supported by multiple lines of evidence. First, phosphorylated KIT is almost always detectable in extracts from GIST cell lines or clinical tumor specimens.[14] Second, mutant KIT is transforming, supporting the growth of stably transfected BA/F3 cells in nude mice.[4] Third, when expressed in transfected cell lines, mutant forms of KIT show constitutive kinase activity in the absence of SCF, as shown by autophosphorylation and activation of downstream signaling pathways.[4,15,16] Fourth, mice engineered to express KIT with mutations of the type found in human GISTs develop diffuse ICC hyperplasia of the stomach and intestine.[17,18] These genetically modified mice also develop GIST-like tumors. This histologic picture is similar to that seen in individuals who inherit germline KIT-activating mutations.[19,20] Fifth, treatment of GIST cell lines or primary GIST cell cultures with KIT kinase inhibitors or interfering RNA against KIT results in decreased proliferation and induction of apoptosis.[16,21] Tyrosine kinase inhibitor (TKI)-resistant KIT-mutant GIST typically have associated secondary kinase mutations that confer drug resistance but maintain kinase activity, suggesting that even in the advanced state, such tumors require KIT kinase activation for tumor proliferation/viability (see later discussion for additional discussion of resistance mutations).[21]

In general, GISTs are heterozygous for a given mutation; however, in approximately 15% of tumors, the remaining WT KIT allele is lost and this is associated with malignant behavior.[22] In serial samples from individual patients, Chen and colleagues[22] have provided evidence that this situation occurs through mitotic nondisjunction, leaving 1 daughter cell with a single chromosome 4 bearing the mutant KIT allele (uniparental monosomy).

As discussed in detail later, correlative studies of outcomes during front-line treatment of metastatic disease have indicated the need to optimize therapy based on tumor genotype. Imatinib dosing recommendations for treatment of KIT-mutant GIST are summarized in **Fig. 1**.

KIT exon 11 mutations

Mutations in KIT exon 11 are the most common oncogenic mutations found in GISTs, occurring in approximately 67% of cases. These mutations include in-frame deletions, insertions, or combinations thereof. Exon 11 encodes the juxtamembrane portion of KIT that normally prevents the kinase activation loop from swinging into the active conformation, thus keeping the receptor in its autoinhibited state. Mutations of KIT exon 11 disrupt this autoinhibition, allowing spontaneous kinase activation.[13]

KIT exon 11-mutant GIST can arise anywhere in the GI tract, with the most common site being the stomach. Tumors with a KIT exon 11 mutation typically have a spindle cell appearance rather than an epithelioid morphology. After complete resection, KIT exon 11-mutant GISTs have a higher rate of recurrence than other genotypic GIST subgroups. Furthermore, GISTs with KIT exon 11 deletions have a worse prognosis than those with exon 11 point mutations, and this is particularly true for deletions involving KIT codons 557 or 558.[23] Conversely, KIT exon 11-mutant GISTs have a more robust and durable response to treatment with the kinase inhibitor imatinib, compared with other types of GIST.

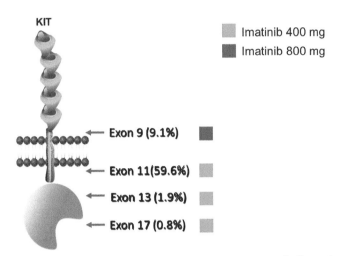

Fig. 1. Dosing recommendations for *KIT*-mutant GIST. Percentages indicate frequency of these specific KIT mutations in GIST. Imatinib dosing recommendations are indicated by the colored box next to the mutation of interest. For example, we recommend imatinib 800 mg per day for KIT exon 9-mutant GIST and 400 mg per day for KIT exon 11-mutant GIST. Standard-dose imatinib typically prescribed as 400 mg taken once daily. High-dose imatinib (800 mg per day) is typically prescribed as 400 mg taken twice daily.

In vitro assays of KIT exon 11-mutant protein have confirmed that these mutations result in constitutive kinase activation.[4] The KIT exon 11-mutant kinase is 10-fold more sensitive to KIT inhibitors, including imatinib, than WT KIT kinase.[24] These in vitro findings are reflected in the clinic, where primary resistance to imatinib treatment (defined by progression within the first 6 months of therapy) is seen in only 5% of cases of advanced KIT exon 11-mutant GIST, compared with 16% in exon-9 mutant or 43% in KIT/PDGFRA WT cases.[25,26] Correspondingly, the objective response rate to imatinib is 67% to 83% for KIT exon 11-mutant GIST versus 35% to 48% for KIT exon 9-mutant GIST.[26,27] The median time to progression on first-line imatinib therapy for KIT exon 11-mutant GIST is approximately 25 months, and the current median overall survival for patients with KIT exon 11-mutant GIST is at least 60 months. The molecular mechanisms leading to drug resistance in KIT exon 11-mutant GISTs are discussed later.

KIT exon 9 mutations

The second most common site of mutation in GISTs is KIT exon 9 (8%–10% of GISTs), which encodes the proximal extracellular domain. More than 95% of the exon 9 mutations consist of an insertion of 6 nucleotides, resulting in duplication of amino acids 502 and 503. Rare cases of amino acid substitutions involving codon 476 have also been reported.[28] Most GISTs harboring an exon 9 mutation are located in the small or large bowel; 25% to 30% of intestinal GISTs harbor an exon 9 mutation. In contrast, KIT exon 9 mutations are found in less than 2% of gastric GISTs.[28]

KIT exon 9 mutations result in constitutive kinase activation and are believed to mimic the conformational change that the extracellular KIT receptor undergoes after ligand binding. The kinase domain in exon 9-mutant KIT is essentially the same as in WT KIT, and shows decreased in vitro sensitivity to imatinib compared with exon 11-mutant KIT.[29,30] In agreement with the in vitro data, results from randomized phase

3 studies showed that patients with KIT exon 9-mutant GIST had a significantly improved progression-free survival when treated with a total daily dose of 800 mg of imatinib compared with patients treated with 400 mg of daily imatinib. Based on a meta-analysis of these results, the median PFS for patients with exon 9-mutant GIST was approximately 1 year longer in the 800-mg imatinib arm versus the 400-mg imatinib arm.[31]

Other KIT mutations

Primary mutation of KIT exon 13, which encodes part of the adenosine triphosphate (ATP)-binding pocket, occurs in approximately 1% of GISTs. The substitution K642E accounts for most of these mutations. Exon 13-mutant GISTs can arise anywhere in the GI tract, but most commonly present as gastric tumors. Tumors with an exon 13 mutation typically have a spindle cell appearance, but occasionally show an epithelioid or mixed histology. The biological basis of kinase activation by this mutation has not been established, but it may interfere with normal autoinhibitory function of the juxtamembrane domain. In vitro and clinical study data indicate that this genotype is sensitive to imatinib.[25,28,32,33]

Primary mutations in exon 17, which encodes the activation loop, are found in approximately 1% of GIST. Substitutions at codons 820, 822, or 823 dominate in this exon. In vitro, some of these mutations are less sensitive to imatinib than KIT exon 11-mutant kinases, but clinical responses to imatinib have been reported for primary KIT exon 17-mutant GIST.[25] Almost all of these tumors have a spindle cell appearance, and most are located in the small bowel, but they can arise in the stomach as well.[32]

PDGFRA-Mutant GIST

Mutations in PDGFRA are the most common non-KIT oncogenic mutations associated with GIST. PDGFRA is a tyrosine kinase receptor that is a close homologue of KIT and uses similar downstream signaling pathways. PDGFRA mutations that are found in GIST result in constitutive kinase activation. These mutations are mutually exclusive with KIT mutations.[34,35] The most common locations for PDGFRA-mutant GISTs are the stomach, mesentery, and omentum, with a strong predilection for the stomach. Histologically, PDGFRA-mutant GISTs usually have an epithelioid or mixed epithelioid/spindle appearance, commonly accompanied by a myxoid stroma.[36] PDGFRA-mutant GISTs have a lower risk of recurrence than KIT-mutant GIST. This finding explains the lower frequency of PDGFRA-mutant GIST in published series of malignant GIST versus population-based series of primary GIST. For example, a population-based series of 492 GISTs in France showed a 15% frequency of PDGFRA-mutant GIST, whereas PDGFRA-mutant GIST comprised only 2.1% of cases in 2 large clinical series of metastatic GIST.[37] These observations have been confirmed in other series.

The biological basis for the decreased malignant potential of many PDGFRA-mutant GISTs is unclear, but these GISTs often have other characteristics of low-risk GIST, including gastric primary site, smaller size, and low mitotic index. Overall, KIT and PDGFRA-mutant GISTs show many similar features, including expression of PKC-θ, DOG-1, and activation of the RAS/MAPK and PI3K pathways.[28] In addition, these tumors also have similar cytogenetic abnormalities, including monosomy of chromosome 14.[34] However, gene expression profiling of KIT-mutant and PDGFRA-mutant GISTs do reveal subtle differences in the underlying tumor biology that may explain some of the differences in clinical behavior between these different entities.[38] As with KIT mutations, rare families with germline PDGFRA mutations and susceptibility to GIST formation have been reported.[39] Overall, the available evidence suggests that PDGFRA mutations can initiate GIST formation.

As with KIT-mutant GIST, correlative studies of outcomes during front-line treatment of metastatic disease have indicated the need to optimize therapy based on tumor genotype. Imatinib dosing recommendations for treatment of PDGFRA-mutant GIST are summarized in **Fig. 2**.

PDGFRA exon 18 mutations

The most common PDGFRA mutations in GISTs occur in exon 18 and are believed to stabilize the kinase activation loop in a conformation that favors kinase activation.[40] A single mutation, D842V, accounts for at least 70% of all PDGFRA mutations seen in GIST.[41] This particular mutation confers biochemical resistance to imatinib and all other approved TKIs.[25] The median time to progression in patients with PDGFRA D842V-mutant GIST was only 2.8 months, compared with 20 to 24 months for other GIST genotypes. In addition, the median overall survival was only 12.8 months, compared with 48 to 60 months in large series of imatinib-treated patients with GIST.[28]

In addition to D842V, several other exon 18 mutations occur in GIST. For clinical purposes, it is useful to classify these mutations as either imatinib-sensitive or imatinib-resistant mutations.[41,42] After D842V, the next most common mutation of exon 18 is deletion of codons 842 to 845 (DIMH), which is imatinib sensitive,[41,42] but other more rare mutations in exon 18 are resistant. Recently, a novel PDGFRA selective kinase inhibitor, crenolanib, was reported to have in vitro potency against D842V and other imatinib-resistant PDGFRA mutations. Based in part on these results, a

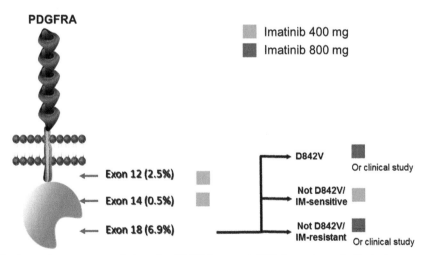

Fig. 2. Dosing recommendations for *PDGFRA*-mutant GIST. Percentages indicate frequency of these specific PDGFRA mutations in GIST. Imatinib dosing recommendations are for the total daily dose. standard-dose imatinib is typically prescribed as 400 mg taken once daily. High-dose imatinib (800 mg per day) is typically prescribed as 400 mg taken twice daily. Dosing recommendations for PDGFRA exon 18-mutant GIST are given for D842-mutant, non-D842V/imatinib-sensitive, or non-D842V/imatinib-sensitive mutations. For example, for D842V-mutant GIST we recommend high-dose imatinib or consideration of experimental therapy (eg, crenolanib). In vitro data on the imatinib sensitivity of non-D842V exon 18 mutations can be found in found in Refs.[41,42]

phase 2 clinical study of this agent to treat advanced GIST with the PDGFRA D842V mutation has been initiated[42] (Clincaltrials.gov identifier NCT01243346).

PDGFRA exon 12 mutations

Exon 12 is the second most commonly mutated PDGFRA exon in GIST. Overall, exon 12 mutations are found in approximately 1% of GISTs.[37,41] PDGFRA exon 12 is homologous to KIT exon 11, and mutations of this region lead to loss of the autoinhibitory function of the juxtamembrane domain.[28,40] In vitro, PDGFRA exon 12 mutant kinases are as sensitive to imatinib as KIT exon-11 mutant kinases. PDGFRA exon 12 mutant GISTs make up only a few metastatic GISTs; however, the available clinical data suggest that this genotype has a good response to imatinib treatment, with high response rates and durable disease control.[25,26,35,41]

PDGFRA exon 14 mutations

Activating mutations of *PDGFRA* exon 14 are found in less than 1% of GISTs, making these tumors one of the rarest types of RTK-mutant GIST. By homology with *KIT* exon 13, mutations in exon 14 may interfere with the autoinhibitory function of the juxtamembrane domain. In vitro and clinical study data suggest that exon 14-mutant kinases respond to imatinib.[41]

RTK-WT *GIST*

Historical perspective

Beginning in 1998, GISTs were classified as KIT-mutant versus WT tumors, based on the original description of KIT exon 11 mutations. Over the next few years, activating mutations of KIT exons 9, 13, and 17 were found in association with GISTs lacking KIT exon 11 mutations. In 2003, PDGFRA-mutant GISTs were described, changing the definition of WT GIST to mean those tumors lacking KIT or PDGFRA mutations. As detailed later, other gain-of-function or loss-of-function mutations have since been uncovered in GISTs lacking KIT or PDGFRA mutations. In light of these newer mutations, categorizing GISTs as WT has become confusing and misleading. Therefore, we suggest that GISTs lacking a KIT or PDGFRA mutation be grouped simply as RTK-WT (see **Table 2**).

SDHB-deficient, RTK-WT GIST

A major breakthrough in the understanding of non-RTK oncogenic mechanisms in GIST arose from studies of patients with Carney-Stratakis syndrome. This autosomal-dominant syndrome manifests as a susceptibility to the development of both paragangliomas and GI stromal tumors. Previous studies of familial paraganglioma syndromes revealed germline inactivating mutations in the genes coding for the succinate dehydrogenase (SDH)-ubiquinone complex II (SDHA, SDHB, SDHC, SDHD). This complex functions in both the Krebs cycle and the mitochondrial respiratory chain, and inactivation of any 1 of the SDH subunits results in its destabilization and loss of enzymatic function.[8] Twelve percent to 16% of patients with apparently sporadic paraganglioma carry germline inactivating mutations in SDH subunits.[43] In a study of patients with Carney-Stratakis syndrome who developed GIST, Pasini and colleagues[44] identified germline mutations in SDHB, SDHC, or SDHD. GISTs in the affected individuals were found to be hemizygous/homozygous for the mutant allele, consistent with the view that the SDH genes have tumor suppressor activity.

Several investigators have shown that absence of immunohistochemical staining for SDHB can be used to identify SDH-deficient GISTs.[45–48] Overall, SDHB-deficient tumors show the following clinical and pathologic characteristics: gastric primary site, epithelioid morphology, a multifocal nodular growth pattern, and frequent involvement of local lymph nodes.[49,50] Miettinen and colleagues[48] reported that 7.5% of 756 gastric GISTs were SDHB immunonegative, but no cases of SDHB deficiency were found among 378 nongastric GISTs. Most SDHB-negative GISTs arise in patients younger than 20 years, although many occur in patients between the ages of 20 and 40 years. In contrast, gastric GIST diagnosed in patients older than 40 years are rarely SDHB deficient.[47,48] SDHB staining is retained in GISTs with KIT or PDGFRA mutations, and in GISTs with other oncogenic mutations, as discussed later.

GISTs that are negative for SDHA immunostaining uniformly harbor SDHA mutations, most of which seem to be inherited.[50–54] Miettinen and colleagues[50] reported that 28% of 127 SDHB-deficient gastric GISTs also lacked SDHA expression, suggesting that SDHA mutations account for more than a quarter of SDH-deficient GISTs. In contrast, 0% of 556 cases of SDHB-positive GISTs lacked SDHA protein expression. Compared with patients with SDHA-positive GISTs, those with SDHA-negative GISTs have an older median age (34 vs 21 years), lower female/male ratio, and a slower course of disease, despite a slightly higher rate of liver metastases. The most common germline SDHA mutation leads to truncation of the protein after codon 31, presumably leading to lack of detectable protein. In rare cases, SDHA staining is retained in an SDHA-mutant tumor that lacks SDHB staining[50]; presumably, this is because the mutant-SDHA protein, although dysfunctional, still reacts with the SDHA antibodies used for immunohistochemistry.

In 50% to 70% of SDHA-positive/SDHB-negative GISTs, no mutations of SDH family members can be identified. These tumors have normal levels of mRNA for SDHB/C/D as assessed by reverse transcription polymerase chain reaction. Thus, the loss of SDHB expression must be related to a posttranscriptional defect, although this has yet to be identified. Theoretically, dysfunction of SDHAF2 or other components of cellular respiration could be responsible.

The mechanisms by which defects in SDH complex activity lead to neoplasia are being explored. Loss of the SDH complex results in defective cellular respiration and mimics the effects of cellular hypoxia. In the case of paragangliomas, it is known that loss of SDH complex activity leads to increased expression of HIF1/2 and VEGF and a high density of tumor-associated microvessels. Other abnormalities in SDH-deficient paragangliomas have also been described, including mitochondrial abnormalities (increased numbers, swollen mitochondria with loss of cristae and inclusion bodies), accumulation of succinate with an increased succinate/fumarate ratio, and inhibition of the prolyl-hydroxylation of HIF1-α and HIF2-α (an essential step in the regulation of these proteins). In addition, in a recent study, IGF1R expression was detected in 71 of 80 SDH-deficient GISTs but only in 9 of 625 (1%) of the SDHB-positive gastric GISTs,[55] indicating that the IGF1R pathway may be activated only in SDH-deficient GISTs. How these abnormalities are related to GIST pathogenesis is unclear.[56]

Identification of SDHB immunonegative GISTs is important for several reasons. First, given the increased frequency of SDH mutations in these tumors, SDH genotyping should be considered. Patients with germline SDH mutations are at risk of developing paragangliomas (or pheochromocytomas) as well as development of additional primary GISTs. Clinical screening guidelines have been described for patients with familial paraganglioma/GIST.[57] Second, conventional risk stratification of SDHB-deficient tumors using tumor size and mitotic index is poorly predictive of tumor behavior. These tumors frequently metastasize but often have an indolent clinical course. In addition, lymph node metastases are common in SDHB-deficient tumors, but extremely rare in SDHB-positive tumors.[49,58] These tumors may respond poorly to imatinib. Pediatric GISTs, which are almost always SDHB deficient, have a poor response to imatinib compared with SDHB-positive GIST arising in adults. However, sunitinib seems to have substantial antitumor activity in pediatric patients,[59] possibly by inhibition of VEGFRs.

The Carney triad represents a distinct clinical entity that is different from Carney-Stratakis syndrome. The Carney triad consists of a nonhereditary association of gastric GIST, paraganglioma, and pulmonary chondroma, usually affecting young females. GISTs in patients with Carney Triad are SDHB negative, but no mutations of KIT, PDGFRA, or SDH family members have been found in these tumors.[28]

RTK-WT/SDHB-positive GIST

GISTs that are RTK-WT/SDHB-positive sometimes harbor mutations that activate the RAS/RAF/MAPK pathway. Among these mutations are tumors arising in patients with neurofibromatosis type I (NF1). Approximately 7% of patients with germline NF1 mutations develop GIST (frequently multiple) of the small bowel, most of which are RTK-WT.[60,61] The NF1 gene product (neurofibromin) is a tumor suppressor that serves to attenuate the activity of the RAS pathway; thus, absence of NF1 can contribute to GIST development through MAPK signaling. Rare NF1-related GISTs have a KIT mutation, possibly as a sporadic, secondary mutation. NF1-associated GISTs are uniformly SDHB positive.[62]

BRAF V600E mutations are present in 7% to 15% of RTK-WT GISTs, or less than 2% of GISTs overall.[63–65] There do not seem to be any anatomic or pathologic distinctions for BRAF-mutant GIST. Rare cases of RAS-mutant GIST have also been described.[28,66] There are few published clinical data on the use of imatinib (or another KIT/VEGFR inhibitor) to treat RAS/RAF-mutant GISTs. However, based on available cell models, these drugs would not be expected to be effective. BRAF or MEK inhibitors might have activity, but future clinical studies are needed to confirm this hypothesis.

The Origins of GIST

ICCs

It is widely hypothesized that ICCs are the cells of origin for GIST. Mice and humans with germline KIT mutations show diffuse ICC hyperplasia within the muscular wall of the stomach and intestine, and are susceptible to development of discrete tumor masses.[17,18] In 1 animal model, putative ICC stem cells and mature myenteric ICCs were both increased in number, indicating that mutant KIT can cause expansion of ICC populations.[67]

The relationship between GIST and ICC is further supported by parallels in gene expression. For example, high levels of PKC-θ, nestin, and DOG-1 are expressed in both GISTs and ICCs. In addition, the ETS family transcription factor ETV1 is highly expressed in both GISTs and in the specific subpopulations of ICCs (myenteric and intramuscular) believed to give rise to GIST.[28]

The observation that some KIT and PDGFRA mutations in GISTs correlate closely with anatomic location (see **Table 2**) might be explained by the originating ICC. For example, GISTs with a KIT exon 9 mutation, which arise primarily in the small intestine, may derive from a different subgroup of ICCs than those with a PDGFRA D842V mutation, which occur only in the stomach, mesentery, and omentum. A similar phenomenon may explain the strong association of SDHB deficiency with the development of gastric GIST. In contrast to these examples, the more common KIT mutations can be found in GISTs throughout the GI tract, perhaps deriving from a more ubiquitous ICC subtype.

Small gastric nodules of ICC/GIST-like cells (1–10 mm) are found up to 35% of the adult population (reported range 2.9%–35%).[68] These so-called micro-GISTs are mitotically inactive and often partially calcified, suggesting growth arrest. In contrast to the diffuse ICC hyperplasia observed in the presence of a germline KIT mutation, micro-GISTs seem to represent a nodular form of ICC overgrowth caused by local, somatic acquisition of a KIT mutation. The type and frequency of KIT mutations in micro-GISTs mirrors that of clinically significant GISTs. These observations suggest that kinase gene mutations occur very early in GIST development; however, these mutations alone are insufficient for progression to a clinically significant lesion. The large pool of micro-GISTs in the general population likely explains reports of patients with 2 or more genotypically distinct GISTs.[68–71] Micro-GISTs further highlight the importance of examining the size and mitotic activity of a given lesion to assess aggressiveness before proceeding with any adjuvant treatment recommendations.[72]

TKI RESISTANCE MECHANISMS
Resistance to TKI Therapy

Primary resistance
Resistance to treatment with KIT/PDGFRA inhibitors such as imatinib can be divided into 2 types: primary and secondary. Approximately 10% of patients with GIST have primary resistance, defined as progression within the first 6 months of treatment. As discussed earlier, clinical responses to imatinib correlate with the primary tumor genotype, with the probability of primary resistance to imatinib for KIT exon 11, KIT exon 9, and RTK-WT GISTs being 5%, 16%, and 23%, respectively.[25,26,31,73]

Based on in vitro data, the most common PDGFRA mutation in GISTs, D842V, is strongly resistant to the effects of imatinib, in vitro.[42] This finding is mirrored by clinical results, with patients with PDGFRA D842V-mutant GIST having low response rates and very short progression-free and overall survival during imatinib treatment. However, there are some PDGFRA mutations that are sensitive to imatinib in vitro, and patients with these mutations have shown durable responses to imatinib.[24,34,41]

As discussed earlier, RTK-WT GISTs include tumors with mutations downstream of KIT or affecting entirely different pathways (eg, SDH).[47,64,65] Hence, these types of GISTs may respond better to other targeted agents, such as VEGFR inhibitors for pediatric/SDH-mutant GIST, and BRAF/MEK inhibitors for BRAF/RAS-mutant GIST.[59] Some patients with RTK-WT GIST have prolonged disease-free and overall survival during front-line imatinib treatment. Whether this situation is caused by an underlying indolent biology or a KIT-dependent subgroup of RTK-WT GIST remains unclear.[26]

Secondary resistance
After an initial benefit from imatinib, most patients develop disease progression or secondary resistance. It is now established that acquired mutations in KIT or PDGFRA account for most secondary resistance in RTK-mutant GIST, and that these mutations occur almost exclusively in the same gene and allele as the primary oncogenic driver mutation.[28]

In a phase II imatinib study for advanced GIST, 67% of the patients whose tumor showed imatinib resistance had a new, or secondary, mutation in KIT. These mutations were common among tumors with a primary exon 11 mutation, but were not observed in RTK-WT GIST tumors.[21] These observations have been confirmed in multiple other studies in which secondary mutations of KIT have never been reported in RTK-WT GIST. Unlike primary mutations that activate KIT, which are predominantly in the juxtamembrane regions encoded by exons 9 and 11, the secondary mutations associated with TKI resistance are typically concentrated in either the ATP-binding pocket (encoded by exons 13 and 14) or the kinase activation loop (encoded by exons 17 and 18).[21] Drug resistance has also been observed in PDGFRA-mutant GISTs, most commonly by acquiring a D842V mutation (activation loop).[21,74] However, there have been no reliable reports of a secondary KIT mutation arising in a GIST with a primary PDGFRA mutation, or vice versa, during treatment with imatinib.

Additional studies using more sensitive assays have identified secondary mutations in more than 80% of drug-resistant GIST lesions.[28] There is a significant heterogeneity of resistance across different metastatic lesions in a patient, and even within different areas of the same lesion.[28] For example, there are reports of up to 5 different drug resistance mutations in different portions of an individual lesion and up to 7 different secondary resistance mutations across multiple tumors in the same patient.[75] This heterogeneity of resistance significantly affects the efficacy of salvage TKI therapy after front-line imatinib, because the diversity of resistant, minority clones precludes the systemic eradication of GIST cells by any particular TKI. Given the problems of tumor heterogeneity and the limited predictive value of lesion genotyping to predict response to changing medical therapy, clinical genotyping of progressive lesions to help guide subsequent TKI therapy is not recommended.

Although secondary mutations in KIT are the most common cause of acquired resistance to imatinib therapy, there are other potential causes for GIST growth in the face of TKI therapy. For example, there can be downregulation or loss of KIT and PKC-θ expression, which is associated with a marked increase in cyclin D1 and JUN.[28] As noted earlier, IGF1R overexpression is seen in most SDH-deficient GIST. Targeting IGF1R may be a novel approach to treatment of SDH-deficient GISTs that are resistant to conventional GIST medical therapy.[76] Focal adhesion kinase may also play a role in the growth and survival of imatinib-resistant GIST cells.[77]

SUMMARY

In the last 15 years, we have moved from a model of GIST as 1 discrete disease to our current understanding that GIST represents a heterogeneous collection of molecular entities, linked by a common histology and presumed cell of origin. Most GISTs are driven by a pathogenic mutant kinase, but other disease-initiating molecular abnormalities have been described, most notably loss of activity of the SDH complex. The type of underlying molecular defect in a given patient's GIST has a significant impact on treatment response and potential mechanisms of primary and secondary resistance.

REFERENCES

1. Long KB, Butrynski JE, Blank SD, et al. Primary extragastrointestinal stromal tumor of the pleura: report of a unique case with genetic confirmation. Am J Surg Pathol 2010;34(6):907–12.
2. Mazur MT, Clark HB. Gastric stromal tumors. Reappraisal of histogenesis. Am J Surg Pathol 1983;7(6):507–19.
3. Isozaki K, Hirota S, Nakama A, et al. Disturbed intestinal movement, bile reflux to the stomach, and deficiency of c-kit-expressing cells in Ws/Ws mutant rats. Gastroenterology 1995;109(2):456–64.
4. Hirota S, Isozaki K, Moriyama Y, et al. Gain-of-function mutations of c-kit in human gastrointestinal stromal tumors. Science 1998;279(5350):577–80.

5. Kindblom LG, Remotti HE, Aldenborg F, et al. Gastrointestinal pacemaker cell tumor (GIPACT): gastrointestinal stromal tumors show phenotypic characteristics of the interstitial cells of Cajal. Am J Pathol 1998;152(5): 1259–69.

6. West RB, Corless CL, Chen X, et al. The novel marker, DOG1, is expressed ubiquitously in gastrointestinal stromal tumors irrespective of KIT or PDGFRA mutation status. Am J Pathol 2004;165(1):107–13.

7. Liegl B, Hornick JL, Corless CL, et al. Monoclonal antibody DOG1.1 shows higher sensitivity than KIT in the diagnosis of gastrointestinal stromal tumors, including unusual subtypes. Am J Surg Pathol 2009;33(3):437–46.

8. van Nederveen FH, Gaal J, Favier J, et al. An immunohistochemical procedure to detect patients with paraganglioma and phaeochromocytoma with germline SDHB, SDHC, or SDHD gene mutations: a retrospective and prospective analysis. Lancet Oncol 2009;10(8):764–71.

9. Joensuu H, Vehtari A, Riihimaki J, et al. Risk of recurrence of gastrointestinal stromal tumour after surgery: an analysis of pooled population-based cohorts. Lancet Oncol 2012;13(3):265–74.

10. Rutkowski P, Bylina E, Wozniak A, et al. Validation of the Joensuu risk criteria for primary resectable gastrointestinal stromal tumour–the impact of tumour rupture on patient outcomes. Eur J Surg Oncol 2011;37(10):890–6.

11. Gold JS, Gonen M, Gutierrez A, et al. Development and validation of a prognostic nomogram for recurrence-free survival after complete surgical resection of localised primary gastrointestinal stromal tumour: a retrospective analysis. Lancet Oncol 2009;10(11):1045–52.

12. Bauer S, Duensing A, Demetri GD, et al. KIT oncogenic signaling mechanisms in imatinib-resistant gastrointestinal stromal tumor: PI3-kinase/AKT is a crucial survival pathway. Oncogene 2007;26(54):7560–8.

13. Mol CD, Dougan DR, Schneider TR, et al. Structural basis for the autoinhibition and STI-571 inhibition of c-Kit tyrosine kinase. J Biol Chem 2004;279(30): 31655–63.

14. Rubin BP, Singer S, Tsao C, et al. KIT activation is a ubiquitous feature of gastrointestinal stromal tumors. Cancer Res 2001;61(22):8118–21.

15. Heinrich MC, Griffith DJ, Druker BJ, et al. Inhibition of c-kit receptor tyrosine kinase activity by STI 571, a selective tyrosine kinase inhibitor. Blood 2000; 96(3):925–32.

16. Tuveson DA, Willis NA, Jacks T, et al. STI571 inactivation of the gastrointestinal stromal tumor c-KIT oncoprotein: biological and clinical implications. Oncogene 2001;20(36):5054–8.

17. Rubin BP, Antonescu CR, Scott-Browne JP, et al. A knock-in mouse model of gastrointestinal stromal tumor harboring kit K641E. Cancer Res 2005;65(15): 6631–9.

18. Sommer G, Agosti V, Ehlers I, et al. Gastrointestinal stromal tumors in a mouse model by targeted mutation of the Kit receptor tyrosine kinase. Proc Natl Acad Sci U S A 2003;100(11):6706–11.

19. Chen H, Hirota S, Isozaki K, et al. Polyclonal nature of diffuse proliferation of interstitial cells of Cajal in patients with familial and multiple gastrointestinal stromal tumours. Gut 2002;51(6):793–6.

20. O'Riain C, Corless CL, Heinrich MC, et al. Gastrointestinal stromal tumors: insights from a new familial GIST kindred with unusual genetic and pathologic features. Am J Surg Pathol 2005;29(12):1680–3.

21. Heinrich MC, Corless CL, Blanke CD, et al. Molecular correlates of imatinib resistance in gastrointestinal stromal tumors. J Clin Oncol 2006;24(29): 4764–74.
22. Chen LL, Holden JA, Choi H, et al. Evolution from heterozygous to homozygous KIT mutation in gastrointestinal stromal tumor correlates with the mechanism of mitotic nondisjunction and significant tumor progression. Mod Pathol 2008; 21(7):826–36.
23. Martin J, Poveda A, Llombart-Bosch A, et al. Deletions affecting codons 557-558 of the c-KIT gene indicate a poor prognosis in patients with completely resected gastrointestinal stromal tumors: a study by the Spanish Group for Sarcoma Research (GEIS). J Clin Oncol 2005;23(25):6190–8.
24. Heinrich MC, Maki RG, Corless CL, et al. Primary and secondary kinase genotypes correlate with the biological and clinical activity of sunitinib in imatinib-resistant gastrointestinal stromal tumor. J Clin Oncol 2008;26(33):5352–9.
25. Heinrich MC, Corless CL, Demetri GD, et al. Kinase mutations and imatinib response in patients with metastatic gastrointestinal stromal tumor. J Clin Oncol 2003;21(23):4342–9.
26. Heinrich MC, Owzar K, Corless CL, et al. Correlation of kinase genotype and clinical outcome in the North American Intergroup Phase III Trial of imatinib mesylate for treatment of advanced gastrointestinal stromal tumor: CALGB 150105 Study by Cancer and Leukemia Group B and Southwest Oncology Group. J Clin Oncol 2008;26(33):5360–7.
27. von Mehren M, Heinrich MC, Joensuu H, et al. Follow-up results after 9 years (yrs) of the ongoing, phase II B2222 trial of imatinib mesylate (IM) in patients (pts) with metastatic or unresectable KIT+ gastrointestinal stromal tumors (GIST). J Clin Oncol 2011;29(Suppl 15):10016.
28. Corless CL, Barnett CM, Heinrich MC. Gastrointestinal stromal tumours: origin and molecular oncology. Nat Rev Cancer 2011;11(12):865–78.
29. Yuzawa S, Opatowsky Y, Zhang Z, et al. Structural basis for activation of the receptor tyrosine kinase KIT by stem cell factor. Cell 2007;130(2):323–34.
30. Heinrich MC, Marino-Enriquez A, Presnell A, et al. Sorafenib inhibits many kinase mutations associated with drug-resistant gastrointestinal stromal tumors. Mol Cancer Ther 2012;11(8):1770–80.
31. Gastrointestinal Stromal Tumor Meta-Analysis Group (MetaGIST). Comparison of two doses of imatinib for the treatment of unresectable or metastatic gastrointestinal stromal tumors: a meta-analysis of 1,640 patients. J Clin Oncol 2010; 28(7):1247–53.
32. Lasota J, Corless CL, Heinrich MC, et al. Clinicopathologic profile of gastrointestinal stromal tumors (GISTs) with primary KIT exon 13 or exon 17 mutations: a multicenter study on 54 cases. Mod Pathol 2008;21(4):476–84.
33. Lux ML, Rubin BP, Biase TL, et al. KIT extracellular and kinase domain mutations in gastrointestinal stromal tumors. Am J Pathol 2000;156(3):791–5.
34. Heinrich MC, Corless CL, Duensing A, et al. PDGFRA activating mutations in gastrointestinal stromal tumors. Science 2003;299(5607):708–10.
35. Hirota S, Ohashi A, Nishida T, et al. Gain-of-function mutations of platelet-derived growth factor receptor alpha gene in gastrointestinal stromal tumors. Gastroenterology 2003;125(3):660–7.
36. Lasota J, Stachura J, Miettinen M. GISTs with PDGFRA exon 14 mutations represent subset of clinically favorable gastric tumors with epithelioid morphology. Lab Invest 2006;86(1):94–100.

37. Emile JF, Brahimi S, Coindre JM, et al. Frequencies of KIT and PDGFRA mutations in the MolecGIST prospective population-based study differ from those of advanced GISTs. Med Oncol 2012;29(3):1765–72.

38. Subramanian S, West RB, Corless CL, et al. Gastrointestinal stromal tumors (GISTs) with KIT and PDGFRA mutations have distinct gene expression profiles. Oncogene 2004;23(47):7780–90.

39. de Raedt T, Cools J, Debiec-Rychter M, et al. Intestinal neurofibromatosis is a subtype of familial GIST and results from a dominant activating mutation in PDGFRA. Gastroenterology 2006;131(6):1907–12.

40. Dibb NJ, Dilworth SM, Mol CD. Switching on kinases: oncogenic activation of BRAF and the PDGFR family. Nat Rev Cancer 2004;4(9):718–27.

41. Corless CL, Schroeder A, Griffith D, et al. PDGFRA mutations in gastrointestinal stromal tumors: frequency, spectrum and in vitro sensitivity to imatinib. J Clin Oncol 2005;23(23):5357–64.

42. Heinrich MC, Griffith D, McKinley A, et al. Crenolanib inhibits the drug-resistant PDGFRA D842V mutation associated with imatinib-resistant gastrointestinal stromal tumors. Clin Cancer Res 2012;18(16):4375–84.

43. Burnichon N, Rohmer V, Amar L, et al. The succinate dehydrogenase genetic testing in a large prospective series of patients with paragangliomas. J Clin Endocrinol Metab 2009;94(8):2817–27.

44. Pasini B, McWhinney SR, Bei T, et al. Clinical and molecular genetics of patients with the Carney-Stratakis syndrome and germline mutations of the genes coding for the succinate dehydrogenase subunits SDHB, SDHC, and SDHD. Eur J Hum Genet 2008;16(1):79–88.

45. Gill AJ, Chou A, Vilain RE, et al. "Pediatric-type" gastrointestinal stromal tumors are SDHB negative ("type 2") GISTs. Am J Surg Pathol 2011;35(8):1245–7 [author reply: 1247–8].

46. Gaal J, Stratakis CA, Carney JA, et al. SDHB immunohistochemistry: a useful tool in the diagnosis of Carney-Stratakis and Carney triad gastrointestinal stromal tumors. Mod Pathol 2011;24(1):147–51.

47. Janeway KA, Kim SY, Lodish M, et al. Defects in succinate dehydrogenase in gastrointestinal stromal tumors lacking KIT and PDGFRA mutations. Proc Natl Acad Sci U S A 2011;108(1):314–8.

48. Miettinen M, Wang ZF, Sarlomo-Rikala M, et al. Succinate dehydrogenase-deficient GISTs: a clinicopathologic, immunohistochemical, and molecular genetic study of 66 gastric GISTs with predilection to young age. Am J Surg Pathol 2011;35(11):1712–21.

49. Doyle LA, Nelson D, Heinrich MC, et al. Loss of succinate dehydrogenase subunit B (SDHB) expression is limited to a distinctive subset of gastric wild-type gastrointestinal stromal tumours: a comprehensive genotype-phenotype correlation study. Histopathology 2012;61(5):801–9.

50. Miettinen M, Killian JK, Wang ZF, et al. Immunohistochemical loss of succinate dehydrogenase subunit A (SDHA) in gastrointestinal stromal tumors (GISTs) signals SDHA germline mutation. Am J Surg Pathol 2013;37(2):234–40.

51. Oudijk L, Gaal J, Korpershoek E, et al. SDHA mutations in adult and pediatric wild-type gastrointestinal stromal tumors. Mod Pathol 2013;26(3):456–63.

52. Belinsky MG, Rink L, Flieder DB, et al. Overexpression of insulin-like growth factor 1 receptor and frequent mutational inactivation of SDHA in wild-type SDHB-negative gastrointestinal stromal tumors. Genes Chromosomes Cancer 2013;52(2):214–24.

53. Dwight T, Benn DE, Clarkson A, et al. Loss of SDHA expression identifies SDHA mutations in succinate dehydrogenase-deficient gastrointestinal stromal tumors. Am J Surg Pathol 2013;37(2):226–33.

54. Wagner AJ, Remillard SP, Zhang YX, et al. Loss of expression of SDHA predicts SDHA mutations in gastrointestinal stromal tumors. Mod Pathol 2013;26(2): 289–94.

55. Lasota J, Wang Z, Kim SY, et al. Expression of the receptor for type i insulin-like growth factor (IGF1R) in gastrointestinal stromal tumors: an immunohistochemical study of 1078 cases with diagnostic and therapeutic implications. Am J Surg Pathol 2013;37(1):114–9.

56. Gill AJ. Succinate dehydrogenase (SDH) and mitochondrial driven neoplasia. Pathology 2012;44(4):285–92.

57. Buffet A, Venisse A, Nau V, et al. A decade (2001-2010) of genetic testing for pheochromocytoma and paraganglioma. Horm Metab Res 2012;44(5):359–66.

58. Celestino R, Lima J, Faustino A, et al. Molecular alterations and expression of succinate dehydrogenase complex in wild-type KIT/PDGFRA/BRAF gastrointestinal stromal tumors. Eur J Hum Genet 2013;21(5):503–10.

59. Janeway KA, Albritton KH, Van Den Abbeele AD, et al. Sunitinib treatment in pediatric patients with advanced GIST following failure of imatinib. Pediatr Blood Cancer 2009;52(7):767–71.

60. Andersson J, Sihto H, Meis-Kindblom JM, et al. NF1-associated gastrointestinal stromal tumors have unique clinical, phenotypic, and genotypic characteristics. Am J Surg Pathol 2005;29(9):1170–6.

61. Kinoshita K, Hirota S, Isozaki K, et al. Absence of c-kit gene mutations in gastrointestinal stromal tumours from neurofibromatosis type 1 patients. J Pathol 2004; 202(1):80–5.

62. Wang JH, Lasota J, Miettinen M. Succinate dehydrogenase subunit B (SDHB) is expressed in neurofibromatosis 1-associated gastrointestinal stromal tumors (GISTs): implications for the SDHB expression based classification of GISTs. J Cancer 2011;2:90–3.

63. Daniels M, Lurkin I, Pauli R, et al. Spectrum of KIT/PDGFRA/BRAF mutations and phosphatidylinositol-3-kinase pathway gene alterations in gastrointestinal stromal tumors (GIST). Cancer Lett 2011;312(1):43–54.

64. Agaram NP, Wong GC, Guo T, et al. Novel V600E BRAF mutations in imatinib-naive and imatinib-resistant gastrointestinal stromal tumors. Genes Chromosomes Cancer 2008;47(10):853–9.

65. Hostein I, Faur N, Primois C, et al. BRAF mutation status in gastrointestinal stromal tumors. Am J Clin Pathol 2010;133(1):141–8.

66. Miranda C, Nucifora M, Molinari F, et al. KRAS and BRAF mutations predict primary resistance to imatinib in gastrointestinal stromal tumors. Clin Cancer Res 2012;18(6):1769–76.

67. Bardsley MR, Horvath VJ, Asuzu DT, et al. Kitlow stem cells cause resistance to Kit/platelet-derived growth factor alpha inhibitors in murine gastrointestinal stromal tumors. Gastroenterology 2010;139(3):942–52.

68. Agaimy A, Wunsch PH, Hofstaedter F, et al. Minute gastric sclerosing stromal tumors (GIST tumorlets) are common in adults and frequently show c-KIT mutations. Am J Surg Pathol 2007;31(1):113–20.

69. Maertens O, Prenen H, Debiec-Rychter M, et al. Molecular pathogenesis of multiple gastrointestinal stromal tumors in NF1 patients. Hum Mol Genet 2006;15(6): 1015–23.

70. Agaimy A, Wunsch PH, Dirnhofer S, et al. Microscopic gastrointestinal stromal tumors in esophageal and intestinal surgical resection specimens: a clinico-pathologic, immunohistochemical, and molecular study of 19 lesions. Am J Surg Pathol 2008;32(6):867–73.

71. Gasparotto D, Rossi S, Bearzi I, et al. Multiple primary sporadic gastrointestinal stromal tumors in the adult: an underestimated entity. Clin Cancer Res 2008; 14(18):5715–21.

72. Joensuu H. Adjuvant treatment of GIST: patient selection and treatment strate-gies. Nat Rev Clin Oncol 2012;9(6):351–8.

73. Debiec-Rychter M, Wasag B, Stul M, et al. Gastrointestinal stromal tumours (GISTs) negative for KIT (CD117 antigen) immunoreactivity. J Pathol 2004; 202(4):430–8.

74. Debiec-Rychter M, Cools J, Dumez H, et al. Mechanisms of resistance to imati-nib mesylate in gastrointestinal stromal tumors and activity of the PKC412 inhib-itor against imatinib-resistant mutants. Gastroenterology 2005;128(2):270–9.

75. Liegl B, Kepten I, Le C, et al. Heterogeneity of kinase inhibitor resistance mech-anisms in GIST. J Pathol 2008;216(1):64–74.

76. Tarn C, Rink L, Merkel E, et al. Insulin-like growth factor 1 receptor is a potential therapeutic target for gastrointestinal stromal tumors. Proc Natl Acad Sci U S A 2008;105(24):8387–92.

77. Sakurama K, Noma K, Takaoka M, et al. Inhibition of focal adhesion kinase as a potential therapeutic strategy for imatinib-resistant gastrointestinal stromal tumor. Mol Cancer Ther 2009;8(1):127–34.

Gastrointestinal Stromal Tumors
Risk Assessment and Adjuvant Therapy

Heikki Joensuu, PhD, MD

KEYWORDS

- Gastrointestinal stromal tumor • Prognostic factor • Risk stratification
- Adjuvant therapy • Imatinib

KEY POINTS

- Approximately 60% of patients with operable gastrointestinal stromal tumor (GIST) are cured by surgery and are not candidates for adjuvant therapy.
- Several tools exist for estimation of the risk of recurrence, including risk-stratification schemes, prognostic heat maps, nomograms, and gene expression profiles.
- Adjuvant imatinib improves recurrence-free survival and probably overall survival of patients with GIST whose tumor harbors an imatinib-sensitive *KIT* or *PDGFRA* mutation.
- Most moderate-risk or high-risk patients may be treated after surgery with imatinib 400 mg daily for 3 years, but the optimal dose and treatment duration are unknown.
- Follow-up of patients is mandatory and should include longitudinal imaging of the abdomen and the pelvis to detect recurrence at a time when the tumor mass is still small.

INTRODUCTION

Gastrointestinal stromal tumors (GISTs) are usually local when first detected, only a few (10%–20%) have given rise to overt metastases.[1,2] GISTs are often cured by surgery.[3] When GIST gives rise to metastases, they are frequently found in the abdominal cavity and the liver, but may sometimes occur also at other sites, including the bone.[4]

Most patients with metastatic GIST achieve durable responses with tyrosine kinase inhibitor therapy,[5–7] but advanced GIST is still frequently lethal.[8] Adjuvant treatment of patients with GIST with imatinib, which inhibits the key molecular drivers of GIST, KIT, and platelet-derived growth factor α (PDGFRA) receptor tyrosine kinases,[9] has emerged as a means to improve recurrence-free survival (RFS) after surgery.[10,11]

Funding Sources: None.
Conflict of Interest: The Clinical Research Institute of Helsinki University Central Hospital has received research funding from Novartis and Bayer.
Department of Oncology, Helsinki University Central Hospital, Helsinki University, Haartmaninkatu 4, Helsinki FIN-00029, Finland
E-mail address: heikki.joensuu@hus.fi

Hematol Oncol Clin N Am 27 (2013) 889–904
http://dx.doi.org/10.1016/j.hoc.2013.07.004   **hemonc.theclinics.com**

Imatinib may improve also overall survival of patients who have undergone surgery for high-risk GIST.[11]

Adjuvant treatment with imatinib of patients who have a significant risk of GIST recurrence after surgery is considered the standard whenever GIST harbors an imatinib-sensitive mutation, but several aspects of the management are still unresolved. Patient selection for adjuvant treatment is important, because patients who are cured by surgery do not benefit from adjuvant therapy but are exposed to drug adverse effects and costs. Despite being generally well tolerated, adjuvant imatinib frequently causes mild or moderate adverse effects.[5–7,10,11] The optimal dose of adjuvant imatinib and the duration of administration are unknown. Follow-up of patients on adjuvant imatinib and after its completion with imaging of the abdomen is likely important, because most patients with recurrent tumor detected after adjuvant imatinib respond to imatinib reinstitution,[12] but little research has been performed on this subject. In this article, the data generated in clinical trials on adjuvant therapy are reviewed, and selection of patients for adjuvant treatment is discussed.

CURE FROM GIST BY SURGERY

The fraction of patients with GIST who are cured by surgery has been challenging to determine. GISTs are rare tumors, and many series on operable GIST have only a limited follow-up time and may be affected by a selection bias. GISTs sometimes recur late, and death from GIST up to 25 to 30 years after the diagnosis has been described.[13,14] The size of the cured fraction likely depends also on delay in GIST detection and the frequency of abdominal imaging in a population. The fraction of patients who are cured by surgery may increase in the future with enhanced access to endoscopy and imaging of the abdomen.

In a pooled analysis of 10 series identified from the literature[3] in which each series consisted of virtually all patients with GIST diagnosed within a defined geographic region and period, the 5-year, 10-year, 15-year, and 20-year RFS rates after surgery were 70.5%, 62.9%, 59.9%, and 57.3%, respectively, among 1625 patients with RFS information available and of whom none had received adjuvant therapy. These findings suggest that GIST recurrence is infrequent after the first 10 years of follow-up after surgery and that some patients with GIST are likely cured by surgery alone. Lower RFS figures have been reported from single centers,[15,16] but patients with small and more indolent GIST might be underrepresented in series of referral centers. Because modern imaging examinations may advance early diagnosis and improve detection of small metastatic deposits compared with historical data, approximately 60% of the patients who now present with operable GIST are probably cured by surgery alone and are thus not candidates for adjuvant therapy.

ASSESSMENT OF THE RISK OF GIST RECURRENCE
Prognostic Factors for GIST Recurrence

The most important independent prognostic factor for GIST recurrence after surgery is probably tumor proliferation rate, as assessed with the mitotic count, despite the several limitations of mitosis counting.[3,13–15] Identification of mitoses may vary between pathologists, and the size of the microscope field of view and tissue fixation time may also influence the reported counts.[17] Immunostaining for the Ki-67 antigen may be a valid alternative to the mitotic count,[18,19] but this remains to be firmly established.

Tumor size and site are also important prognostic factors.[3,20] Gastric GISTs have generally more favorable outcome than those arising from the small intestine, colon, or rectum, although the risks associated with colonic and rectal GISTs have been difficult to define because of their rarity.[3,15,20–24] GISTs may rarely arise from tissues outside the gastrointestinal tract. Such GISTs, frequently referred to as extragastrointestinal GISTs (E-GISTs), are generally associated with unfavorable outcome, but some E-GISTs may be metastases from an unidentified primary tumor in the gastrointestinal tract.[3] Tumor rupture before surgery or at surgery is an adverse prognostic factor, probably independent of tumor size, site, and mitotic count,[3] and is associated with a risk of recurrence greater than 80%.[23,25,26] Besides tumor mitotic count, size, site, and rupture, numerous other clinical, biological, and histologic factors have been found to be associated with survival.[27]

Risk-Stratification Schemes

Several risk-stratification schemes have been devised for estimating the risk of GIST recurrence after surgery.[2,20,23,27,28] The first one of these schemes was the US National Institutes of Health (NIH) consensus criteria, which stratify the risk as very low, low, intermediate, or high based on tumor size and mitotic count (Table 1).[28]

Table 1
Three commonly used schemes for estimating the risk of GIST recurrence after surgery

	GIST Characteristic		
Risk Group	Diameter (cm)	Mitotic Count/50 HPFs	Site
NIH consensus criteria			
Very low risk	<2	<5	Tumor site not considered
Low risk	2–5	<5	in risk stratification
Intermediate risk	<5	6–10	
	5–10	<5	
High risk	>10	Any count	
	Any size	>10	
	>5	>5	
Modified NIH consensus criteria			
Very low risk	<2.0	≤5	Any site
Low risk	2.1–5.0	≤5	Any site
Intermediate risk	≤5.0	6–10	Gastric
	5.1–10.0	≤5	Gastric
High risk	>10.0	Any count	Any site
	Any size	>10	Any site
	>5.0	>5	Any site
	≤5.0	>5	Nongastric
	5.1–10.0	≤5	Nongastric
	Any size, site, or mitotic count if tumor rupture present		
AFIP criteria for size and mitosis count			
Group 1	<2.0	≤5	Criteria available for gastric,
Group 2	2.1–5.0	≤5	duodenal, jejunal/ileal, and
Group 3a	5.1–10.0	≤5	rectal GISTs[20]
Group 3b	>10.0	≤5	
Group 4	<2.0	>5	
Group 5	2.1–5.0	>5	
Group 6a	5.1–10.0	>5	
Group 6b	>10.0	>5	

Abbreviations: AFIP, Armed Forces Institute of Pathology; HPF, high-power field of the microscope.

The NIH consensus criteria were confirmed to have prognostic validity in several clinical series,[27] but they suffer from a limitation of not taking into account tumor site.

The Armed Forces Institute of Pathology (AFIP) criteria were the first to acknowledge the importance of tumor site as a prognostic factor besides tumor size and mitotic count. They were developed based on large patient series with long follow-up from a single center.[13,14,20,24] Tumor mitosis count was grouped into 2 categories (≤5 or >5 mitoses per 50 high-power fields [HPFs]) and size into 4 categories (<2.0 cm, 2.1–5.0 cm, 5.1–10.0 cm, and >10.0 cm) resulting in 8 prognostic groups (see **Table 1**). These criteria were studied separately in series of GISTs arising from different sites of the gastrointestinal tract, the stomach,[13] duodenum,[29] ileum or jejunum,[14] or rectum.[24] The AFIP stratification does not recognize tumor rupture as a prognostic factor. Because only 1 cutoff value is available for the mitotic count, substantially different risk estimations may be obtained for patients whose count is close to 5 mitotic figures per 50 HPFs. For example, a patient with 6 cm gastric GIST with 5 mitoses per 50 HPFs has group 3a GIST with 3.6% risk of progressive disease, whereas a similar tumor with 6 mitoses qualifies for group 6a and has 55% risk of progressive tumor.[20] The AFIP risk stratification has been validated.[3]

The NIH classification was modified based on the AFIP classification and a literature review.[27] Besides tumor size, site, and mitotic count, the modified NIH classification considers also tumor rupture for risk stratification. Nongastric GISTs 5.0 cm or smaller in diameter with more than 5 mitoses per 50 HPFs, and nongastric tumors 5.1 to 10.0 cm in size with few mitoses (<5/50 HPFs) are considered high-risk lesions (see **Table 1**).[27] The modified NIH scheme has been validated.[3,23] A potential advantage of the modified NIH classification is that GISTs classified in the very-low-risk, low-risk, and intermediate-risk categories have generally favorable and similar outcomes, leaving the high-risk category as the only group to be considered for adjuvant treatment (**Table 2**).[3] Although 2 cutoff points are used for categorization of the mitotic

Table 2
RFS after surgery of patients with GIST with operable tumor by the AFIP and the modified NIH schemes[a]

		Time from Surgery			
Risk Group	**Group Size (%)**	**5-y RFS (%)**	**10-y RFS (%)**	**15-y RFS (%)**	**20-y RFS (%)**
AFIP scheme					
1	12.7	97	95	95	95
2	29.3	91	90	90	90
3a	19.0	86	80	78	78
3b	8.9	68	62	62	64
4	0.5	86	46	—	—
5	7.7	61	49	39	—
6a	12.1	33	25	19	19
6b	9.9	21	9	9	0
Modified NIH scheme					
Very low	11.9	97	95	95	95
Low	28.7	91	90	90	90
Intermediate	13.5	91	87	87	87
High	45.8	46	36	32	25

[a] The data on the group size and RFS are derived from Ref.[3]

count, small differences in the mitotic counts close to these cutoff values may affect substantially the predicted outcomes as in the AFIP classification.

The prognostic accuracy of the NIH scheme, the modified NIH scheme, and the AFIP risk-stratification scheme may be roughly similar. In the pooled data from 10 population-based series consisting of patients who had undergone surgery for local GIST, the area under the curve (AUC) values addressing 10-year RFS for the NIH scheme, the modified NIH scheme, and the AFIP scheme were 0.79, 0.78, and 0.82, respectively, in a receiver operating characteristics (ROC) curve analysis, and the AUC values were similar also in an independent series consisting of 920 patients with GIST (0.76, 0.76, and 0.77, respectively).[3] These AUC values suggest that each method predicts RFS reasonably well.

A tumor-grade-metastasis classification has been proposed for GIST.[2] In this classification, the M (metastasis) category includes both regional lymph node metastases and distant metastases. The tumor-grade-metastasis classification is infrequently used, because mitotic counting is frequently preferred to histologic grading, and GIST only rarely gives rise to lymph node metastases (approximately 1%) except for pediatric GISTs, syndromic GISTs, and in pediatric-type GISTs in young adults, in whom lymph nodes are involved in 20% to 59% of the patients.[30–32]

Prognostic Nomograms

Two nomograms, reported by Gold and colleagues[21] and Rossi and colleagues,[22] are available for estimation of outcome of patients with operable GIST. In the nomograms, scores are first provided for tumor size, mitotic count, and tumor site, after which the overall score thus generated is used to predict outcome. In the Gold nomogram, tumor size is a continuous variable, whereas mitotic count is categorized into 2 groups (<5 vs ≥5 mitoses/50 HPFs). This situation leads to marked differences in RFS estimations for patients with the tumor mitotic count exactly 5 or just more than 5 compared with patients with tumor mitotic count just less than 5. In the Rossi nomogram, both size and mitotic count are continuous variables, circumventing the problem created by a single cutoff value for the mitotic count, but the Rossi nomogram is limited to patients 65 years or younger at the time of the diagnosis and predicts 10-year overall survival instead of RFS.[22] The Gold nomogram suggests that patients with colonic or rectal GIST have better RFS than those with small bowel GIST, whereas the Rossi nomogram suggests their outcome to be worse. The Gold nomogram has been validated.[21]

Prognostic Heat Maps

The prognostic heat maps consider tumor size, site, mitotic count, and rupture in prognostication of RFS after surgery. The risk of GIST recurrence is depicted in the maps with different colors, the shades of red corresponding to high risks of recurrence and the shades of blue to a small risk. The maps were developed based on the pooled data from all population-based series on operable GIST in which patients had not been treated with adjuvant therapy identified from the literature.[3] Tumor size and mitotic count were treated as continuous parameters that have a nonlinear effect on the risk of GIST recurrence when generating the maps.

When the prognostic accuracy of the heat maps was compared with the NIH scheme, the modified NIH scheme, and the AFIP criteria, the maps provided more accurate estimations for the 10-year risk of GIST recurrence, with an AUC of 0.88 in an ROC analysis versus values ranging from 0.78 to 0.82 with the 3 risk-stratification schemes.[3] Because tumor size and mitotic count are treated as continuous variables in the maps, no abrupt changes in RFS estimations occur at any parameter value. The maps can be applied to all GISTs regardless of their site or origin, including E-GISTs.

Gene Expression Profiles

The CINSARC (Complexity Index in SARComas) gene expression array, which consists of 67 genes involved in the maintenance of chromosome integrity and mitotic control, was effective in segregation of 60 operable GISTs into low-risk and high-risk groups.[33] The resulting low-risk group consisted of 32 patients, of whom none developed distant metastases during the follow-up, whereas the high-risk group with 28 patients had only 38% 5-year metastasis-free survival. One of the array component genes, Aurora kinase A (AURKA), which encodes a mitotic centrosomal protein kinase, was effective as a single factor in identifying patients with unfavorable outcome. Overexpression of AURKA induces centrosome duplication and segregation abnormalities, leading to aneuploidy,[33,34] and its overexpression has been found to be associated with poor prognosis also in another GIST patient cohort.[35] A prognostic Genomic Index (GI), defined as the ratio of the square of the total number of genomic alterations detected (gains or losses in a comparative genomic hybridization array, A^2) and the number of chromosomes involved (C; $GI = A^2/C$), effectively segregated patients with intermediate-risk GIST by the AFIP classification into 2 distinct prognostic groups. The GI can be determined from formalin-fixed paraffin-embedded tissue.[33]

A recent study[36] compared 4 gene expression signatures with the AFIP classification in prediction of RFS in a series of 146 localized GISTs treated with surgery alone. In this study the Genomic Grade Index (GGI), which involves expression of 108 genes,[37] outperformed a gene expression signature consisting of 275 genes, the CINSARC signature, 16-kinase signature, and the AFIP classification, and could split the AFIP intermediate-risk/high-risk samples into 2 groups with different outcomes.

Gene expression profiles are promising new methods for estimating the risk of GIST recurrence, but it has not been established whether these methods are superior to the prognostication tools that rely on the standard clinical and histopathologic prognostic factors.

Selection of Patients for Adjuvant Therapy: Key Messages

- Any of the validated prognostication schemes (see **Table 1**) may be used for estimation of the risk of GIST recurrence after surgery and to select patients for adjuvant therapy.
- The AFIP scheme segregates the GIST patient population into several groups with widely varying risk, whereas the modified NIH scheme results essentially in only 2 groups with either low or high risk for GIST recurrence, the high-risk group being the target population for adjuvant therapy (see **Table 2**).
- The prognostic heat maps have an advantage that a small change in tumor size or mitotic count does not produce a large change in outcome estimation, allowing risk estimation of those patients whose tumor size or mitotic count is close to a cutoff value with more confidence. The heat maps seem to be at least as accurate as the conventional prognostic schemes in outcome estimation.
- The prognostic gene profiles are promising but need further validation.

CLINICAL TRIALS ON ADJUVANT THERAPY IN GIST

Imatinib is the only agent that has been evaluated as adjuvant treatment of operable GIST. The key evidence regarding its safety and efficacy stems from 2 prospective randomized phase 3 trials: the ACOSOG (American College of Surgeons Oncology

Group) trial Z9001[10] and the SSG (Scandinavian Sarcoma Group) XVIII/AIO (Arbeitsgemeinschaft Internistische Onkologie) trial (**Table 3**).[11] In Z9001, 713 patients who had undergone surgery for GIST 3 cm or larger in diameter were randomly assigned to either imatinib 400 mg daily orally or placebo for 1 year after surgery.[10] The trial Data and Safety Monitoring Committee halted patient accrual once a planned interim analysis showed a substantial difference between the groups in favor of the imatinib arm, which resulted in a short median duration of follow-up of only 19.7 months. One-year RFS was 98% in the imatinib group and 83% in the placebo group, and the hazard ratio [HR] between the arms was 0.35 (95% confidence interval [CI] 0.22–0.53; $P<.0001$). There was no difference in overall survival between the groups at the time of reporting; crossover from the placebo group to the imatinib group was allowed after detection of GIST recurrence. The US Food and Drug Administration approved adjuvant imatinib for the treatment of KIT-positive GIST based on the Z9001 findings in 2008, and the European Medicines Agency for the treatment of KIT-positive GIST with a significant risk of relapse in 2009.

The SSGXVIII/AIO trial compared 2 durations of adjuvant imatinib. In this study, 400 patients considered to have high risk of GIST recurrence based on the NIH consensus classification or who had tumor rupture either before surgery or at surgery were assigned to imatinib 400 mg daily for either 12 or 36 months.[11] Many (20%) of the patients had ruptured GIST. The median duration of follow-up was 54 months at the time when the preplanned number of RFS events had accumulated and the study was

Table 3
Reported prospective randomized phase 3 trials evaluating adjuvant imatinib for GIST

	ACOSOG Z9001	SSGXVIII/AIO
Study characteristic		
Design	Placebo-controlled	Open-label
Allocation groups	Imatinib 400 mg/d for 12 mo	Imatinib 400 mg/d for 12 mo
	Placebo for 12 mo	Imatinib 400 mg/d for 36 mo
Primary objective	RFS	RFS
Key inclusion criteria	KIT-positive GIST, ≥3 cm in diameter; age ≥18 y; ECOG performance status ≤2	KIT-positive GIST, high-risk GIST by the NIH consensus criteria or tumor rupture; age ≥18 y; ECOG performance status ≤2
Setting	United States, Canada	Finland, Germany, Norway, Sweden
Accrual period	2002–2007	2004–2008
Main results		
Randomized patients	713	400
Median follow-up time	19.7 mo	54 mo
RFS		
Number of events	Imatinib, 30; placebo, 70	36 mo, 50; 12 mo, 84
HR	0.35 (95% CI, 0.22–0.53)	0.46 (95% CI, 0.32–0.65)
P	<.0001	<.0001
Overall survival		
Number of events	Imatinib, 5; placebo, 8	36 mo, 12; 12 mo, 25
HR	0.66 (95% CI, 0.22–2.03)	0.45 (95% CI, 0.22–0.89)
P	.47	.02

Abbreviation: ECOG, Eastern Cooperative Oncology Group.

analyzed. Patients assigned to the 3-year group had 5-year RFS of 65.6% compared with 47.9% in the 1-year group (HR 0.46; 95% CI 0.32–0.65; $P<.0001$). Overall survival was a secondary end point in the study, and the trial was not powered to assess overall survival, but the analysis of overall survival also favored the 3-year group over the 1-year group (5-year survival 92.0% vs 81.7%, respectively; HR 0.45, 95% CI 0.22–0.89; $P = .019$). The National Comprehensive Cancer Network (NCCN) of the United States now recommends consideration of adjuvant imatinib for at least 3 years for patients with intermediate or high risk of GIST recurrence,[38] and the European Society for Medical Oncology (ESMO) for 3 years when risk of relapse is high.[39]

The European Organization for Research and Treatment of Cancer–sponsored randomized trial 62024 (NCT00103168) compares 2 years of imatinib with observation in a patient population with intermediate or high risk of GIST recurrence. The first results, based on 908 patients randomized and a median follow-up time of 4.7 years, confirmed that imatinib prolongs the time to GIST recurrence, but no significant difference was found in the time to imatinib failure once GIST had recurred between the 2 groups.[40]

Most patients tolerate adjuvant imatinib relatively well and most adverse effects are graded mild to moderate (grade 1 or 2). Yet, virtually all patients have some adverse effects.[10,11] Many of the side effects can be alleviated with symptomatic treatments,[41] but sometimes dose reduction is required. The most frequent adverse effects include anemia, periorbital edema and watery eyes, diarrhea, muscle cramps (typically in hands and legs), fatigue, and nausea.[11] In Z9001, 96 (27%) and 46 (13%) of the study participants discontinued imatinib early for reasons other than GIST recurrence in the imatinib and placebo groups, respectively, and in the SSGXVIII/AIO trial 25 (13%) and 51 (26%) of patients assigned to the 12-month and 36-month groups discontinued imatinib early for a similar reason.[10,11] Adverse events graded as severe (grade 3 or higher) were recorded in the Z9001 trial relatively frequently; 104 (31%) patients assigned to imatinib and 63 (18%) of those assigned to placebo had such events. Grade 3 or higher adverse events occurred in 39 (20%) and 65 (33%) of the patients in the 1-year and the 3-year groups in the SSGXVIII/AIO trial, respectively.

A few nonrandomized registered phase 2 trials[42–44] and cohort studies[45–49] have evaluated adjuvant imatinib as the treatment of operable GIST. In general, the results of these studies are in agreement with the findings of the randomized trials and suggest that adjuvant imatinib prolongs RFS.

Adjuvant imatinib administered at a daily dose of 400 mg after surgery prolonged RFS in 2 large randomized trials, and 36 months of adjuvant imatinib improved survival compared with 12 months of imatinib in 1 trial. However, the effect on adjuvant imatinib on overall survival was based on a limited number of events (see **Table 3**) and requires confirmation. The data suggest that 3 years of imatinib is a reasonable choice for adjuvant systemic therapy whenever the risk of GIST recurrence is significant and GIST harbors an imatinib-sensitive mutation.

PREOPERATIVE IMATINIB

Five nonrandomized studies[50–54] have investigated the role of preoperative imatinib as a treatment of locally advanced GIST. Imatinib was usually administered for 2 to 6 months before surgery, and sometimes continued as adjuvant treatment after surgery.

Most GISTs shrink or stabilize in size on preoperative imatinib. This finding may facilitate surgical tumor resection and may allow organ sparing.[55] Preoperative imatinib may be considered for selected patients, in particular for those who have rectal or duodenal GIST, to avoid resections that adversely influence the quality of life, and for patients with a large gastric GIST, which likely requires gastrectomy unless preoperative imatinib is given. Patients treated with preoperative imatinib should have tumor mutation analysis performed from a tissue biopsy and tumor response to imatinib carefully monitored with imaging at intervals of a few weeks, because not all GISTs are responsive to imatinib. A biopsy does not allow full evaluation of the tumor mitotic rate, which may make decisions on the need of adjuvant imatinib after surgery challenging, and concerns have been raised regarding contamination of the serosal surfaces with tumor cells at biopsy. Yet, many GISTs treated with neoadjuvant therapy are large lesions that qualify for the high-risk category because of size alone.

THE ROLE OF TUMOR MUTATION ANALYSIS

Tumor mutation analysis provides both prognostic and predictive information when adjuvant therapy is considered. GISTs with *KIT* exon 9 mutation or exon 11 deletion mutation involving the codons 557 to 558 are associated with unfavorable outcome when treated with surgery alone, whereas patients with *PDGFRA* exon 18 mutation D842V generally have favorable outcome.[15,56,57] Almost all *KIT* exon 9 mutations are duplication mutations of the codons 502 to 503 leading to duplication of the alanine and tyrosine amino acid residues in the protein, whereas the deletions involving *KIT* exon 11 codons 557 to 558 have variable lengths and may consist of a deletion combined with an insertion. Although mutations of *KIT* and *PDGFRA* carry prognostic significance, they have not been incorporated into the current risk-stratification schemes, because numerous different *KIT* and *PDGFRA* mutations have been identified in GIST[1] and it is not clear whether the mutations confer information independent from other prognostic factors.

Besides prognostication, tumor mutation analysis is of importance in identifying mutations that confer insensitivity to imatinib. The D842V mutation occurs in up to 10% of GISTs and may be the most frequent single mutation in GIST.[1] This mutation confers insensitivity to imatinib in vitro,[58,59] and no responses were achieved among 31 patients with the D842V mutation when advanced GIST was treated with imatinib.[60] Most of the other mutations that infrequently occur at the *PDGFRA* locus D842, such as RD841-842KI, DI842-843IM, D842Y, D842I, and deletion I843, are also imatinib resistant.[58,61]

Adjuvant treatment of patients with GIST that is wild-type with respect of *KIT* and *PDGFRA* is controversial. In the subgroup analyses of the Z9001 and SSGXVIII/AIO trials, the numbers of wild-type GISTs were likely too small to reach firm conclusions.[11,62] Patients with neurofibromatiosis 1 (NF1) are at a substantially increased risk of being diagnosed with GIST,[63] which is usually wild-type in mutation analysis[63,64] and rarely responds to imatinib.[64] Therefore, patients with NF1-associated wild-type GIST should probably not be treated with adjuvant imatinib. There are no data available to show that patients with succinate dehydrogenase (SDH)-deficient GIST or *BRAF*-mutated GIST benefit from adjuvant imatinib.

IMATINIB DOSE

Only the imatinib dose of 400 mg daily has been evaluated in the adjuvant setting. Patients with advanced GISTs with *KIT* exon 9 mutation generally benefit from treatment with higher than the 400 mg daily dose of imatinib,[65] but whether such doses are beneficial in the adjuvant setting remains to be shown.

When treating advanced GIST, low imatinib trough levels (<1100 ng/mL) in samples taken 4 weeks after imatinib initiation were associated with a short time to disease progression.[66] In the advanced setting, the bioavailability of imatinib was found to decrease during the first 3 months on treatment by approximately 30%,[67] and subtotal and total gastrectomy were associated with low imatinib trough plasma levels.[68] Measurement of imatinib trough plasma concentrations and increase of the dosage might thus be reasonable to consider in selected cases to avoid underdosing,[69] but no research data are available to support such an approach.

PATIENT FOLLOW-UP DURING AND AFTER ADJUVANT THERAPY

Follow-up of patients during and after adjuvant treatment is mandatory to detect and manage treatment-related adverse effects and to discover GIST recurrence early. Most GISTs that recur after completion of adjuvant treatment either respond or stabilize on imatinib reinstitution,[12] but the duration of such responses is unknown. Because recurrences are frequently detected at longitudinal follow-up imaging examinations, the tumor bulk is often still small. Data from advanced GIST suggest that patients whose tumor mass is small at the time of initiation of imatinib have the longest times to the development of secondary resistance to imatinib,[8,70] and, therefore, early detection of GIST recurrence after adjuvant therapy could contribute to overall survival.

The optimal follow-up schemes are unknown, and different schedules have not been compared in prospective studies. Imaging of the abdomen and the pelvis is usually sufficient, because bone and lung metastases are uncommon. Computed tomography (CT) is often preferred in the follow-up because access to magnetic resonance imaging or positron emission tomography CT may be limited, and small metastases in the abdominal cavity may not be readily detectable with ultrasonography.

The NCCN suggests performing abdominal/pelvic CT 3 to 6 monthly for 3 to 5 years, then annually,[38] which results in 13 to 25 abdominal/pelvic CT scans within the first 10 years of follow-up (Table 4). The ESMO 2012 guidelines suggest abdominal/pelvic CT to be performed 3 to 6 monthly for the first 3 years, then 3 monthly for 2 years, then 6 monthly for 3 years, then annually, acknowledging that the hazard of GIST recurrence is the greatest within the 2 years that follow discontinuation of the 3-year period of adjuvant imatinib.[39] Assuming that 1 CT delivers a dose of 8 mSv,[71] imaging according to the NCCN and the ESMO guidelines results in a cumulative radiation dose of 104 to 200 mSv and 176 to 224 mSv during the first 10 years of follow-up, respectively, which approaches the lifetime dose received from background radiation.[71] Most GIST recurrences occur during the first 10 years from surgery when no adjuvant therapy is given,[3] and follow-up for 10 years after surgery may thus suffice. In the randomized trials that evaluated adjuvant imatinib,[10,11] physical examination and measurement of the blood cell counts and blood biochemistry were performed at 1-month to 3-month intervals during administration of adjuvant imatinib.

Table 4		
Follow-up of patients with GIST after surgery with CT		
Guideline	Follow-Up Frequency with Abdominal/Pelvic CT	Total Number of CT Scans Within the First 10 y After Surgery
NCCN, 2013	3–6 monthly for 3–5 y, then annually	13–25
ESMO, 2012	3–6 monthly for 3 y, then 3 monthly for 2 y, then 6 monthly for 3 y, then annually	22–28

MANAGEMENT OF PATIENTS WHOSE GIST RECURS DURING ADJUVANT THERAPY

GISTs that recur during adjuvant imatinib may be managed as GIST progressing on imatinib in the advanced setting, although no trial has yet addressed this patient population. Dose escalation of imatinib may thus be considered, especially when GIST with *KIT* exon 9 mutation progresses on adjuvant imatinib at the dose of 400 mg daily, or initiation of sunitinib may be considered.

FUTURE DEVELOPMENTS

More than 10 novel agents are being investigated in the treatment of advanced GIST, but only imatinib is being studied in the adjuvant setting.[72,73] Because many GISTs recur soon after discontinuing adjuvant imatinib, some patients might benefit from longer than 3 years of adjuvant imatinib. Adjuvant treatments of long duration seem intuitively attractive in subgroups of patients with a very high risk of GIST recurrence, such as patients with ruptured GIST or those with large nongastric GISTs with many mitoses, in whom the risk of recurrence after surgery alone approaches 100%, but durations longer than 3 years have not been studied in randomized trials and carry a risk for overtreatment.

Adjuvant trials focusing on important molecular subgroups, such as *KIT* exon 9-mutated GIST, SDH-deficient GIST, and D842-mutated GIST are warranted, but are challenging because of the rarity of these tumors and their sometimes variable clinical behavior. The optimal dosing of imatinib in the adjuvant setting is unknown, and warrants further evaluation. Novel agents that might have efficacy also for the putative GIST stem cells that may be resistant to KIT inhibitors and thus survive adjuvant imatinib, may be needed to increase the fraction of patients who are cured from GIST.[74] Methods to detect GIST recurrence early during and after adjuvant therapy need to be explored.

SUMMARY

GIST has usually not given rise to overt distant metastases when first detected, and approximately 60% of patients with local tumor are cured by surgery. The remaining 40% are potential candidates for adjuvant imatinib, provided that the tumor carries a mutation that is sensitive to imatinib. Patients who have *PDGFRA* locus D842 mutation are excluded from adjuvant therapy because such tumors are insensitive to imatinib, as are many patients with wild-type GIST, including those with NF1-associated GIST, and possibly patients with SDH-deficient or *BRAF*-mutated GIST.

The risk of GIST recurrence may be estimated with one of the validated risk-stratification schemes, which include the NIH consensus criteria, the modified NIH criteria, and the AFIP criteria. Patients with a high estimated risk of recurrence are usually selected for treatment with adjuvant imatinib, but whether patients with an intermediate risk should be offered adjuvant imatinib is controversial.[38,39] When the modified NIH classification is used for risk stratification, the intermediate-risk group has roughly similar outcome to the low-risk group, leaving only the high-risk group for consideration of adjuvant systemic treatment. Many risk-stratification methods use cutoff values for tumor size and mitosis count, which may result in a large change in the estimated outcome when tumor size or mitotic count is close to a cutoff value. The prognostic heat maps treat size and mitotic counts as continuous variables and may be more accurate than the NIH and AFIP risk-stratification schemes in estimation of the risk of recurrence. Gene expression profiles are effective in outcome estimation, and further study comparing gene expression profiles with the conventional methods is warranted.

Adjuvant imatinib at the dose of 400 mg/d improves RFS, and according to 1 randomized trial, 3 years of adjuvant imatinib improves RFS and overall survival compared with 1 year of adjuvant imatinib. The optimal dose of adjuvant imatinib and the optimal duration of treatment remain unknown, but treating patients with a moderate or high estimated risk of GIST recurrence for 3 years with adjuvant imatinib is a reasonable choice. Whether a duration of adjuvant imatinib longer than 3 years confers further benefits over 3 years of imatinib is an important research topic, particularly for the subgroup of patients who have a very high risk of GIST recurrence, such as patients with ruptured tumor, or large nongastric GIST with frequent mitoses.

Clinical follow-up of patients during and after adjuvant imatinib is mandatory for detection and management of treatment-related adverse effects, for adjustment of imatinib dose when necessary, and to detect recurrence early. Imaging is usually performed with longitudinal CT scans of the abdomen and the pelvis. Most GISTs that recur after completion of adjuvant therapy respond to imatinib reinstitution. Hypothetically, detection of GIST recurrence at the time when the tumor bulk is still small may increase the likelihood of achieving a durable response on imatinib reinstitution, because the latency of a secondary resistance mutation to emerge is likely associated with size of the tumor mass.

REFERENCES

1. Emile JF, Brahini S, Coindre JM, et al. Frequencies of KIT and PDGFRA mutations in the MolecGIST prospective population-based study differ from those of advanced GISTs. Med Oncol 2012;29(3):1765–72.
2. Woodall CE 3rd, Brock GN, Fan J, et al. An evaluation of 2537 gastrointestinal stromal tumors for a proposed clinical staging system. Arch Surg 2009; 144(7):670–8.
3. Joensuu H, Vehtari A, Riihimäki J, et al. Risk of gastrointestinal stromal tumour recurrence after surgery: an analysis based on pooled population-based cohorts. Lancet Oncol 2012;13(3):265–74.
4. DeMatteo RP, Lewis JJ, Leung D, et al. Two hundred gastrointestinal stromal tumors: recurrence patterns and prognostic factors for survival. Ann Surg 2000; 231(1):51–8.
5. Demetri GD, von Mehren M, Blanke CD, et al. Efficacy and safety of imatinib mesylate in advanced gastrointestinal stromal tumors. N Engl J Med 2002;347(7): 472–80.
6. Verweij J, Casali PG, Zalcberg J, et al. Progression-free survival in gastrointestinal stromal tumours with high-dose imatinib: randomised trial. Lancet 2004; 364(9440):1127–34.
7. Blanke CD, Demetri GD, von Mehren M, et al. Long-term results from a randomized phase II trial of standard- versus higher-dose imatinib mesylate for patients with unresectable or metastatic gastrointestinal stromal tumors expressing KIT. J Clin Oncol 2008;26(4):620–5.
8. Von Mehren M. Follow-up results after 9 years of the ongoing, phase II B2222 trial of imatinib mesylate in patients with metastatic or unresectable KIT+ gastrointestinal stromal tumors (GIST). J Clin Oncol 2011;29(Suppl): 609s.
9. Buchdunger E, Cioffi CL, Law N, et al. Abl protein-tyrosine kinase inhibitor STI571 inhibits in vitro signal transduction mediated by c-kit and platelet-derived growth factor receptors. J Pharmacol Exp Ther 2000;295(1):139–45.

10. DeMatteo RP, Ballman KV, Antonescu CR, et al. Adjuvant imatinib mesylate after resection of localised, primary gastrointestinal stromal tumour: a randomised, double-blind, placebo-controlled trial. Lancet 2009;373(9669):1097–104.

11. Joensuu H, Eriksson M, Sundby Hall K, et al. One vs three years of adjuvant imatinib for operable gastrointestinal stromal tumor: a randomized trial. JAMA 2012;307(12):1265–72.

12. Reichardt P, Hartmann J, Sundby Hall K, et al. Response to imatinib rechallenge of GIST that recurs following completion of adjuvant imatinib treatment–the first analysis in the SSGXVIII/AIO trial patient population. Eur J Cancer 2011; 47(Suppl 2):15.

13. Miettinen M, Sobin LH, Lasota J. Gastrointestinal stromal tumors of the stomach. A clinicopathologic, immunohistochemical, and molecular genetic study of 1765 cases with long-term follow-up. Am J Surg Pathol 2005;29(1):52–68.

14. Miettinen M, Makhlouf H, Sobin LH, et al. Gastrointestinal stromal tumors of the jejunum and ileum. A clinopathologic, immunohistochemical, and molecular genetic study of 906 cases before imatinib with long-term-follow-up. Am J Surg Pathol 2006;30(4):477–89.

15. DeMatteo RP, Gold JS, Saran L, et al. Tumor mitotic rate, size, and location independently predict recurrence after resection of primary gastrointestinal stromal tumor (GIST). Cancer 2008;112(3):608–15.

16. Crosby JA, Catton CN, Davis A, et al. Malignant gastrointestinal stromal tumors of the small intestine: a review of 50 cases from a prospective database. Ann Surg Oncol 2001;8(1):50–9.

17. Gal R, Rath-Wolfson L, Rosenblatt Y, et al. An improved technique for mitosis counting. Int J Surg Pathol 2005;13(2):161–5.

18. Jiang J, Jin MS, Suo J, et al. Evaluation of malignancy using Ki-67, p53, EGFR and COX-2 expressions in gastrointestinal stromal tumors. World J Gastroenterol 2012;18(20):2569–75.

19. Liang YM, Li XH, Li WM, et al. Prognostic significance of PTEN, Ki-67 and CD44s expression patterns in gastrointestinal stromal tumors. World J Gastroenterol 2012;18(14):1664–71.

20. Miettinen M, Lasota J. Gastrointestinal stromal tumors: pathology and prognosis at different sites. Semin Diagn Pathol 2006;23(2):70–83.

21. Gold JS, Gönen M, Gutiérrez A, et al. Development and validation of a prognostic nomogram for recurrence-free survival after complete surgical resection of localised primary gastrointestinal stromal tumour: a retrospective analysis. Lancet Oncol 2009;10(11):1045–52.

22. Rossi S, Miceli R, Messerini L, et al. Natural history of imatinib-naive GISTs: a retrospective analysis of 929 cases with long-term follow-up and development of a survival nomogram based on mitotic index and size as continuous variables. Am J Surg Pathol 2011;35(11):1646–56.

23. Rutkowski P, Bylina E, Wozniak A, et al. Validation of the Joensuu risk criteria for primary resectable gastrointestinal stromal tumour–the impact of tumour rupture on patient outcomes. Eur J Surg Oncol 2011;37(10):890–6.

24. Miettinen M, Furlong M, Sarlomo-Rikala M, et al. Gastrointestinal stromal tumors, intramural leiomyomas, and leiomyosarcomas in the rectum and anus: a clinicopathologic, immunohistochemical, and molecular genetic study of 144 cases. Am J Surg Pathol 2001;25(9):1121–33.

25. Takahashi T, Nakajima K, Nishitani A, et al. An enhanced risk-group stratification system for more practical prognostication of clinically malignant gastrointestinal stromal tumors. Int J Clin Oncol 2007;12(5):369–74.

26. Hohenberger P, Ronellenfitsch U, Oladeji O, et al. Pattern of recurrence in patients with ruptured primary gastrointestinal stromal tumour. Br J Surg 2010; 97(12):1854–9.

27. Joensuu H. Risk stratification of patients diagnosed with gastrointestinal stromal tumor. Hum Pathol 2008;39(10):1411–9.

28. Fletcher CD, Berman JJ, Corless C, et al. Diagnosis of gastrointestinal stromal tumors: a consensus approach. Hum Pathol 2002;33(5):459–65.

29. Miettinen M, Kopczynski J, Makhlouf HR, et al. Gastrointestinal stromal tumors, intramural leiomyomas, and leiomyosarcomas in the duodenum: a clinicopathologic, immunohistochemical, and molecular genetic study of 167 cases. Am J Surg Pathol 2003;27(5):625–41.

30. Agaimy A, Wünsch PH. Lymph node metastasis in gastrointestinal stromal tumours (GIST) occurs preferentially in young patients < or = 40 years: an overview based on our case material and the literature. Langenbecks Arch Surg 2009;394:375–81.

31. Zhang L, Smyrk TC, Young WF Jr, et al. Gastric stromal tumors in Carney triad are different clinically, pathologically, and behaviorally from sporadic gastric gastrointestinal stromal tumors: findings in 104 cases. Am J Surg Pathol 2010; 34:53–64.

32. Rege TA, Wagner AJ, Corless CL, et al. "Pediatric-type" gastrointestinal stromal tumors in adults: distinctive histology predicts genotype and clinical behavior. Am J Surg Pathol 2011;35:495–504.

33. Lagarde P, Pérot G, Kauffmann A, et al. Mitotic checkpoints and chromosome instability are strong predictors of clinical outcome in gastrointestinal stromal tumors. Clin Cancer Res 2012;18(3):826–38.

34. Zhou H, Kuang J, Zhong L, et al. Tumour amplified kinase STK15/BTAK induces centrosome amplification, aneuploidy and transformation. Nat Genet 1998; 20(2):189–93.

35. Yen CC, Yeh CN, Cheng CT, et al. Integrating bioinformatics and clinicopathological research of gastrointestinal stromal tumors: identification of aurora kinase A as a poor risk marker. Ann Surg Oncol 2012;19(11):3491–9.

36. Bertucci F, Finetti P, Ostrowski J, et al. Genomic Grade Index predicts postoperative clinical outcome of GIST. Br J Cancer 2012;107(8):1433–41.

37. Sotiriou C, Wirapati P, Loi S, et al. Gene expression profiling in breast cancer: understanding the molecular basis of histologic grade to improve prognosis. J Natl Cancer Inst 2006;98(4):262–72.

38. National Comprehensive Cancer Network. Clinical practice guidelines in oncology. Soft tissue sarcoma. V. 2.2011. Available at: http://www.nccn.org/professionals/physician_gls/. Accessed January 31, 2013.

39. ESMO/European Sarcoma Network Working Group. Gastrointestinal stromal tumors: ESMO Clinical Practice Guidelines for diagnosis, treatment and follow-up. Ann Oncol 2012;23(Suppl 7):vii49–55.

40. Casali P. Imatinib failure-free survival in patients with localized gastrointestinal stromal tumors (GIST) treated with adjuvant imatinib: The EORTC/AGITG/FSG/GEIS/ISG randomized controlled phase III trial. J Clin Oncol 2013;31(Suppl): 632s.

41. Joensuu H, Trent JC, Reichardt P. Practical management of tyrosine-kinase inhibitor-associated side effects in GIST. Cancer Treat Rev 2011;37(1):75–88.

42. DeMatteo RP, Owzar K, Antonescu CR, et al. Efficacy of adjuvant imatinib mesylate following complete resection of localized, primary gastrointestinal stromal tumor (GIST) at high risk of recurrence: the U.S. Intergroup phase II trial ACOSOG

Z9000. Presented at American Society of Clinical Oncology 2008 Gastrointestinal Cancers Symposium. Orlando, January 25–27, 2008 [abstract 8].

43. Kanda T, Nishida T, Wada N, et al. Adjuvant therapy with imatinib mesylate after resection of primary high-risk gastrointestinal stromal tumors in Japanese patients. Int J Clin Oncol 2013;18(1):38–45.

44. Kang B, Lee J, Ryu M, et al. A phase II study of imatinib mesylate as adjuvant treatment for curatively resected high-risk localized gastrointestinal stromal tumors. J Clin Oncol 2009;27(Suppl):e21515.

45. Zhan WH. Efficacy and safety of adjuvant post-surgical therapy with imatinib in patients with high risk of relapsing GIST. J Clin Oncol 2007;25(Suppl):556s.

46. Nilsson B, Sjölund K, Kindblom LG, et al. Adjuvant imatinib treatment improves recurrence-free survival in patients with high-risk gastrointestinal stromal tumours (GIST). Br J Cancer 2007;96(11):1656–8.

47. Huang H, Liang H, Zhan ZL, et al. Surgical outcomes of gastrointestinal stromal tumors of the stomach: a single unit experience in the era of targeted drug therapy. Med Oncol 2012;29(2):941–7.

48. Jiang WZ, Guan GX, Lu HS, et al. Adjuvant imatinib treatment after R0 resection for patients with high-risk gastrointestinal stromal tumors: a median follow-up of 44 months. J Surg Oncol 2011;104(7):760–4.

49. Li J, Gong JF, Wu AW, et al. Post-operative imatinib in patients with intermediate or high risk gastrointestinal stromal tumor. Eur J Surg Oncol 2011;37(10): 319–24.

50. Wang D, Zhang Q, Blanke CD, et al. Phase II trial of neoadjuvant/adjuvant imatinib mesylate for advanced primary and metastatic/recurrent operable gastrointestinal stromal tumors: long-term follow-up results of Radiation Therapy Oncology Group 0132. Ann Surg Oncol 2012;19(4):1074–80.

51. Andtbacka RH, Ng CS, Scaife CL, et al. Surgical resection of gastrointestinal stromal tumors after treatment with imatinib. Ann Surg Oncol 2007;14(1):14–24.

52. McAuliffe JC, Hunt KK, Lazar JF, et al. A randomized, phase II study of preoperative plus postoperative imatinib in GIST: evidence of rapid radiographic response and temporal induction of tumor cell apoptosis. Ann Surg Oncol 2009;16(4):910–9.

53. Hohenberger P, Oladeji O, Licht T, et al. Neoadjuvant imatinib and organ preservation in locally advanced gastrointestinal stromal tumors (GIST). J Clin Oncol 2009;27(Suppl):548s.

54. Blesius A, Cassier PA, Bertucci F, et al. Neoadjuvant imatinib in patients with locally advanced non metastatic GIST in the prospective BRF 14 trial. BMC Cancer 2011;11:72.

55. Eisenberg BL, Trent JC. Adjuvant and neoadjuvant imatinib therapy: current role in the management of gastrointestinal stromal tumors. Int J Cancer 2011; 129(11):2533–42.

56. Wardelmann E, Losen I, Hans V, et al. Deletion of Trp-557 and Lys-558 in the juxtamembrane domain of the c-kit protooncogene is associated with metastatic behavior of gastrointestinal stromal tumors. Int J Cancer 2003;106(6):887–95.

57. Martin J, Poveda A, Llombart-Bosch A, et al. Deletions affecting codons 557-558 of the c-KIT gene indicate a poor prognosis in patients with completely resected gastrointestinal stromal tumors: a study by the Spanish Group for Sarcoma Research (GEIS). J Clin Oncol 2005;23(25):6190–8.

58. Corless CL, Schroeder A, Griffith D, et al. PDGFRA mutations in gastrointestinal stromal tumors: frequency, spectrum and in vitro sensitivity to imatinib. J Clin Oncol 2005;23(23):5357–64.

59. Weisberg E, Wright RD, Jiang J, et al. Effects of PKC412, nilotinib, and imatinib against GIST-associated PDGFRA mutants with differential imatinib sensitivity. Gastroenterology 2006;131(6):1734–42.

60. Cassier PA, Fumagilli E, Rutkowski P, et al. Outcome of patients with platelet-derived growth factor receptor alpha-mutated gastrointestinal stromal tumors in the tyrosine kinase inhibitor era. Clin Cancer Res 2012;18(16):4458–64.

61. Heinrich MC, Griffith D, McKinley A, et al. Crenolanib inhibits the drug-resistant PDGFRA D842V mutation associated with imatinib-resistant gastrointestinal stromal tumors. Clin Cancer Res 2012;18(16):4375–84.

62. Corless C, Ballman KV, Antonescu C, et al. Relation of tumor pathologic and molecular features to outcome after surgical resection of localized primary gastrointestinal stromal tumor (GIST): results of the intergroup phase III trial ACOSOG Z9001. J Clin Oncol 2010;28(Suppl):699s.

63. Miettinen M, Fetsch JF, Sobin LH, et al. Gastrointestinal stromal tumors in patients with neurofibromatosis 1: a clinicopathologic and molecular genetic study of 45 cases. Am J Surg Pathol 2006;30(1):90–6.

64. Mussi C, Schildhaus HU, Gronchi A, et al. Therapeutic consequences from molecular biology for gastrointestinal stromal tumor patients affected by neurofibromatosis type 1. Clin Cancer Res 2008;14(14):4550–5.

65. Debiec-Rychter M, Sciot R, Le Cesne A, et al. EORTC Soft Tissue and Bone Sarcoma Group; Italian Sarcoma Group; Australasian GastroIntestinal Trials Group. KIT mutations and dose selection for imatinib in patients with advanced gastrointestinal stromal tumours. Eur J Cancer 2006;42(8):1093–103.

66. Demetri GD, Wang Y, Wehrle E, et al. Imatinib plasma levels are correlated with clinical benefit in patients with unresectable/metastatic gastrointestinal stromal tumors. J Clin Oncol 2009;27(19):3141–7.

67. Eechoute K, Fransson MN, Reyners AK, et al. A long-term prospective population pharmacokinetic study on imatinib plasma concentrations in GIST patients. Clin Cancer Res 2012;18(20):5780–7.

68. Yoo C, Ryu MH, Kang BW, et al. Cross-sectional study of imatinib plasma trough levels in patients with advanced gastrointestinal stromal tumors: impact of gastrointestinal resection on exposure to imatinib. J Clin Oncol 2010;28(9):1554–9.

69. Judson IR. Therapeutic drug monitoring of imatinib–new data strengthen the case. Clin Cancer Res 2012;18(20):517–9.

70. Blesius A. Who are the long responders to imatinib in patients with advanced GIST? Results of the BRF14 prospective French Sarcoma Group randomized phase III trial. J Clin Oncol 2011;29(Suppl):616s.

71. Davies HE, Wathen CG, Gleeson FV. The risks of radiation exposure related to diagnostic imaging and how to minimise them. BMJ 2011;342:d947.

72. ClinicalTrials.gov. Available at: http://www.clinicaltrials.gov/. Accessed January 31, 2013.

73. ISRCTN register. Available at: http://isrctn.org/. Accessed January 31, 2013.

74. Bardsley MR, Horváth VJ, Asuzu DT, et al. Kitlow stem cells cause resistance to Kit/platelet-derived growth factor alpha inhibitors in murine gastrointestinal stromal tumors. Gastroenterology 2010;139(3):942–52.

Gastrointestinal Stromal Tumors
Management of Metastatic Disease and Emerging Therapies

Joseph Vadakara, MD, Margaret von Mehren, MD*

KEYWORDS

- GIST • Tyrosine kinase inhibitors • SDH-deficient GIST • KIT • PDGFRA • IGF-1R
- HSP90

KEY POINTS

- GIST represents a family of tumors with similar histologic features but different molecular drivers.
- The routine use of TKI therapies for the management of advanced GIST has led to increased survival for many patients.
- There are three approved agents for the treatment of GIST, and several other agents in which data support their use.
- Tumors that are refractory to TKIs remain a challenge and novel combination therapies being tested in the phase I setting may lead to new therapeutic options.

TYROSINE KINASE INHIBITORS

Activating mutations in the KIT and platelet-derived growth factor-α (PDGFRA) genes have been implicated in the pathogenesis of gastrointestinal stromal tumors (GIST) (**Box 1**). Most GIST have an activating mutation in the KIT gene commonly in exon 11 followed by exons 9, 13, and 17, which constitutively activates the gene product, a cell surface protein kinase receptor.[1] Activating mutations in the PDGFRA gene occur in one-third of GIST tumors that lack KIT mutations.[2] Tyrosine kinase inhibitors (TKIs) target mutated KIT and PDGFRA. Currently, imatinib is the agent of choice in the first-line setting followed by sunitinib in patients who are imatinib intolerant or resistant. Reports of GIST with alternate kinase mutations in B-RAF and RAS have been

Disclosures: None (J. Vadakara); M. von Mehren served as a scientific advisor to Novartis and Pfizer; M. von Mehren supported in part by R21 CA150381 and R01 CA106588.
Department of Medical Oncology, Fox Chase Cancer Center, 333 Cottman Avenue, Philadelphia, PA 19111, USA
* Corresponding author.
E-mail address: Margaret.vonMehren@fccc.edu

Box 1
Currently approved and investigational agents for the management of GIST

Tyrosine Kinase Inhibitors

Imatinib[a]

Sunitinib[a]

Regorafenib[a]

Nilotinib[a]

Sorafenib[a]

Masitinib

Vatalanib

Dovitinib

Pazopanib[a]

Cedarinib

Crenolanib

Hsp90 Inhibitors

BIIB021

AT13387

AUY922

Ganestespib (STA-9090)

PI3K-AKT-mTOR Inhibitors

Perifosine

Everolimus[a]

Sirolimus[a]

Temsirolimus[a]

Monoclonal Antibodies

Olaratumab

Insulin-like Growth Factor 1 Receptor Inhibitors

OSI-906 (Linsitinib)

[a] Commercially available.

---

described.[3] GIST without kinase mutations, classically called wild-type, represents a family of tumors associated with loss of succinate dehydrogenase (SDH) B protein expression with or without mutations in the SDH family of genes, occur in patients with neurofibromatosis, or may have a novel mechanism not yet identified.[4,5] The mechanism of action of currently approved and investigational TKIs is summarized in **Table 1**.

FOOD AND DRUG ADMINISTRATION–APPROVED AGENTS FOR GIST
Imatinib

Imatinib (Gleevec) is a small-molecule TKI that exhibits inhibitory activity against ABL kinase, and KIT and PDGFRA receptor. Imatinib was first tested in a proof of principle

Table 1
GIST targets of currently approved and investigational TKIs

	KIT	PDGFR α, β	VEGFR 1, 2, 3	RET	FGFR 1, 3
Imatinib	+	+			
Sunitinib	+	+	+		
Regorafenib	+	+	+	+	+
Nilotinib	+	+			
Sorafenib	+	+	+		
Masitinib	+	+			
Vatalanib	+	+	+		
Dovitinib	+	+	+		+
Papzopanib	+	+	+		+
Cedarinib			+		
Crenolanib		+			

Abbreviation: VEGFR, vascular endothelial growth factor receptor.

trial in a patient with KIT exon 11 mutated metastatic GIST; the patient experienced a dramatic and durable response to therapy.[6] Subsequent phase I-III studies demonstrated significant objective responses summarized in **Table 2**.[7–10] Phase I studies determined the maximum tolerated dose for imatinib to be 800 mg daily, with edema, including periorbital edema, diarrhea, nausea, vomiting, and myelosuppression being the main adverse events. The studies evaluated a range of doses: 400 mg daily, 600 mg daily, and 400 mg twice daily, with all studies demonstrating a high rate of objective responses. Two phase III studies compared 400 mg daily with 400 mg twice daily in advanced disease with similar overall response rate (ORR), complete response rate (CR), partial response rate (PR), and stable disease (SD) rates between the two arms.[11,12] Patients were allowed to cross over from the 400-mg daily dose to 400-mg twice daily for progression; in one study 3% of patients who crossed over to the high-dose imatinib arm at the time of progression achieved a partial response and 28% achieved disease stabilization, albeit for a median progression-free survival (PFS) of 5 months.[12] A meta-analysis of the phase III studies evaluated dosage of imatinib and showed that there was a PFS advantage for patients treated at the higher dose with a hazard ratio (HR) of 0.89 (95% confidence interval [CI], 0.79–1.00; $P = .04$); however, there was no difference seen in overall survival (OS) between the two arms. On subset analysis patients with KIT exon 9 mutations had a better ORR (47% vs 21%; $P = .0037$) and a significantly better PFS with an adjusted HR of 0.58 (95% CI, 0.38–0.91), again without a difference in OS between the two dose levels.[13] The PFS benefit seen at the higher dose level in the meta-analysis was attributed to the benefit in patients with exon 9 tumors. Based on these data the current standard of care for advanced GIST is initiation of imatinib at a dose of 400 mg daily for all patients except for those with an exon 9 mutation and those who progressed on the lower dose of imatinib; these patients do better at a dose of 800 mg daily.

Approximately 14% of GIST tumors have primary resistance to imatinib, progressing within 6 months of initiating therapy.[9] These tumors most commonly are those with mutations in PDGFRA in exon 18, D842V, or those lacking mutations in either KIT or PDGFRA. Secondary resistance occurs in patients on long-term imatinib, greater than 6 months. Most of this resistance occurs because of clonal evolution. These clones express the primary mutation along with additional mutations that render

Table 2
Clinical trials of imatinib in metastatic GIST

Study	Study Type	Dosages Studied	Number of Patients	Results
van Oosterom et al,[7] 2001	Phase I	400 mg qd, 300 mg bid, 400 mg bid, 500 mg bid	40	54% PR 37% SD
Demetri et al,[9] 2002	Phase II	400 mg qd vs 600 mg qd	147	No statistically significant differences in toxicity or response between the two doses Response rate in the 400-mg qd arm 49.3% PR, 31.5% SD, and 16.4% PD Response rate in the 600-mg qd arm 58.1% PR, 24.3% SD, and 10.8% PD
Verweij et al,[10] 2003	Phase II	400 mg bid	27	4% CR, 67% PR, 19% SD, 11% PD 73% free from disease at 1 y
Verweij et al,[11] 2004	Phase III	400 mg qd vs 400 mg bid	946	Response rate in the 400-mg qd arm 4% CR, 45% PR, 32% SD, 13% PD Response rate in the 400-mg bid arm 6% CR, 48% PR, 32% SD, 9% PD After a median follow-up of 760 d, 263 (56%) of 473 patients in the once-a-day arm had progressed compared with 235 (50%) of 473 in the twice-a-day arm (HR, 0.82; 95% CI, 0.69–0.98; $P = .026$) OS was 85% at 1 y and 69% at 2 y in patients treated once a day, and 86% at 1 y and 74% at 2 y in those treated twice a day Increased dose reductions (77 [16%] vs 282 [60%]) and interruptions (189 [40%] vs 302 [64%]) in the twice-a-day arm
Blanke et al,[12] 2008	Phase III	400 mg qd vs 400 mg bid	694	Response rate in the 400-mg qd arm 5% CR, 40% PR, 25% SD, 12% PD Response rate in the 400-mg bid arm 3% CR, 42% PR, 22% SD, 10% PD Median PFS was 18 and 20 mo in the once-daily and twice-daily arms, respectively Median OS was 55 and 51 mo in the once-daily and twice-daily arms, respectively No statistically significant differences in objective response rates, PFS, or OS

Abbreviations: CR, complete response rate; OS, overall survival; PD, progressive disease; PFS, progression-free survival, PR, partial response rate; SD, stable disease.
Data from Refs.[7–12]

them resistant to imatinib, leading to treatment failure and relapse; the secondary mutations occur within the same gene. The most common secondary mutations seen are in exons 13, 14, and 17 of the KIT gene and the D842V mutation in exon 18 of PDGFRA.[14–16] The median time to progression on imatinib is approximately 2 years; however, some patients remain free of progression for greater than 10 years. Factors associated with long-term disease stability are good performance status and low base line neutrophil count. Factors that are associated with better OS include younger age, female gender, low neutrophil count, normal albumin, and good performance status.[12] In addition, smaller tumor volume has also been associated with longer PFS.[17]

Sunitinib

Sunitinib (Sutent) is a small-molecule TKI that inhibits vascular endothelial growth factor receptor (VEGFR) 1, 2, and 3; PDGFRA; PDGFR-β (PDGFRB); KIT; Flt3; RET; and CSF1R.[18] In an early phase I study that looked at the use of sunitinib in patients with advanced malignancies, 6 of 22 evaluable patients had an objective response including one patient with imatinib-resistant GIST.[19] A subsequent phase I-II study tested sunitinib in 97 patients who were intolerant to or had progressed on imatinib. A clinical benefit rate (CBR) defined as PR or SD lasting for more than 6 months was seen in 58%, 34%, and 56% of KIT exon 9 and 11, and KIT-PDGFRA wild-type mutations, respectively. The chances of achieving a PR with sunitinib was greater in tumors with an exon 9 KIT mutation compared with exon 11 KIT mutations (37% vs 5%). The median PFS was better for patients with exon 9 mutant and KIT-PDGFRA wild-type tumors compared with those with exon 11 mutations (19.4, 19, and 5.1 months, respectively). Median OS was also longer for patients with exon 9 mutants and KIT-PDGFRA wild-type tumors compared with the exon 11 mutants (26.9, 30.5, and 12.3 months, respectively) indicating that imatinib-insensitive mutations were more responsive to sunitinib in the second-line setting. Although those with KIT exon 11 mutations had less benefit, these patients represent a different population than those with imatinib-naive disease; rather, they represented those patients with clonal evolution and imatinib-insensitive secondary mutations. When secondary mutations were considered, the PFS for mutant KIT exon 11 patients with secondary KIT exon 13 or 14 mutation was 7.8 months with a median OS of 13 months and a CBR of 61% compared with a PFS of 2.3 months and a median OS of 4 months with a CBR of 15% for those with a KIT exon 17 or 18 mutation.[20–22]

The pivotal phase III trial of sunitinib was a double-blind placebo-controlled study that enrolled patients with advanced GIST that had failed therapy with imatinib or who were intolerant to imatinib. Patients were treated with sunitinib at a dose of 50 mg daily for 4 weeks followed by a 2-week break in 6-week cycles. The primary end point of the study was time to tumor progression; secondary endpoints included PFS, OS, confirmed ORR, time to tumor response, duration of response, and duration of performance status maintenance. The results were impressive with the time to tumor progression for the sunitinib arm being 27.3 weeks, versus 6.4 weeks in the placebo arm with an HR of 0.33 (95% CI, 0.23–0.47; P<.0001). The study was unblinded at the first interim analysis and all patients on placebo were allowed to cross over to sunitinib. Even with crossover there was an OS advantage in the sunitinib arm with an HR of 0.49 (95% CI, 0.29–0.83; P = .007). The main toxicities were hematologic including anemia, thrombocytopenia and leucopenia, fatigue, diarrhea, nausea, vomiting, anorexia, stomatitis, and hand-foot syndrome.[23]

The phase III trial of sunitinib administered sunitinib for 4 weeks followed by 2 weeks off drug. A schedule with intermittent breaks is less flexible and convenient for patients than a continuous dosing schedule. In addition, some patients experienced symptomatic progression or metabolic progression by fluorodeoxyglucose positron emission tomography scans during the time off drug. A phase II single arm study looked at the feasibility of daily dosing of sunitinib at a dose of 37.5 mg daily given continuously. The study demonstrated a CBR of 53%, including 13% PR and 40% SD. The median PFS was 34 weeks and the median OS was 107 weeks. The toxicity profile was similar to the phase III study.[24] Based on these studies sunitinib is now the standard of care in patients with GIST who have failed imatinib, and is commonly given in a daily fashion.

Regorafenib

Regorafenib (Stivarga, BAY 73-4506) is a small-molecule TKI that inhibits VEGFR 1, 2, and 3; PDGFRB; FGFR1; KIT; RET; and BRAF among others.[25] In a phase II trial of regorafenib, 33 patients with GIST tumors resistant to imatinib and sunitinib, but sorafenib-naive, showed a CBR of 75% (4 PR + 22 SD); the median PFS was 10 months and the median OS was not achieved at the time of reporting. Patients with a primary exon 11 mutation had a better PFS than patients with exon 9 mutations; however, there was no difference when they were compared with patients with wild-type GIST. The major toxicities that were reported were hypertension, hand-foot syndrome, hypophosphatemia, rash, fatigue, and diarrhea.[26] In the recently reported phase III randomized controlled double-blind placebo-controlled GRID trial of regorafenib in patients with GIST tumors resistant to imatinib and sunitinib, the median PFS of patients on the regorafenib arm was 4.8 months and 0.9 months for those on placebo with an HR of 0.27 (95% CI, 0.18–0.39; $P<.0001$).[27] Both these studies show promising results and regorafenib was approved in February 2013 as the third-line drug of choice.

OTHER THERAPIES EVALUATED FOR THERAPY IN GIST
VEGFR-targeted TKIs

Sorafenib

Sorafenib (Nexavar) is a small-molecule TKI that inhibits Raf-1; VEGFR 1, 2, and 3; Flt3; KIT; and PDGFRB among others.[28] Structurally, this agent is similar to regorafenib. Preclinical studies of sorafenib in imatinib-resistant cell lines showed that it was similar in potency to sunitinib in cell lines harboring KIT mutations affecting the ATP binding domain, but importantly, more potent than sunitinib in cell lines harboring KIT mutations affecting the ATP binding domain, exons 13 and 14.[29] A retrospective study of 32 patients treated with sorafenib in the fourth-line setting after failing imatinib, sunitinib, and nilotinib showed a 63% benefit (19% PR and 44% SD). The median PFS was 20 weeks and the median OS was 42 weeks.[30] A subsequent phase II trial of sorafenib in resistant GIST that enrolled 38 patients (6 were imatinib resistant and 32 were imatinib and sunitinib resistant) showed a disease control rate of 68% (13% PR + 55% SD). The main toxicities seen were hand-foot syndrome, hypertension, diarrhea, hypophosphatemia, gastrointestinal bleeding and perforation, thrombosis, and intracranial hemorrhage.[31] Based on these studies sorafenib is a reasonable drug for the third- and fourth-line setting; however, it is not known if patients that have received regorafenib before sorafenib derive benefit.

Vatalanib

Vatalanib (PTK787/ZK 222584) is a small-molecule TKI that inhibits VGEFR 1, 2, and 3; KIT; c-Fms; and PDGFR-β.[32] In a phase II study of the agent in 45 patients with imatinib-resistant metastatic GIST, 18 (40%) had a clinical benefit with 2 (4.4%) achieving PR and 16 (35.6%) achieving SD. The clinical benefit and median time to progression was higher in those who received only imatinib in the past (46.2% and 5.8 months) compared with those who received imatinib and sunitinib (31.6% and 3.2 months). The drug was relatively well tolerated with the common side effects being hypertension, nausea, dizziness, proteinuria, abdominal pain, and diarrhea.[33]

Dovitinib
Dovitinib (TKI258, CHR-258) is a small-molecule TKI of KIT; PDGFRA; PDGFRB; FGFR; and VEGFR 1, 2, and 3 among others.[34] A phase I study of this agent in patients with advanced solid tumors showed that this drug was safe. A patient with refractory GIST in this study achieved stable disease that lasted for 8 months.[35] Dovitinib is currently in phase II clinical trials in patients who are refractory or intolerant to imatinib (NCT01478373) and in patients who are refractory to imatinib and sunitinib (NCT01440959).

Pazopanib
Pazopanib (Votrient, GW786034) is an oral multikinase inhibitor and inhibits VEGFR 1, 2, and 3; PDGFRA; PDGFRB; KIT; and FGFR among others.[36] The drug is currently approved in the United States for patients with renal cell carcinoma and advanced soft tissue sarcoma. Currently, pazopanib is being evaluated in phase II studies in the imatinib-resistant setting (NCT01391611) and in the third-line setting after failure of imatinib and sunitinib (NCT01524848, NCT01323400).

Cedarinib
Cedarinib (AZD2171) is an oral TKI of VEGFR 2.[37] A phase II clinical trial looking at the activity of cedarinib in patients with imatinib-resistant GIST and soft tissue sarcoma has been completed and results are awaited (NCT00385203).

Non–VEGFR-targeted TKIs

Nilotinib
Nilotinib (Tasigna) is a small-molecule TKI that was designed specifically to inhibit bcr-abl for the treatment of chronic myelogenous leukemia. However, it has additional biologic targets including ARG, KIT, PDGFRA, and PDGFRB.[38] In a phase I study that evaluated the combination of nilotinib with imatinib and nilotinib alone in patients with imatinib-resistant GIST, the drug was found to be safe with evidence of benefit. The primary therapeutic benefit was SD (72%) with PR seen in (4%).[39] In phase II and retrospective studies, summarized in **Table 3**, responses ranged from PR 10% to 12%,

Table 3
Phase II and retrospective studies of nilotinib in metastatic and recurrent GIST

Study	Study Type	Number of Patients	Results
Cauchi et al,[40] 2012	Phase II	13	Most responses were stable disease: 7.7% (1) PR by Choi criteria; 61% (8) PD by RECIST; and 38.5% (5) PD by Choi criteria.
Sawaki et al,[41] 2011	Phase II	35	3% PR, 66% SD. Median PFS of 113 d and OS of 310 d.
Montemurro et al,[42] 2009	Retrospective analysis	52	47 evaluable patients. 10% had SD, 2% CR, 8.5% PR. Median PFS 12 wk. Median OS 34 wk. Median survival from the first diagnosis of GIST was 72 mo.

Data from Refs.[40–42]

with SD of 37% to 59%.[40–42] Two of the studies demonstrated response and prolonged stable disease in patients with KIT exon 11 mutations with secondary exon 17 mutations (D820G, N822K, and Y823D). The phase III study of nilotinib versus best supportive care did not demonstrate an improvement in PFS on central review with a median of 109 days in the nilotinib arm versus 111 days in the control arm; it should be noted that in this study patients could have received other investigational TKIs or therapies before study entry and that best supportive care included the use of imatinib or sunitinib in the control arm. Of the patients in the control arm, 93% continued to receive imatinib or sunitinib as part of best supportive care. A post hoc analysis of patients who were receiving nilotinib in the true third-line setting (ie, after failure of imatinib and sunitinib) demonstrated an OS advantage with a median OS of 405 days versus 280 days (HR, 0.67; P = .02 difference). This difference was not seen in the intent-to-treat population where the median OS was 361 days versus 300 days (HR, 0.84; P = .28).[43]

Masitinib

Masitinib mesylate (AB1010) is a small-molecule TKI that inhibits KIT (wild-type and activated with juxtamembrane mutations); PDGFRA; PDGFRB; Lyn kinase; FGFR3; and FAK pathway.[44] In a phase I study of patients with advanced malignancies, including 19 with GIST, the drug was found to have an acceptable tolerability profile. Masitinib showed a clinical benefit in the imatinib-naive and the imatinib-resistant cohort of patients. One of two imatinib-intolerant patients achieved a PR and the other SD. In the imatinib-resistant group (N = 17), five patients achieved stable disease.[44] In a phase II study of the agent in 30 imatinib-naive patients with locally advanced or metastatic GIST, 96.7% of the patients had a clinical benefit (3.3% CR + 50% PR + 43.3% SD); 4-year follow-up results of the study showed that the median PFS was 41 months and median OS was not reached. The mutation status of the patients was known in 53% (16) of the patients; most had a mutation in exon 11 (56%), followed by wild-type KIT-PDGFRA (19%), exon 11 and exon 13 (13%), and PDGFRA (6%).[45,46] Masitinib has also been studied in the second-line setting in imatinib-resistant GIST in a phase II randomized trial between masitinib and sunitinib in patients with imatinib-resistant GIST. Masitinib was better tolerated than sunitinib with a lower rate of severe adverse events (17% vs 52%). The median PFS was 3.9 months for the masitinib arm versus 3.8 months for the sunitinib arm with a median OS of 15 months for the sunitinib, whereas that for masitinib was not reached. At 24 months the OS was 53% and 0% in the masitinib and sunitinib arms, respectively.[47] This study was not powered to determine a statistical difference in outcome and further data are needed to assess the benefit of masitinib in this setting. It is likely that patients on the masitinib treatment arm received sunitinib at the time of progression. Additional phase III studies are underway comparing masitinib with imatinib in the frontline setting (NCT00812240) and with sunitinib in the imatinib-resistant setting (NCT01694277).

NON–TKI-TARGETED THERAPIES
Hsp90 Inhibitors

Heat shock protein 90 (Hsp90) belongs to a family of proteins that function as molecular chaperons and bind other proteins denoted as client proteins. They play an important role in the folding, transport, and degradation of client proteins. There are many client proteins for Hsp90, including KIT and PDGFRA. Inhibition of Hsp90 in vitro leads to cell death in GIST cell lines that express KIT, including cell lines with secondary KIT mutations resistant to imatinib.[48] Therefore, targeting Hsp90 may be an effective strategy in GIST. One challenge with this class of agents is that most agents have intravenous formulations, which is a change for patients who have been taking an oral agent for therapy.

IPI-504

The first agent of this class to be tested was IPI-504, a water-soluble HSP-90 inhibitor.[49,50] Phase I testing revealed dose-limiting toxicities of headache and myalgias. In a group of 36 patients with advanced GIST, there was one partial response and an additional 24 patients with stable disease. A phase III placebo-controlled double-blind study was initiated using 400 mg/m^2 intravenously twice weekly for 2 out of every 3 weeks. The study was terminated before meeting its accrual goals because of increased mortality in the patients receiving IPI-504.[50]

BIIB021

BIIB021 is an oral synthetic inhibitor of Hsp90 and binds to the ATP binding pocket of Hsp90.[51] BIIB021 was studied in a phase II trial in patients with imatinib- and sunitinib-resistant GIST. A total of 10 (43%) patients out of 23 achieved stable disease by RECIST criteria. One patient had a metabolic partial response (>25% reduction in mean standard uptake value [SUV]max) and six patients achieved SD by this criteria. The agent was well tolerated and had minimal toxicities with dizziness and syncope being dose-limiting toxicities.[52]

AT13387

AT13387 is a synthetic Hsp90 inhibitor and has been shown to be active in imatinib-sensitive and -resistant GIST cell lines and xenograft models.[53] A phase II open-labeled randomized study is looking at intravenous AT13387 as monotherapy or in combination with imatinib in patients with advanced GIST who have progressed on a maximum of three TKIs (NCT01294202).

AUY922

AUY922 is also a synthetic Hsp90 inhibitor and has shown activity in preclinical studies in GIST.[54] The agent has been found to be safe in phase I clinical trials.[55] AUY922 is now being studied in a phase II clinical trial in patients with imatinib- and sunitinib-resistant GIST (NCT01404650).

Ganestespib

Ganestespib (STA-9090) is also a synthetic Hsp90 inhibitor. Preclinical studies have shown that ganestespib has activity in imatinib-sensitive and -resistant cell lines.[56] A phase II study looking at ganestespib in patients who are refractory to imatinib and sunitinib has shown some benefits but has not yet been reported.[57]

PI3K-AKT-mTOR Inhibitors

The PI3K-AKT-mTOR pathway is downstream of KIT and plays an important role in cell signaling and survival in imatinib-resistant GIST.[58] Animal models have shown that inhibition of this pathway inhibits cell proliferation.[59]

Perifosine

Perifosine is an oral alkylphospholipid and inhibits the phosphorylation of AKT.[60] It has been studied in a phase II trial along with imatinib in patients with imatinib-resistant GIST. Perifosine did not show significant clinical activity with no partial or complete responses. Most benefit was in the form of SD.[61]

mTOR Inhibitors

Everolimus (RAD001; Afinitor) is an oral mTOR inhibitor. Preclinical studies of everolimus in combination with imatinib have shown some benefit.[62,63] A phase I-II study looked at the use of everolimus in combination with imatinib in patients who had progressed on imatinib and both imatinib and sunitinib or another TKI. Up to 37% of patients achieved stable disease for 4 months or greater. The PFS for patients in the second-line setting was 1.9 months, and 3.5 months in those who had progressed after sunitinib or another TKI.[62] Another phase II study looked at the combination of imatinib and everolimus in imatinib-resistant GIST; none of 27 patients in the study achieved SD.[63] Both studies have shown an acceptable toxicity profile with modest clinical benefit. Currently a phase II-III trial is ongoing that is looking at the combination of everolimus and imatinib in imatinib-resistant GIST (NCT00510354).

Sirolimus is an mTOR inhibitor and has also shown benefit when combined with other TKIs, such as imatinib or PKC412 (a multitargeted TKI that inhibits KIT among other targets) in patients with the PDGFRA-D842V mutations.[64,65]

Temsirolimus is yet another mTOR inhibitor that is approved for the management of metastatic renal cell cancer. A phase II study looking at temsirolimus in GIST and other soft tissue sarcomas has been completed and results are awaited (NCT00087074).

AGENTS FOR SPECIAL GIST POPULATIONS
Crenolanib

Crenolanib (CP-868,596) is an oral TKI with potent activity against PDGFRA and PDGFRB. Preclinical studies have shown that crenolanib is significantly more potent than imatinib in inhibiting imatinib-resistant mutant PDGFRA kinases including the D842V mutants.[66] Phase I studies had shown that this agent is safe with gastrointestinal side effects being the major adverse effects observed.[67] Based on the in vitro data in PDGFRA D842V, a phase II trial is currently evaluating its efficacy in patients with advanced PDGFRA D842-related mutations and deletions GIST tumors (NCT01243346).

Olaratumab

Olaratumab (IMC-3G3) is a fully human IgG1 monoclonal antibody that in vitro binds to PDGFRA and blocks its activation. It can also mediate immune-mediated cell destruction by means of antibody-dependent cellular cytotoxicity and complement-dependent cytotoxicity. A phase II study of IMC3G3 has been completed in patients with GIST who progressed on imatinib and sunitinib; results are awaited (NCT01316263).

Insulin-like Growth Factor 1 Receptor Inhibitors

Approximately 10% of GIST tumors do not have mutations of KIT or PDGFRA and are termed wild-type GIST. In addition to these adult patients, GIST that arises in the pediatric population is also usually without mutations in these two genes. These tumors have been shown to have mutations in SDH genes and to have high expression of IGF-1R, albeit without any mutations.[4,68-75] Mutations in SDH genes (A, B, C, and D) result in loss of the formation of a complex made by the four protein products. This is identified by loss of SDHB expression by immunohistochemistry, which has led these tumors to be called SDH-deficient GIST.[76] Loss of the SDH complex leads to activation of HIF transcriptional programs promoting angiogenesis, glycolysis, and cell proliferation.[77] This is the likely mechanism for the overexpression of IGF-1R in SDH-deficient GIST.

IGF-1R is a receptor tyrosine kinase and binds to its ligand IGF1 and IGF2 and mediates intracellular signaling through the Ras-Raf-ERK-MAPK and PI3K-AKT-mTOR pathways. The IGF-1R mediated signaling is implicated in many cancers and is important in its development and progression.[78] In preclinical studies it has been shown that inhibition of IGF-1R in GIST cell lines induced apoptosis.[75] Linsitinib

(OSI-906), an oral IGF-1R inhibitor, is being investigated in a phase II clinical trial in patients with pediatric GIST and adult wild-type GIST (NCT01560260).

SUMMARY

Over a decade has elapsed since the routine use of TKI therapies for the management of advanced GIST. This has led to increased survival for many patients in a disease that was universally lethal within 1 year if disease was unresectable. Today, there are three approved agents for the treatment of GIST, and several other agents in which data support its use. Tumors that are refractory to TKIs remain a challenge and novel combination therapies being tested in the phase I setting will likely lead to new therapeutic options; in particular agents targeting downstream pathways, which have been shown to remain active despite KIT-PDGFRA targeting, such as AKT, are of great interest. In addition, clinicians have come to appreciate that GIST represents a family of tumors with similar histologic features but different molecular drivers. As agents targeting specific mutations or mechanisms are developed it will become increasingly important to genotype patients so as to prescribe appropriate therapies.

REFERENCES

1. Rubin BP, Singer S, Tsao C, et al. KIT activation is a ubiquitous feature of gastrointestinal stromal tumors. Cancer Res 2001;61:8118–21.
2. Heinrich MC, Corless CL, Duensing A, et al. PDGFRA activating mutations in gastrointestinal stromal tumors. Science 2003;299:708–10.
3. Miranda C, Nucifora M, Molinari F, et al. KRAS and BRAF mutations predict primary resistance to imatinib in gastrointestinal stromal tumors. Clin Cancer Res 2012;18:1769–76.
4. Belinsky MG, Rink L, Flieder D, et al. Overexpression of insulin-like growth factor 1 receptor and frequent mutational inactivation of SDHA in wild-type SDHB-negative gastrointestinal stromal tumors. Genes Chromosomes Cancer 2013; 52:214–24.
5. Mussi C, Schildhaus HU, Gronchi A, et al. Therapeutic consequences from molecular biology for gastrointestinal stromal tumor patients affected by neurofibromatosis type 1. Clin Cancer Res 2008;14:4550–5.
6. Joensuu H, Roberts PJ, Sarloma-Rikala M, et al. Effect of the tyrosine kinase inhibitor STI571 in a patient with a metastatic gastrointestinal stromal tumor. N Engl J Med 2001;344:1052–6.
7. van Oosterom AT, Judson I, Verwelj J, et al. Safety and efficacy of imatinib (STI571) in metastatic gastrointestinal stromal tumours: a phase I study. Lancet 2001;358:1421–3.
8. van Oosterom AT, Judson IR, Verwelj J, et al. Update of phase I study of imatinib (STI571) in advanced soft tissue sarcomas and gastrointestinal stromal tumors: a report of the EORTC Soft Tissue and Bone Sarcoma Group. Eur J Cancer 2002;38(Suppl 5):S83–7.
9. Demetri GD, von Mehren M, Blanke CD, et al. Efficacy and safety of imatinib mesylate in advanced gastrointestinal stromal tumors. N Engl J Med 2002; 347:472–80.
10. Verweij J, van Oosterom A, Blay JY, et al. Imatinib mesylate (STI-571 Glivec®, Gleevec™) is an active agent for gastrointestinal stromal tumours, but does not yield responses in other soft-tissue sarcomas that are unselected for a molecular target. Results from an EORTC Soft Tissue and Bone Sarcoma Group phase II study. Eur J Cancer 2003;39:2006–11.

11. Verweij J, Casali PG, Zalcberg J, et al. Progression-free survival in gastrointestinal stromal tumours with high-dose imatinib: randomised trial. Lancet 2004; 364:1127–34.
12. Blanke CD, Rankin C, Demetri GD, et al. Phase III randomized, intergroup trial assessing imatinib mesylate at two dose levels in patients with unresectable or metastatic gastrointestinal stromal tumors expressing the kit receptor tyrosine kinase: S0033. J Clin Oncol 2008;26:626–32.
13. Gastrointestinal Stromal Tumor Meta-Analysis Group. Comparison of two doses of imatinib for the treatment of unresectable or metastatic gastrointestinal stromal tumors: a meta-analysis of 1,640 patients. J Clin Oncol 2010;28:1247–53.
14. Heinrich MC, Corless CL, Blanke CD, et al. Molecular correlates of imatinib resistance in gastrointestinal stromal tumors. J Clin Oncol 2006;24:4764–74.
15. Wardelmann E, Thomas N, Merkelbach-Bruse S, et al. Acquired resistance to imatinib in gastrointestinal stromal tumours caused by multiple KIT mutations. Lancet Oncol 2005;6:249–51.
16. Debiec-Rychter M, Cools J, Dumez H, et al. Mechanisms of resistance to imatinib mesylate in gastrointestinal stromal tumors and activity of the PKC412 inhibitor against imatinib-resistant mutants. Gastroenterology 2005;128:270–9.
17. Blanke CD, Rankin C, Demetri GD, et al. Long term results from a randomized phase II trial of standard versus higher dose imatinib mesylate for patients with unresectable or metastatic gastrointestinal stromal tumors expressing KIT. J Clin Oncol 2008;26:626–32.
18. Faivre S, Demetri G, Sargent W, et al. Molecular basis for sunitinib efficacy and future clinical development. Nat Rev Drug Discov 2007;6:734–45.
19. Faivre S, Delbaldo C, Vera K, et al. Safety, pharmacokinetic, and antitumor activity of SU11248, a novel oral multitarget tyrosine kinase inhibitor, in patients with cancer. J Clin Oncol 2006;24:25–35.
20. Heinrich MC, Maki RG, Corless CL, et al. Primary and secondary kinase genotypes correlate with the biological and clinical activity of sunitinib in imatinib-resistant gastrointestinal stromal tumor. J Clin Oncol 2008;26:5352–9.
21. Heinrich M, Maki RG, Corless CR, et al. Sunitinib (SU) response in imatinib-resistant (IM-R) GIST correlates with KIT and PDGFRA mutation status. J Clin Oncol 2006;24(Suppl 18):a9502.
22. Maki RG, Fletcher JA, Heinrich MC, et al. Results from a continuation trial of SU11248 in patients (pts) with imatinib (IM)-resistant gastrointestinal stromal tumor (GIST). Proc Am Soc Clin Oncol 2005;9011.
23. Demetri GD, van Oosterom AT, Garrett CR, et al. Efficacy and safety of sunitinib in patients with advanced gastrointestinal stromal tumour after failure of imatinib: a randomised controlled trial. Lancet 2006;368:1329–38.
24. George S, Blay JY, Casali PG, et al. Clinical evaluation of continuous daily dosing of sunitinib malate in patients with advanced gastrointestinal stromal tumour after imatinib failure. Eur J Cancer 2009;45:1959–68.
25. Wilhelm SM, Dumas J, Adnane L, et al. Regorafenib (BAY 73-4506): a new oral multikinase inhibitor of angiogenic, stromal and oncogenic receptor tyrosine kinases with potent preclinical antitumor activity. Int J Cancer 2011;129:245–55.
26. George S, Wang Q, Heinrich MC, et al. Efficacy and safety of regorafenib in patients with metastatic and/or unresectable GI stromal tumor after failure of imatinib and sunitinib: a multicenter phase II trial. J Clin Oncol 2012;30:2401–7.
27. Demetri GD, Reichardt P, Kang YK, et al. Randomized phase III trial of regorafenib in patients (pts) with metastatic and/or unresectable gastrointestinal

stromal tumor (GIST) progressing despite prior treatment with at least imatinib (IM) and sunitinib (SU): GRID trial. J Clin Oncol (ASCO Meeting Abstracts) 2012;30(Suppl 18):LBA10008.

28. Wilhelm SM, Adnane L, Newell P, et al. Preclinical overview of sorafenib, a multi-kinase inhibitor that targets both Raf and VEGF and PDGF receptor tyrosine kinase signaling. Mol Cancer Ther 2008;7:3129–40.

29. Heinrich MC, Carden R, Griffith D, et al. In vitro activity of sorafenib against imatinib- and sunitinib-resistant kinase mutations associated with drug-resistant GI stromal tumors. J Clin Oncol (ASCO Meeting Abstracts) 2009; 27(Suppl 15):10500.

30. Reichardt P, Montemurro M, Gelderblom H, et al. Sorafenib fourth-line treatment in imatinib-, sunitinib-, and nilotinib-resistant metastatic GIST: a retrospective analysis. J Clin Oncol (ASCO Meeting Abstracts) 2009;27(Suppl 15):10564.

31. Kindler H, Campbell NP, Wroblewski K, et al. Sorafenib (SOR) in patients (pts) with imatinib (IM) and sunitinib (SU)-resistant (RES) gastrointestinal stromal tumors (GIST): final results of a University of Chicago Phase II Consortium trial. J Clin Oncol (ASCO Meeting Abstracts) 2011;29(Suppl 15):10009.

32. Wood JM, Bold G, Buchdunger E, et al. PTK787/ZK 222584, a novel and potent inhibitor of vascular endothelial growth factor receptor tyrosine kinases, impairs vascular endothelial growth factor-induced responses and tumor growth after oral administration. Cancer Res 2000;60:2178–89.

33. Joensuu H, De Braud F, Grignagni G, et al. Vatalanib for metastatic gastrointes-tinal stromal tumour (GIST) resistant to imatinib: final results of a phase II study. Br J Cancer 2011;104:1686–90.

34. Lee SH, Lopes de Menezes D, Vora J, et al. In vivo target modulation and biological activity of CHIR-258, a multitargeted growth factor receptor kinase inhibitor, in colon cancer models. Clin Cancer Res 2005;11:3633–41.

35. Sarker D, Molife R, Evans TR, et al. A phase I pharmacokinetic and pharma-codynamic study of TKI258, an oral, multitargeted receptor tyrosine kinase inhibitor in patients with advanced solid tumors. Clin Cancer Res 2008;14: 2075–81.

36. Kumar R, Knick VB, Rudolph SK, et al. Pharmacokinetic-pharmacodynamic cor-relation from mouse to human with pazopanib, a multikinase angiogenesis inhib-itor with potent antitumor and antiangiogenic activity. Mol Cancer Ther 2007;6: 2012–21.

37. Wedge SR, Kendrew J, Hennequin LF, et al. AZD2171: a highly potent, orally bioavailable, vascular endothelial growth factor receptor-2 tyrosine kinase inhib-itor for the treatment of cancer. Cancer Res 2005;65:4389–400.

38. Weisberg E, Manley PW, Breiltenstein W, et al. Characterization of AMN107, a selective inhibitor of native and mutant Bcr-Abl. Cancer Cell 2005;7:129–41.

39. Demetri GD, Casali PG, Blay JY, et al. A phase I study of single-agent nilotinib or in combination with imatinib in patients with imatinib-resistant gastrointestinal stromal tumors. Clin Cancer Res 2009;15:5910–6.

40. Cauchi C, Somaiah N, Engstrom PF, et al. Evaluation of nilotinib in advanced GIST previously treated with imatinib and sunitinib. Cancer Chemother Pharma-col 2012;69:977–82.

41. Sawaki A, Nishida T, Doi T, et al. Phase 2 study of nilotinib as third-line therapy for patients with gastrointestinal stromal tumor. Cancer 2011;117:4633–41.

42. Montemurro M, Schöffski P, Reichardt P, et al. Nilotinib in the treatment of advanced gastrointestinal stromal tumours resistant to both imatinib and sunitinib. Eur J Cancer 2009;45:2293–7.

43. Reichardt P, Blay JY, Gelderblom H, et al. Phase III study of nilotinib versus best supportive care with or without a TKI in patients with gastrointestinal stromal tumors resistant to or intolerant of imatinib and sunitinib. Ann Oncol 2012;23:1680–7.

44. Soria JC, Massard C, Magné N, et al. Phase 1 dose-escalation study of oral tyrosine kinase inhibitor masitinib in advanced and/or metastatic solid cancers. Eur J Cancer 2009;45:2333–41.

45. Blay J, Le Cesne A, Bin N, et al. Overall survival benefit with masitinib mesylate in imatinib-naive, locally advanced, or metastatic gastrointestinal stromal tumor (GIST): 4-years follow-up of the French Sarcoma Group phase II trial. ASCO Meeting Abstracts 2011;85.

46. Le Cesne A, Blay JY, Bui BN, et al. Phase II study of oral masitinib mesilate in imatinib-naïve patients with locally advanced or metastatic gastro-intestinal stromal tumour (GIST). Eur J Cancer 2010;46:1344–51.

47. Adenis A, Le Cesne A, Nguyen BB, et al. Masitinib mesylate in imatinib-resistant advanced GIST: a randomized phase II trial. ASCO Meeting Abstracts 2012; 30(Suppl 15):10007.

48. Bauer S, Yu LK, Demetri GD, et al. Heat shock protein 90 inhibition in imatinib-resistant gastrointestinal stromal tumor. Cancer Res 2006;66:9153–61.

49. Demetri GD, Le Cesne A, von Mehren M, et al. Final results from a phase III study of IPI-504 (retsapimycin hydrochloride) versus placebo in patients (pts) with gastrointestinal stromal tumors (GIST) following failure of kinase inhibitor therapies. In: ASCO Gastrointestinal Cancers Symposium. Orlando, FL; January 22–24, 2010. [abstract 64].

50. Muhlenberg T, Zhang Y, Wagner AJ, et al. Inhibitors of deacetylases suppress oncogenic KIT signalling, acetylate HSP90, and induce apopotosis in gastrointestinal stromal tumors. Cancer Res 2009;69:6941–50.

51. Lundgren K, Zhang H, Brekken J, et al. BIIB021, an orally available, fully synthetic small-molecule inhibitor of the heat shock protein Hsp90. Mol Cancer Ther 2009;8:921–9.

52. Dickson MA, Okuno SH, Keohan ML, et al. Phase II study of the HSP90-inhibitor BIIB021 in gastrointestinal stromal tumors. Ann Oncol 2013;24:252–7.

53. Smyth T, Van Looy T, Curry JE, et al. The HSP90 inhibitor, AT13387, is effective against imatinib-sensitive and -resistant gastrointestinal stromal tumor models. Mol Cancer Ther 2012;11:1799–808.

54. Hsueh YS, Yen CC, Shih NY, et al. Autophagy is involved in endogenous and NVP-AUY922-induced KIT degradation in gastrointestinal stromal tumors. Autophagy 2013;9:220–33.

55. Samuel T, Sessa C, Britten C, et al. AUY922, a novel HSP90 inhibitor: final results of a first-in-human study in patients with advanced solid malignancies. J Clin Oncol 2010;28(Suppl 15):2528.

56. Fletcher J, Debiec-Rychter M, Swank S, et al. HSP90 inhibitor STA-9090 potently suppresses heterogeneous KIT kinase-domain mutations responsible for gastrointestinal stromal tumor progression during imatinib therapy. AACR-NCI-EORTC International Conference on Molecular Targets and Cancer Therapeutics. Mol Cancer Ther 2009;8(Suppl 12):B184.

57. Demetri G, Heinrich MC, Chmielowski B, et al. An open-label phase II study of the Hsp90 inhibitor ganetespib (STA-9090) in patients (pts) with metastatic and/or unresectable GIST. ASCO Meeting Abstracts 2011;10011.

58. Bauer S, Duensing A, Demetri GD, et al. KIT oncogenic signaling mechanisms in imatinib-resistant gastrointestinal stromal tumor: PI3-kinase/AKT is a crucial survival pathway. Oncogene 2007;26:7560–8.

59. Rossi F, Ehlers I, Agosti V, et al. Oncogenic KITsignaling and therapeutic intervention in a mouse model of gastrointestinal stromal tumor. Proc Natl Acad Sci U S A 2006;103:12843-8.

60. Kondapaka SB, Singh SS, Dasmahapatra GP, et al. Perifosine, a novel alkylphospholipid, inhibits protein kinase B activation. Mol Cancer Ther 2003;2: 1093-103.

61. Conley A, Araujo D, Ludwig J, et al. A randomized phase II study of perifosine (P) plus imatinib for patients with imatinib-resistant gastrointestinal stromal tumor (GIST). J Clin Oncol (ASCO Meeting Abstracts) 2009;27(Suppl 15):10563.

62. Schöffski P, Reichardt P, Blay JY, et al. A phase I-II study of everolimus (RAD001) in combination with imatinib in patients with imatinib-resistant gastrointestinal stromal tumors. Ann Oncol 2010;21:1990-8.

63. Hohenberger P, Bauer S, Gruenwald V, et al. Multicenter, single-arm, two-stage phase II trial of everolimus (RAD001) with imatinib in imatinib-resistant patients (pts) with advanced GIST. ASCO Meeting Abstracts. J Clin Oncol 2010;28: 10048.

64. Palassini E, Fumagalli E, Coco P, et al. Combination of PKC412 and sirolimus in a metastatic patient with PDGFRA-D842V gastrointestinal stromal tumor (GIST). ASCO Meeting Abstracts. J Clin Oncol 2008;21515.

65. Piovesan C, Fumagalli E, Coco P, et al. Response to sirolimus in combination to tirosine kinase inhibitors (TKI) in three cases of PDGFRA-D842V metastatic gastrointestinal stromal tumor (GIST). J Clin Oncol (ASCO Meeting Abstracts) 2009;27(Suppl 15):10565.

66. Heinrich MC, Griffith D, McKinley A, et al. Crenolanib inhibits the drug-resistant PDGFRA D842V mutation associated with imatinib-resistant gastrointestinal stromal tumors. Clin Cancer Res 2012;18:4375-84.

67. Lewis NL, Lewis LD, Eder JP, et al. Phase I study of the safety, tolerability, and pharmacokinetics of oral CP-868,596, a highly specific platelet-derived growth factor receptor tyrosine kinase inhibitor in patients with advanced cancers. J Clin Oncol 2009;27:5262-9.

68. Wagner AJ, Remillard SP, Zhang YX, et al. Loss of expression of SDHA predicts SDHA mutations in gastrointestinal stromal tumors. Mod Pathol 2013;26:289-94.

69. Italiano A, Chen CL, Sung YS, et al. SDHA loss of function mutations in a subset of young adult wild-type gastrointestinal stromal tumors. BMC Cancer 2012;12: 408.

70. Oudijk L, Gaal J, Korpershoek E, et al. SDHA mutations in adult and pediatric wild-type gastrointestinal stromal tumors. Mod Pathol 2013;26:456-63.

71. Dwight T, Benn DE, Clarkson A, et al. Loss of SDHA expression identifies SDHA mutations in succinate dehydrogenase-deficient gastrointestinal stromal tumors. Am J Surg Pathol 2013;37:226-33.

72. Miettinen M, Killian JK, Wang ZF, et al. Immunohistochemical loss of succinate dehydrogenase subunit A (SDHA) in gastrointestinal stromal tumors (GISTs) signals SDHA germline mutation. Am J Surg Pathol 2013;37:234-40.

73. Carney JA, Stratakis CA. Familial paraganglioma and gastric stromal sarcoma: a new syndrome distinct from the Carney triad. Am J Med Genet 2002;108:132-9.

74. Pantaleo MA, Nannini M, Astolfi A, et al. A distinct pediatric-type gastrointestinal stromal tumor in adults: potential role of succinate dehydrogenase subunit A mutations. Am J Surg Pathol 2011;35:1750.

75. Tarn C, Rink L, Merkel E, et al. Insulin-like growth factor 1 receptor is a potential therapeutic target for gastrointestinal stromal tumors. Proc Natl Acad Sci U S A 2008;105:8387-92.

76. Miettinen M, Wang ZF, Sarlomo-Rikala M, et al. Succinate dehydrogenase-deficient GISTs: a clinicopathologic, immunohistochemical, and molecular genetic study of 66 gastric GISTs with predilection to young age. Am J Surg Pathol 2011;35:1712–21.

77. Cervera AM, Apostolova N, Crespo FL, et al. Cells silenced for SDHB expression display characteristic features of the tumor phenotype. Cancer Res 2008; 68:4058–67.

78. Larsson O, Girnita A, Girnita L. Role of insulin-like growth factor 1 receptor signalling in cancer. Br J Cancer 2005;92:2097–101.

Treatment of Localized Sarcomas

Alessandro Gronchi, MD[a], Chandrajit P. Raut, MD, MSc[b],*

KEYWORDS

- Sarcoma • GIST • Surgery • Radiation therapy • Chemotherapy
- Tyrosine kinase inhibitors • Survival • Outcome

KEY POINTS

- Sarcomas may arise in a variety of body sites and within a variety of tissues. The management of soft tissue sarcomas (STSs) and gastrointestinal stromal tumors (GISTs) requires a thorough understanding of the biology of the different histologies and molecular subtypes as well as the constraints of specific anatomic site.
- Limb-sparing and function-sparing approaches should be used when feasible for STSs located in the extremities and girdles, but extent of surgery should not be compromised for ease of closure. Margins of resection and use of adjuvant/neadjuvant radiation therapy and chemotherapy are contingent on accurate histologic diagnosis. Adjuvant therapy after a marginal resection, however, is not an appropriate substitute for a margin negative operation.
- Extended resections, including adjacent viscera, which may be adherent but not invaded, should be the goal in retroperitoneal sarcoma (RPS), to minimize microscopic intralesional margins and maximize local tumor control and possibly improve survival. The use of neo-adjuvant radiation therapy is under investigation. Adjuvant (postoperative) radiation therapy is of limited value. Chemotherapy is not routinely used, save for specific sensitive subtypes.
- Complete tumor resection avoiding tumor rupture should be the goal in GIST. Preoperative imatinib should be considered whenever the expected morbidity is not minimal or surgery is not expected to be microscopically complete.
- Treatment planning should include multidisciplinary consultation to determine optimal therapy, taking into consideration tumor histology, site, and extent of the disease; its natural history and sensitivity to available treatments; surgical challenges; and the wishes of patients.

INTRODUCTION

Surgery remains the standard and only potentially curative therapy in the management of localized STSs of the adult and GISTs. Although belonging to the same family of

Disclosures: The authors have nothing to disclose.
[a] Department of Surgery, Sarcoma Service, Fondazione IRCCS Istituto Nazionale dei Tumori, Via Venezian 1, Milan 20133, Italy; [b] Department of Surgery, Brigham and Women's Hospital, Center for Sarcoma and Bone Oncology, Dana-Farber Cancer Institute, Harvard Medical School, 75 Francis Street, Boston, MA 02115, USA
* Corresponding author.
E-mail address: craut@partners.org

Hematol Oncol Clin N Am 27 (2013) 921–938
http://dx.doi.org/10.1016/j.hoc.2013.07.006
0889-8588/13/$ – see front matter © 2013 Elsevier Inc. All rights reserved.

tumors, surgical principles and sensitivity to locoregional and systemic therapies are completely different between the 2 entities; therefore, they are discussed separately. The treatment of pediatric sarcomas (including primitive peripheral neuroectodermic tumors, alveolar/embryonal rhabdomyosarcomas, and desmoplastic small round cell tumors) is different; systemic chemotherapy is the primary treatment and surgery may sometimes be omitted. The discussion of pediatric sarcomas is beyond the scope of this review.

SOFT TISSUE SARCOMAS

The basic principle for surgery is that the tumor must be resected en bloc with a cuff of healthy tissue, to avoid contamination of the residual tissue from the tumor surface and remove tumor microsatellites, which may be present in the healthy tissues surrounding the pseudocapsule. The extent of resection and adequacy of margins depends on a variety of factors, including histology and presence of an intact biologic barrier, such as muscular fascia, vascular adventitia, periosteum, or epineurium.[1] Every attempt should be made to avoid positive microscopic margins (tumor at the border of the specimen), because this is independently associated with a worse survival.[2]

Patients with STS should undergo evaluation at a sarcoma center, because the administration of neoadjuvant or adjuvant therapy may be indicated. Generally, this involves multidisciplinary evaluation by a surgical oncologist and, depending on histology, a medical oncologist and a radiation oncologist. Re-evaluation of pathology slides by a pathologist specializing in sarcomas is critical, to confirm the exact histology and determine the most appropriate treatment. Approximately 24% of all sarcomas are initially designated with the incorrect histology, usually by pathologists who do not have extensive experience with evaluating sarcomas, and approximately 16% are assigned the wrong histology in a clinically significant manner, having an impact on treatment plan.[3] STSs are a family of more than 50 different diseases that can arise anywhere in the body. Principles of local treatment may vary according to histologic subtype and site. Surgical margins that may be adequate for one histologic subtype may be inadequate for another, and the sensitivity to and goals of chemotherapy and radiation therapy vary considerably between different histologies.

Histology-Specific Treatment

Atypical lipomatous tumor/well-differentiated liposarcoma

Atypical lipomatous tumor (ALT) and well-differentiated liposarcoma (WDLPS) are histologically the same entity. By convention, the term ALT is used when referring to low-grade lipomatous neoplasms confined to the trunk or extremity, where margin-negative resections are possible, and WDLPS is used when referring to deeper cavity tumors in the abdomen, retroperitoneum, and chest, where margin-negative resections are generally not possible. When arising in the extremity, this tumor has a low rate of recurrence, may not recur for some time, and has no risk of distant metastatic spread and death, unless dedifferentiation occurs over its natural history.[4] Dedifferentiation, if it occurs, entails a risk of metastatic spread as high as 20%. In contrast, low-grade, locally recurrent ALT may grow slowly for years. Therefore, such tumors arising in the extremity can be resected with a limited negative or even a positive margin, especially when preserving limb function is an issue. Radiographically, ALT may be difficult to distinguish from an intramuscular lipoma, a benign entity that can also arise in deep muscle tissue. WDLPS is a more threatening neoplasm when located in the retroperitoneum, even in absence of areas of dedifferentiation. As discussed later, local control is a challenging issue at this site, and patients often die of locoregional failure, without developing distant metastases.[5]

Dermatofibrosarcoma protuberans

Dermatofibrosarcoma protuberan (DFSP) is a superficial tumor that infiltrates soft tissue for centimeters beyond the obvious margins of the lesion and can recur locally after an inadequate resection.[6] The more common variety of DFSP does not display metastatic behavior. Therefore, the goal of surgery should be negative margins, often necessitating reconstruction by plastic surgery. Once negative margins are obtained, the risk of failure is virtually none. When cosmesis is an issue, limited positive margins may be accepted, and a wider resection postponed until DFSP locally recurs. Moreover, a limited positive margin does not automatically translate into local recurrence and does not increase the risk of metastatic spread. Radiation therapy (described later) is not routinely considered, even in the presence of positive margins. Approximately 5% to 10% of patients with DFSP have a more aggressive fibrosarcomatous variant, which may recur locally and metastasize.[6] Those individuals should be treated as patients affected by a conventional sarcoma with more aggressive local therapy (including radiation) and followed with systematic imaging.

Myxofibrosarcoma

Myxofibrosarcoma, when located superficially, infiltrates through soft tissue (subcutaneous fat and investing fascia) centimeters beyond the ostensible margins of the visible or palpable mass. When located intramuscularly, the extension of the infiltration is usually limited by anatomic barriers, although it has a higher propensity to invade into those anatomic boundaries compared with other histologic subtypes. Myxofibrosarcoma most commonly arises in the extremities of elderly individuals. It demonstrates a 30% rate of local recurrence and 16% rate of distant recurrence.[7,8] Multiple local recurrences have been associated with eventual amputation. Therefore, it is critical to pursue aggressive local therapy. Wide surgical margins (2–4 cm radial margins beyond the clinical boundaries of the palpable mass, especially in more superficial tumors) should be the goal of surgery, which often requires complex wound closure or flap reconstruction by a plastic and reconstructive surgeon as well as resection and reconstruction of vessels and/or nerves. Radiation therapy, either preoperatively or postoperatively (described later), may be considered, although the direct impact on this specific histology remain unknown.

Angiosarcoma

Scalp angiosarcoma is a particularly insidious malignancy.[9] Scalp angiosarcomas are commonly multifocal, by both clinical examination and CT or MRI imaging. Although radical surgery is possible (requiring complex flap reconstructions), it is not uncommon for patients to develop local recurrences immediately outside the margins of resection even if the margins of the initial resection were widely negative and with or without radiation therapy. Angiosarcoma is sensitive to systemic chemotherapy and to radiation therapy. Because surgery is rarely curative, it should not be considered first-line therapy for scalp angiosarcoma. Surgery may be reserved for patients who are experiencing problems with local control (bleeding from a fungating tumor) or who only appear to have a solitary site of disease by both clinical examination and imaging while undergoing systemic therapy. Similar considerations apply to angiosarcoma arising at other superficial sites. When it occurs in the deep tissues, multifocality is less of an issue and the outcome is usually dominated by distant spread. The approach includes chemotherapy, radiation therapy, and surgery (discussed previously),[9] although reconstruction by plastic surgery rarely is required. Vascular angiosarcoma has a particularly dismal prognosis and usually is also treated by a multimodality approach.[9] For tumors not suitable to complete surgical resection, definitive radiation therapy, possibly with heavy particles, can be considered. Management of primary and radiation-induced (secondary) angiosarcoma of the breast is later.

Radiation-induced soft tissue sarcomas

Radiation-induced STSs are rare and include a variety of histologic subtypes, the most common of which are unclassified pleomorphic sarcoma, angiosarcoma, malignant peripheral nerve sheath tumors, and leiomyosarcoma.[10] In addition to the intrinsic characteristics of each histologic subtype, they are all characterized by a high propensity to locally recur, given the difficulty of obtaining clear margins. This is due in part to the difficulty in distinguishing tumor infiltration of healthy tissues from radiation-induced soft tissue changes around the tumor site and in part to the discontiguous and multifocal involvement of tissue within the radiation field.[10] The tumor should be excised with as much tissue around it as possible. This often, if not always, requires reconstruction and coverage by a plastic surgeon and potentially a more liberal policy of neurovascular resection and reconstruction. Systemic chemotherapy and re-irradiation are often considered, given the overall dismal prognosis, although the use of the latter must be weighed with caution.

Malignant peripheral nerve sheath tumors

Malignant peripheral nerve sheath tumors tumors often arise from a major peripheral nerve, which can be identified macroscopically. They can occur sporadically or in the context of neurofibromatosis type 1 (von Recklinghausen disease).[11] The high-grade variant is marked by an early propensity for distant metastases.[11] When originating from a peripheral nerve, malignant peripheral nerve sheath tumors tumors also may spread along the nerve fibers proximally or distally. Wider margins at this level should be obtained (if possible at least 4 cm of macroscopic healthy nerve), in order to limit locoregional failure, which eventually may reach the spinal cord. Intraoperative frozen section analysis may help ensure clear margins. Systemic chemotherapy is used on an individualized basis.

Site-Specific Treatment

Extremity and trunk wall soft tissue sarcoma

Diagnosis Imaging alone is rarely diagnostic of the specific sarcoma histology, with the exception of WDLPS (ie, ALT). ALTs have a radiographic density similar to normal surrounding fat but tend to be well encapsulated with thick internal septations. Such tumors may be treated with limited resection (complete excision with a minimal margin of normal surrounding muscle, fat, or fascia to minimize risk of local recurrence) and do not require a biopsy.

Other neoplasms suspicious for sarcoma should be biopsied. Core needle biopsy is the preferred method.[12] It can be done either under radiographic guidance or without imaging directly in the clinic depending on location. Although biopsy tract recurrences are rare, the site selected for the core needle biopsy should be planned such that it can be included in the incision used during the subsequent definitive resection or at least in the radiation field. If a core needle biopsy fails to yield a diagnosis, an open incisional or excisional biopsy should be obtained. Although incisional biopsies commonly are used for diagnosis, they are often performed improperly in inexperienced hands. Incisional biopsies for extremity lesions should be performed through longitudinally oriented incisions placed such that the incision can be included in the final resection when a definitive resection is planned. If a transverse incision is used, then when subsequent re-excision is required, challenges for reconstruction and risk of lymphatic disruption (depending on location) are magnified. Excisional biopsies should be confined to lesions less than 2 cm in size and superficial in location.

Surgical treatment Currently, the goal of surgery is limb sparing and function sparing, while achieving appropriate biologic margins. Surgical resection should be carefully planned based on preoperative imaging. Resections should include not only the entire tumor (without rupture or violation of the surrounding pseudocapsule) but also an adequately wide margin (1–2 cm) of normal, non-neoplastic tissue (**Fig. 1**).[1,13] Resections performed with positive margins do result in higher risk of local recurrences and, to a lesser extent, of distant metastases and death (**Table 1**).[2,14–16] Tumors abutting bone may include the periosteum as a margin if the bone is not directly invaded. If necessary, vascular resection and reconstruction should be considered for involved vessels. If a critical nerve is encased, reconstruction with an interposition nerve graft should be considered. Such reconstructions may be compromised if radiation is administered postoperatively, and, therefore, preoperative radiation may be warranted. Furthermore, it is critical to take into account the specific histology (described previously). For instance, resection for myxofibrosarcoma requires wider margins than resection for ALT. Thus, it is important for surgeons to understand the different sarcoma histologies, confirm the accuracy of the diagnosis, and review the treatment plan in a multidisciplinary consultation.

Adjuvant/neoadjuvant radiation therapy and chemotherapy Limb-sparing surgery generally relies on adjuvant/neoadjuvant radiation therapy to minimize risk of local recurrence, as demonstrated in a landmark National Cancer Institute (NCI) trial.[17] The goal of radiation is to treat the margin to minimize the risk of recurrence, not

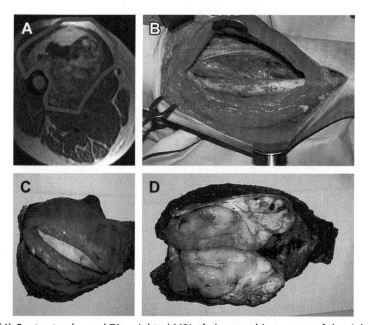

Fig. 1. (A) Contrast-enhanced T1-weighted MRI of pleomorphic sarcoma of the right thigh, originating in the anterior compartment. The planned resection line is outlined. (B) Surgical field after removal of the tumor. (C) Surgical specimen. (D) Specimen cut through the longest diameter. The tumor is surrounded by a clean margin of healthy tissue all around.

Table 1
Incidence of local recurrence, distant metastases, and death in major published series of extremities soft tissue sarcoma, according to microscopic surgical margins

	5-y LR		5-y DM		5-y CSD		10-y LR		10-y DM		10-y CSD	
	M+ (%)	M− (%)	M+ (%)	M− (%)	M+ (%)	M− (%)	M+ (%)	M− (%)	M+ (%)	M− (%)	M+ (%)	M− (%)
Trovik et al,[14] 2000	36	18	28	28	NR	NR	NR	NR	NR	NR	NR	NR
Stojadinovic et al,[15] 2002	35	18	32	24	30	20	NR	NR	NR	NR	NR	NR
Zagars et al,[16] 2003	36	12	25	28	31	25	44	14	33	33	39	34
Gronchi et al,[2] 2010	26	10	20	21	29	16	30	12	24	24	38	19

Abbreviations: DM, incidence of distant metastases; LR, incidence of local recurrence; M+, positive microscopic surgical margins; M−, negative microscopic surgical margins; NR, not reported.
Data from Refs.[2,14–16]

necessarily to reduce the size of the tumor per se. Radiation therapy reduces the risk of local recurrence from greater than 30% to less than 10% in most series but does not have an impact on distant failure or overall survival (OS).

Radiation therapy may be delivered as external beam radiation therapy (EBRT), brachytherapy, or intraoperative radiation therapy (IORT). EBRT may be delivered preoperatively or postoperatively. One randomized trial, by O'Sullivan and colleagues and sponsored by the Canadian NCI,[18] compared preoperative EBRT to postoperative EBRT. There was no difference in local recurrence rates. Preoperative EBRT was associated with a doubling in the rate of wound complications (35% vs 17%) but importantly with a lower rate of late complications and tissue fibrosis and better functional outcomes. Postoperative EBRT generally covers a larger field (including drain sites) and is higher dose than preoperative EBRT. This is particularly important in young adults of childbearing age with proximal thigh STS; preoperative EBRT may spare the gonads whereas postoperative radiation may not. Moreover, the implementation of preoperative EBRT in a multimodality approach to high-risk extremity STS has also been shown to improve overall oncologic outcome in large retrospective series.[19] Thus, it is the preferred approach at many experienced centers. A recent retrospective study identified diabetes, tumor size greater than 10 cm, tumor less than 3 mm from the skin surface, and need for reconstruction as independent predictors of major wound complications on multivariate analysis.[20] Therefore, in patients potentially at higher risk of wound complications, judicious use of neoadjuvant EBRT, generous resection of at-risk superficial soft tissue, and proactive wound care measures may reduce complication rates.

Brachytherapy, delivered through afterloading catheters placed across the tumor bed at the end of surgery, or IORT, delivered during surgery via a cone applicator to the tumor bed after tumor removal, are options usually reserved to deliver additional radiation to a precisely defined close margin (including neurovascular structures) with minimal treatment to surrounding tissue, particularly when further EBRT is no longer feasible. Both brachytherapy and IORT may be used selectively with acceptable toxicity, but neither is generally used alone with either preoperative or postoperative EBRT. Brachytherapy offers the advantage of awaiting final margin analysis before determine which margins are indeed close, because catheters are not typically loaded with radioisotope for a minimum of 5 days postoperatively. They are not considered as routinely as EBRT, especially when preoperative therapy has been delivered.[21,22]

Patients with small (<5 cm), superficial, well-circumscribed STS resected with an appropriately wide margin (>1 cm) of non-neoplastic tissue or biologic barrier (fascia) may not require RT, provided that the patient can be reliably followed.[23]

Approximately 25% to 50% of patients with extremity STSs develop distant metastatic disease. Those with large (>5 cm), deep, high-grade STSs may be considered for preoperative or postoperative chemotherapy, usually with active agents, such as doxorubicin and ifosfamide.

The benefit of such an approach is limited, however, because it can at best provide an absolute improvement of OS of 5% at 10 years, and the data are inconsistent.[24,25] Therefore, there is no consensus among sarcoma experts about the routine use of chemotherapy in the adjuvant setting for extremity sarcomas. Nevertheless, recent data have shown that when chemotherapy is selected for high-risk STS patients, a short full-dose regimen consisting of 3 cycles of anthracyclines plus ifosfamide may be considered. Toxicity is limited. It can also be delivered preoperatively and combined with RT, depending on the surgical needs, especially for tumors of borderline resectability or when preservation of function is a goal.[26,27]

Hyperthermic isolated limb perfusion (ILP) has been investigated in several institutions because treatment of patients with locally advanced STS in whom limb-sparing, function-sparing surgery may not be possible.[28] This procedure involves placing vascular access catheters into the main artery and vein of the affected extremity and perfusing with high-dose chemotherapy (usually melphalan) and tumor necrosis factor α under hyperthermic conditions. Although safe in experienced hands, early and late complication rates of more than 20% have been reported.[29] More recently, isolated limb infusion (ILI) has been evaluated.[30] Similar to ILP, ILI circulates high-dose chemotherapy in an isolated extremity but in contrast is generally performed through catheters placed percutaneously (rather than through an open approach) and under hypoxic conditions. Although high rate of complete responses (15%–30%) and further limb-sparing procedures (80%) are achieved by ILP and ILI, no randomized trials have ever compared either technique over aggressive limb-sparing resection with EBRT for STS. Arguably, patients under consideration for ILP usually have locally advanced or multifocal STS and are not necessarily candidates for surgery with EBRT at first evaluation. ILP and/or ILI should be considered as potential therapy in appropriately selected patients, and eligible patients should be referred to centers where this therapy is available.

RPS

Clinical and diagnostic evaluation Imaging alone is rarely diagnostic of the specific sarcoma histology, with the exception of WDLPS. As described previously, WDLPSs have a radiographic density similar to normal surrounding fat but tend to be well encapsulated with thick internal septations. Giant lipomas are identified only anecdotally in the retroperitoneum; therefore, any mass consisting of very well-differentiated fatty tissue should be considered a WDLPS and treated as such. These tumors do not require a biopsy. Other lesions suspicious for RPS should be biopsied. The authors prefer to obtain core needle biopsies under radiographic guidance. Biopsy tract recurrences are rare and do not need to be re-excised during definitive surgery. Furthermore, if preoperative EBRT is planned, the biopsy site is usually included within the radiation field.

Surgical treatment Proper resection of RPS requires appreciation of the anatomic boundaries of the tumor.[31] CT imaging should be reviewed to identify landmarks defining the extent of the mass to determine which structures may be safely resected and which ones cannot. The anterior margin of an RPS is generally the ipsilateral colon and mesocolon, pancreas, liver, or stomach. The posterior margin is generally the psoas and iliacus muscles inferiorly, the ipsilateral kidney and diaphragm superiorly, and the ipsilateral ureter and gonadal vessels medially. These margins may vary, however, from tumor to tumor, and some or all of these structures could be anterior to the mass, in which case they would constitute a portion of the anterior margin. The medial margin usually includes the spine and paraspinous muscles, the inferior vena cava (for right-sided tumors), and the aorta (for left-sided tumors). The lateral margin is constituted by the lateral or flank musculoskeletal sidewall, although depending on the size and location of the tumor, the kidney and/or colon could also border the lateral portion of the mass. The superior margin is similarly dependent on the size and location of the mass and may include the diaphragm on either side, the right lobe of the liver, the duodenum, and the head/uncinate process of the pancreas for right-sided tumors and the pancreatic tail, spleen, and splenic vessels for left-sided tumors. The inferior margin may include the iliopsoas muscle; the femoral nerve; the common, internal, and external iliac vessels;

and the pelvic sidewall. The size and specific location of the mass determine which of these many structures constitute which specific margin.

In general, the ipsilateral kidney, colon, mesocolon and at least a portion of the psoas can be safely and relatively easily resected. Resection of the, pancreatic tail and spleen can usually be performed with low short-term morbidity. Resection of other structures, including but not limited to the aorta, inferior vena cava, iliac vessels, femoral nerve, diaphragm, duodenum, pancreatic head or uncinate process, and liver, entail more significant resections, with ensuing greater morbidity.[32]

The goal of surgery should be an aggressive multiorgan resection, removing involved or attached surrounding organs and retroperitoneal fat en bloc with the tumor in an effort to maximally clear the margins and avoid spilling tumor (**Fig. 2**). This extended approach has shown to benefit patients affected by RPS, especially when the systemic risk was not high (**Table 2**).[33–39] A macroscopically incomplete resection is no more beneficial than nonoperative management.

Radiation therapy The role of RT is controversial, in the absence of phase III randomized controlled trial data. Radiation therapy unequivocally reduces the risk of local recurrence in patients with extremity STS, but this has not been proved in RPS.[40–42] Furthermore, the proximity of radiosensitive tissues and organs, such as liver and

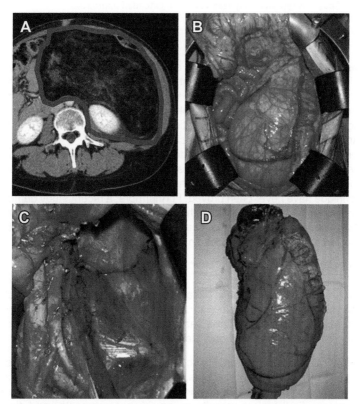

Fig. 2. (*A*) Contrast-enhanced CT scan of left retroperitoneal liposarcoma. The planned resection line is outlined. (*B*) Tumor at laparotomy. (*C*) Surgical field after tumor removal. (*D*) Surgical specimen. The tumor is covered by left kidney and colon (and psoas muscle in the back, not shown).

Table 2
Local recurrence-free survival and overall survival in major published series of retroperitoneal sarcoma

	Study Period	Median FU	Patients (N)	Complete Resection (%)	5-y LRFS	5-y OS
Lewis et al,[35] 1998	1982–1997	28	231	80	59	54
Stoeckle et al,[36] 2001	1980–1994	47	165	65	42	49
Ferrario & Karakousis,[37] 2003	1977–2001	41	79	99	43	65
Hassan et al,[38] 2004	1983–1995	36	97	78	56	51
Lehnert et al,[39] 2009	1998–2002	89	71	70	59	65
Bonvalot et al,[32] 2010	**2000–2008**	**37**	**249**	**93**	**78**	**65**
Gronchi et al,[34] 2012	**2002–2008**	**48**	**136**	**94**	**79**	**68**

Bold, series of patients systematically resected by an extended approach.
Abbreviations: FU, follow-up; LRFS, local recurrence-free survival.
Data from Refs.[32,34–39]

small intestine, together with the large size of the radiation field limits its utility in some patients. The sarcoma surgeons and radiation oncologists who use radiation therapy generally favor delivering it preoperatively, when the bulk of the tumor itself displaces uninvolved organs out of the radiation field. There is one ongoing randomized trial evaluating the utility of preoperative radiation therapy in patients with RPS, based in Europe and open in selected North American centers.[43]

Another controversial issue with respect to RT and RPS is the concept of dose escalation using intensity-modulated RT to presumed high-risk tumor margins in order to reduce locoregional recurrence rates. Although conceptual interesting, the benefits of this technique have never been proved. Furthermore, a recent study demonstrated that among patients with RPS treated with standard field preoperative RT, only 25% of patients who developed locoregional recurrences failed within the radiation field, thus calling into question the utility of such an approach.[44]

Breast sarcoma

The most common sarcoma histologies arising in the breast are angiosarcoma and phyllodes. Angiosarcoma may arise either primarily within the breast parenchyma or secondarily within the breast skin as a consequence of lymphedema or more commonly radiation therapy delivered as a part of breast conservation therapy for breast cancer. Each of these malignancies is considered individually.

Primary angiosarcoma Primary angiosarcoma is a disease of the breast parenchyma arising in young women.[45] Angiosarcoma, irrespective of site, is in general responsive to systemic chemotherapy. Once chemotherapy is stopped, however, the disease tends to regrow. Furthermore, despite its sensitivity to chemotherapy, there is no proved survival benefit from systemic therapy. The only potentially curative therapy is surgery. Although breast cancer may be treated with breast conservation, limited surgery due to the proved benefit of radiation therapy and hormonal therapy, there are no such proved beneficial adjuvant therapies for primary breast angiosarcoma. Therefore, patients should be offered a simple mastectomy instead of lumpectomy. Partial resection of pectoralis major may be necessary to achieve negative margins. The skin may be closed primarily. The contralateral breast may be a site for metastatic disease, but to date, there is no proved benefit from a contralateral prophylactic mastectomy.

Secondary breast angiosarcoma
Secondary breast angiosarcoma is a disease affecting older women.[46,47] Historically, secondary angiosarcoma arose in the setting of lymphedema. Now, it is more commonly seen as a consequence of RT. RT-induced angiosarcoma is a cutaneous malignancy that may extend into breast parenchyma, whereas primary angiosarcoma is a disease of the breast parenchyma. Thus, the operation for secondary angiosarcoma is different than that for primary angiosarcoma. Patients with secondary RT-induced angiosarcoma should undergo not only a total mastectomy but, more importantly, resection of the affected organ—all of the breast skin. This disease is often multifocal and, therefore, as much of the irradiated skin should be removed en bloc with the breast as possible. This is critical—a simple mastectomy alone does not remove the organ (skin) involved, and recurrences may be noted within weeks to months. If tumor extends to pectoralis major, then the muscle should be removed as well. All patients require extensive reconstruction, including skin grafting just to restore a flat, closed chest wall.

Phyllodes tumor
Phyllodes tumors of the breast can grow to be quite large.[48] Surgery alone is the primary therapy. Tumors should be resected with a negative margin; for smaller tumors, a lumpectomy may be possible, but for larger tumors, a simple mastectomy may be necessary. Lymph node biopsy is not necessary. Recurrences may be observed in approximately 15% of patients, including local recurrences in the ipsilateral breast and distant recurrences in locations, such as lung and liver. Contralateral breast recurrences are exceedingly rare; thus, contralateral prophylactic mastectomy is not indicated.

GASTROINTESTINAL STROMAL TUMORS

GISTs are rare neoplasms, representing only 0.1% to 3% of all gastrointestinal malignancies.[49] They are the most common sarcoma, however, and account for 80% of gastrointestinal mesenchymal neoplasms.[49] In the past 12 years, understanding and treatment of GIST has witnessed remarkable advances due to 2 key developments: (1) the identification of constitutively active signals (oncogenic mutation of the c-KIT and platelet-derived growth factor alpha [PDGFRA] genes encoding receptor tyrosine kinases) and (2) the development of therapeutic agents that suppress tumor growth by specifically targeting and inhibiting this signal resulting in improved outcomes (imatinib mesylate, sunitinib malate, and regorafenib). These developments in the management of GIST represent a proof of principle of translational therapeutics in oncology, confirming that specific inhibition of tumor-associated receptor tyrosine kinase activity may be an effective cancer treatment. The advent of effective therapy has dramatically improved outcomes for patients with GIST. Nevertheless, surgery remains the only potentially curative therapy for patients with GIST.

GISTs commonly arise in the stomach (50%–70%), small intestine (25%–35%), colon and rectum (5%–10%), mesentery or omentum (7%), and esophagus (<5%). Occasionally, GISTs may arise in the duodenal ampulla, appendix, gallbladder, and urinary bladder. A preoperative biopsy is not routinely necessary for a primary, resectable neoplasm suspicious for GIST. If, however, the differential diagnosis includes entities, such as lymphoma, that would be treated differently, if neoadjuvant therapy is under consideration, or if there is metastatic disease, biopsy is appropriate.

Surgery for Localized GIST

Surgery remains the standard of care and only potentially curative therapy for patients with primary, resectable, localized GIST. At laparotomy, the abdomen should be thoroughly explored to identify and remove any previously undetected peritoneal metastatic deposits. Although primary GISTs may demonstrate inflammatory adhesions to surrounding organs, they do not generally invade other organs beyond the site of origin despite CT appearance. The goal of the operation is an R0 resection. The ideal margin of resection is unknown. A macroscopically complete resection with negative or positive microscopic margins (R0 or R1 resection, respectively) is associated with a better prognosis than a macroscopically incomplete resection (R2 resection). Post hoc analysis of a randomized trial evaluating the utility of 1 year of adjuvant imatinib mesylate therapy after resection of primary GISTs at least 3 cm in size demonstrated that there was no significant difference in recurrence-free survival (RFS) for patients undergoing an R0 versus R1 resection with or without the use of adjuvant imatinib.[50] Data on OS are unknown. What is known is that tumor rupture or violation of the tumor capsule during surgery is associated with an increased risk of recurrence and, therefore, should be avoided. Lymphadenectomy is not required because lymph nodes are rarely involved (in adult patients).

In general, the extent of surgery is usually a wedge or segmental resection of the involved stomach or bowel without the wide margins necessary for adenocarcinoma. Rarely, a more extensive resection (total gastrectomy for a large proximal gastric GIST, pancreaticoduodenectomy for a periampullary GIST, or abdominoperineal resection for a low rectal GIST) may be necessary (**Fig. 3**). Several recent

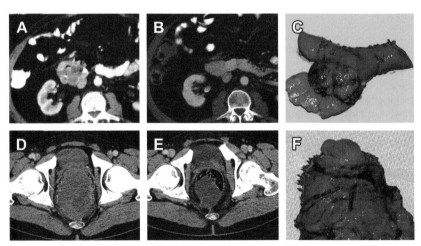

Fig. 3. Contrast-enhanced CT of a duodenal GIST arising at the second portion of the duodenum before (A) and after (B) imatinib therapy for 1 year. Surgical specimen of the tumor and the segmental resection of the duodenum (C). Contrast-enhanced CT of a rectal GIST arising from the lower third before (D) and after (E) imatinib for 1 year. Surgical specimen of the rectum, with the tumor close to the distal end (F), margins microscopically clear.

multi-institutional retrospective series have questioned the need for extensive re-sections, such as pancreaticoduodenectomy or abdominoperineal resection in the setting of well-tolerated, orally available targeted therapies.[51–56] Specifically, neo-adjuvant imatinib may shrink a periampullary or rectal GIST sufficiently to allow a more localized resection (local excision of periampullary GIST or transanal resection of rectal GIST), and adjuvant imatinib may be continued postoperatively. Thus, if an extensive operation is expected for complete tumor removal, neoadjuvant imatinib should be strongly considered.

Not uncommonly, margins after local resections after such downstaged operations may be close or microscopically positive. There are no data, however, indicating that patients who have an R1 resection require re-excision, and the lack of any difference in RFS between patients undergoing R0 versus R1 resection suggests that re-excision or more radical resections may be avoided. Furthermore, margins may retract after resection, or a pathologist may trim away the staple line (converting a technically negative microscopic margin into a positive one). Therefore, all cases of positive microscopic margins should be carefully reviewed by a multidisciplinary team, including surgical oncologist, pathologist, and medical oncologist, to assess the need for re-excision or adjuvant therapy with imatinib.

All GISTs 2 cm in size or greater should be resected when possible, because none of these can be considered benign. The natural history of GISTs under 2 cm in size is un-known, however, and thus their management is more debatable. Although the low risk of progression of GISTs under 2 cm may support a more conservative approach, an accurate mitotic index cannot be determined by biopsy or fine-needle aspiration. Therefore, observation for GISTs 1 cm to 2 cm is difficult to recommend. As such, resection of GISTs measuring 1 cm to 2 cm should be considered, and the risks and benefits of surgery versus observation should be reviewed with patients. Given the higher risk of aggressive behavior of small bowel and colon GISTs, any tumor in such locations should be resected irrespective of size. In contrast, most gastric GISTs under 1 cm in size may be followed. Two studies suggest that subcentimeter gastric GISTs are common, detected in 22.5% of autopsies in adults over age 50 in Germany and in 35% of patients undergoing gastrectomy for gastric cancer in Japan.[57,58] Despite their relative frequency, few of these neoplasms seem clinically relevant. Until further data are available, the most appropriate management of such small tumors re-mains uncertain. Although endoscopic resection of small gastric GISTs has been re-ported by gastroenterologists, this cannot be recommended routinely. Unlike early gastric cancers (mucosal malignancies) amenable to endoscopic mucosal resection, GISTs involve the muscularis propria, so attempts at endoscopic resection risk leaving a positive margin and, due to the depth of the lesion, could result in perforation. Regardless of their size, any small GISTs that are symptomatic (eg, hemorrhage from erosion through the mucosa) or increase in size on serial follow-up should be resected.

Laparoscopic or laparoscopy-assisted resection of primary GISTs may be per-formed following standard oncologic principles. Two early studies confirmed both the safety and feasibility of a laparoscopic approach. Otani and colleagues[59,60] re-ported a series of 35 gastric GISTs (2–5 cm) resected laparoscopically; no local or distant recurrences were observed for tumors under 4 cm in size with a median follow-up of 53 months. Novitsky and colleagues[61] reported a study of 50 patients with gastric GISTs (1.0–8.5 cm) resected laparoscopically or using laparoscopy-assistance, with 92% of patients disease-free with a mean follow-up of 3 years. Several subsequent studies have corroborated the safety and feasibility of laparo-scopic resections.

Given the safety of laparoscopic resections of localized GIST, a more contemporary approach, particularly for gastric GISTs, is to aim for laparoscopic resection. If a tumor is small enough to be easily removed laparoscopically, then the patient may be considered for surgery up front. If not, then consider neoadjuvant imatinib and continue it until laparoscopy is feasible, which may require 6 months or more. Laparoscopy does not usually change the extent of organ resection (for instance, the amount of stomach that needs to be resected) but may allow the surgeon to convert from an open procedure to a minimally invasive one.

Despite a macroscopically complete resection, as many as 50% of individuals may develop recurrent disease at a median of 24 months after surgery. An R0 or R1 resection is associated with 5-year OS rates of 34% to 63% whereas R2 resection is associated with 5-year OS as low as 8%. Adjuvant therapy with imatinib, as described in a separate article by Joensuu elsewhere in this issue, improves both progression-free survival and OS after R0/R1 resection.[62,63]

SUMMARY

Sarcomas may arise in a variety of body sites and within a variety of tissues. The management of STSs and GISTs requires a thorough understanding of the biology of the different histologies and molecular subtypes as well as the constraints of specific anatomic site. Limb-sparing and function-sparing approaches should be used when feasible for STSs located in the extremities and girdles, but extent of surgery should not be compromised to for ease of closure. Margins of resection and use of adjuvant/neadjuvant radiation therapy and chemotherapy are contingent on accurate histologic diagnosis. Adjuvant therapy after a marginal resection, however, is not an appropriate substitute for a margin negative operation. Extended resections, including adjacent uninvolved viscera, should be the goal in RPS, to minimize microscopic intralesional margins and maximize local tumor control and possibly improve survival. The use of neoadjuvant radiation therapy is under investigation. Adjuvant (postoperative) radiation therapy is of limited value. Chemotherapy is not routinely used, save for specific sensitive subtypes. Complete tumor resection avoiding tumor rupture should be the goal in GIST. Preoperative imatinib should be considered whenever the expected morbidity is not minimal or surgery is not expected to be microscopically complete. Treatment planning should include multidisciplinary consultation to determine optimal therapy, taking into consideration tumor histology, site, and extent of the disease; its natural history and sensitivity to available treatments; surgical challenges; and, of course, the wishes of patients.

REFERENCES

1. Kawaguchi N, Ahmed AR, Matsumoto S, et al. The concept of curative margin in surgery for bone and soft tissue sarcoma. Clin Orthop 2004;419:165–72.
2. Gronchi A, Lo Vullo S, Colombo C, et al. Extremity soft tissue sarcoma in a series of patients treated at a single institution: local control directly impacts survival. Ann Surg 2010;251:512–7.
3. Raut CP, George S, Hornick JL, et al. High rates of histopathologic discordance in sarcoma with implications for clinical care. J Clin Oncol 2011; 29(suppl) [abstract 10065].
4. Sommerville SM, Patton JT, Luscombe JC, et al. Clinical outcomes of deep atypical lipomas (well-differentiated lipoma-like liposarcomas) of the extremities. ANZ J Surg 2005;75(9):803–6.

5. Dalal KM, Kattan MW, Antonescu CR, et al. Subtype specific prognostic nomogram for patients with primary liposarcoma of the retroperitoneum, extremity, or trunk. Ann Surg 2006;244(3):381–91.

6. Fiore M, Miceli R, Mussi C, et al. Dermatofibrosarcoma protuberans treated at a single institution: a surgical disease with a high cure rate. J Clin Oncol 2005; 23(30):7669–75.

7. Haglund KE, Raut CP, Nascimento AF, et al. Recurrence patterns and survival for patients with intermediate- and high-grade myxofibrosarcoma. Int J Radiat Oncol Biol Phys 2012;82(1):361–7.

8. Sanfilippo R, Miceli R, Grosso F, et al. Myxofibrosarcoma: prognostic factors and survival in a series of patients treated at a single institution. Ann Surg Oncol 2011;18(3):720–5.

9. Fayette J, Martin E, Piperno-Neumann S, et al. Angiosarcomas, a heterogeneous group of sarcomas with specific behavior depending on primary site: a retrospective study of 161 cases. Ann Oncol 2007;18(12):2030–6.

10. Gladdy RA, Qin LX, Moraco N, et al. Do radiation-associated soft tissue sarcomas have the same prognosis as sporadic soft tissue sarcomas? J Clin Oncol 2010;28(12):2064–9.

11. Anghileri M, Miceli R, Fiore M, et al. Malignant peripheral nerve sheath tumors: prognostic factors and survival in a series of patients treated at a single institution. Cancer 2006;107(5):1065–74.

12. Strauss DC, Qureshi YA, Hayes AJ, et al. The role of core needle biopsy in the diagnosis of suspected soft tissue tumours. J Surg Oncol 2010;102(5): 523–9.

13. Enneking WF, Spanier SS, Goodman MA. A system for the surgical staging of musculoskeletal sarcoma. Clin Orthop Relat Res 1980;(153):106–20.

14. Trovik CS, Bauer HCF, Alvegard TA, et al. Surgical margins, local recurrence and metastasis in soft tissue sarcomas: 599 surgically-treated patients from the Scandinavian Sarcoma Group register. Eur J Cancer 2000;36:710–6.

15. Stojadinovic A, Leung DH, Hoos A, et al. Analysis of the prognostic significance of microscopic margins in 2,084 localized primary adult soft tissue sarcomas. Ann Surg 2002;235(3):424–34.

16. Zagars GK, Ballo MT, Pisters PW, et al. Surgical margins and re-excision in the management of patients with soft tissue sarcoma using conservative surgery and radiation therapy. Cancer 2003;97:2530–43.

17. Yang JC, Chang AE, Baker AR, et al. Randomized prospective study of the benefit of adjuvant radiation therapy in the treatment of soft tissue sarcomas of the extremity. J Clin Oncol 1998;16(1):197–203.

18. O'Sullivan B, Davis AM, Turcotte R, et al. Preoperative versus postoperative radiotherapy in soft-tissue sarcoma of the limbs: a randomised trial. Lancet 2002;359:2235–41.

19. Gronchi A, Miceli R, Colombo C, et al. Primary extremity soft tissue sarcomas: outcome improvement over time at a single institution. Ann Oncol 2011;22: 1675–81.

20. Baldini EH, Lapidus MR, Wang Q, et al. Predictors for major wound complications following preoperative radiotherapy and surgery for soft-tissue sarcoma of the extremities and trunk: importance of tumor proximity to skin surface. Ann Surg Oncol 2013;20(5):1494–9.

21. Dagan R, Indelicato DJ, McGee L, et al. The significance of a marginal excision after preoperative radiation therapy for soft tissue sarcoma of the extremity. Cancer 2012;118(12):3199–207.

22. Al Yami A, Griffin AM, Ferguson PC, et al. Positive surgical margins in soft tissue sarcoma treated with preoperative radiation: is a postoperative boost necessary. Int J Radiat Oncol Biol Phys 2010;77(4):1191–7.

23. Baldini EH, Goldberg J, Jenner C, et al. Long-term outcomes after function-sparing surgery without radiotherapy for soft tissue sarcoma of the extremities and trunk. J Clin Oncol 1999;17(10):3252–9.

24. Pervaiz N, Colterjohn N, Farrokhiar F, et al. A systematic met-analysis of randomized controlled trials for adjuvant chemotherapy for localized resectable soft tissue sarcoma. Cancer 2008;113(3):573–81.

25. Frustaci S, Gherlinzoni F, De Paoli A, et al. Adjuvant chemotherapy for adult soft tissue sarcomas of the extremities and girdles: results of the Italian randomized cooperative trial. J Clin Oncol 2001;19:1238–47.

26. Gronchi A, Frustaci S, Mercuri M, et al. Short, full-dose adjuvant chemotherapy in high-risk adult soft tissue sarcomas: a randomized clinical trial from the Italian Sarcoma Group and the Spanish Sarcoma Group. J Clin Oncol 2012; 10:850–6.

27. Gronchi A, Verderio P, De Paoli A, et al. Quality of surgery and neoadjuvant combined therapy in the ISG-GEIS trial on soft tissue sarcomas of limbs and trunk wall. Ann Oncol 2013;24(3):817–23.

28. Deroose JP, Eggermont AM, van Geel AN, et al. Long-term results of tumor necrosis factor alpha- and melphalan-based isolated limb perfusion in locally advanced extremity soft tissue sarcomas. J Clin Oncol 2011;29(30):4036–44.

29. Cherix S, Speiser M, Matter M, et al. Isolated limb perfusion with tumor necrosis factor and melphalan for non-resectable soft tissue sarcomas: long-term results on efficacy and limb salvage in a selected group of patients. J Surg Oncol 2008; 98(3):148–55.

30. Wong J, Chen YA, Fisher KJ, et al. Isolated limb infusion in a series of over 100 infusions: a single-center experience. Ann Surg Oncol 2013;20(4):1121–7.

31. Bonvalot S, Raut CP, Pollock RE, et al. Technical considerations in surgery for retroperitoneal sarcomas: position paper from E-surge, a master class in sarcoma surgery, and EORTC-STBSG. Ann Surg Oncol 2012;19(9):2981–91.

32. Bonvalot S, Miceli R, Berselli M, et al. Aggressive surgery in retroperitoneal soft tissue sarcoma carried out at high-volume centers is safe and is associated with improved local control. Ann Surg Oncol 2010;17:1507–14.

33. Gronchi A, Lo Vullo S, Fiore M, et al. Aggressive surgical policies in a retrospectively reviewed single-institution case series of retroperitoneal soft tissue sarcoma patients. J Clin Oncol 2009;27:24–30.

34. Gronchi A, Miceli R, Colombo C, et al. Frontline extended surgery is associated with improved survival in retroperitoneal low-intermediate grade soft tissue sarcomas. Ann Oncol 2012;23(4):1067–73.

35. Lewis JJ, Leung D, Woodruff JM. Retroperitoneal soft-tissue sarcoma: analysis of 500 patients treated and followed at a single institution. Ann Surg 1998;228: 355–65.

36. Stoeckle E, Coindre JM, Bonvalot S, et al. Prognostic factors in retroperitoneal sarcoma: a multivariate analysis of a series of 165 patients of the French Cancer Center Federation Sarcoma Group. Cancer 2001;92:359–68.

37. Ferrario T, Karakousis CP. Retroperitoneal sarcomas: grade and survival. Arch Surg 2003;138:248–51.

38. Hassan I, Park SZ, Donohue JH, et al. Operative management of primary retroperitoneal sarcomas: a reappraisal of an institutional experience. Ann Surg 2004;239:244–50.

39. Lehnert T, Cardona S, Hinz U, et al. Primary and locally recurrent retroperitoneal soft-tissue sarcoma: local control and survival. Eur J Surg Oncol 2009;35: 986–93.

40. Le Péchoux C, Musat E, Baey C, et al. Should adjuvant radiotherapy be administered in addition to front-line aggressive surgery (FAS) in patients with primary retroperitoneal sarcoma? Ann Oncol 2012. http://dx.doi.org/10.1093/annonc/mds516.

41. Ballo MT, Zagars GK, Pollock RE, et al. Retroperitoneal soft tissue sarcoma: an analysis of radiation and surgical treatment. Int J Radiat Oncol Biol Phys 2007; 67(1):158–63.

42. Pawlik TM, Pisters PW, Mikula L, et al. Long-term results of two prospective trials of preoperative external beam radiotherapy for localized intermediate- or high-grade retroperitoneal soft tissue sarcoma. Ann Surg Oncol 2006;13(4): 508–17.

43. Available at: http://www.eortc.be/protoc/Details.asp?protocol=62092. Accessed August 27, 2013.

44. McBride SM, Raut CP, Lapidus M, et al. Locoregional recurrence after preoperative radiation therapy for retroperitoneal sarcoma: adverse impact of multifocal disease and potential implications of dose escalation. Ann Surg Oncol 2013; 20(7):2140–7.

45. Scow JS, Reynolds CA, Degnim AC, et al. Primary and secondary angiosarcoma of the breast: the Mayo Clinic experience. J Surg Oncol 2010;101(5): 401–7.

46. Morgan EA, Kozono DE, Wang Q, et al. Cutaneous radiation-associated angiosarcoma of the breast: poor prognosis in a rare secondary malignancy. Ann Surg Oncol 2012;19(12):3801–8.

47. Seinen JM, Styring E, Verstappen V, et al. Radiation-associated angiosarcoma after breast cancer: high recurrence rate and poor survival despite surgical treatment with R0 resection. Ann Surg Oncol 2012;19(8):2700–6.

48. Jang JH, Choi MY, Lee SK, et al. Clinicopathologic risk factors for the local recurrence of phyllodes tumors of the breast. Ann Surg Oncol 2012;19(8): 2612–7.

49. Demetri GD, von Mehren M, Antonescu CR, et al. NCCN Task Force report: update on the management of patients with gastrointestinal stromal tumors. J Natl Compr Canc Netw 2010;8(Suppl 2):S1–41.

50. McCarter MD, Antonescu CR, Ballman KV, et al. Microscopically positive margins for primary gastrointestinal stromal tumors: analysis of risk factors and tumor recurrence. J Am Coll Surg 2012;215(1):53–9.

51. Colombo C, Ronellenfitsch U, Yuxin Z, et al. Clinical, pathological and surgical characteristics of duodenal gastrointestinal stromal tumor and their influence on survival: a multi-center study. Ann Surg Oncol 2012;19(11):3361–7.

52. Jakob J, Mussi C, Ronellenfitsch U, et al. Gastrointestinal stromal tumor of the rectum: results of surgical and multimodality therapy in the era of imatinib. Ann Surg Oncol 2013;20(2):586–92.

53. Gronchi A, Raut CP. The combination of surgery and imatinib in GIST: a reality for localized tumors at high risk, an open issue for metastatic ones. Ann Surg Oncol 2012;19(4):1051–5.

54. Wang D, Zhang Q, Blanke CD, et al. Phase II trial of neoadjuvant/adjuvant imatinib mesylate for advanced primary and metastatic/recurrent operable gastrointestinal stromal tumors: long-term follow-up results of Radiation Therapy Oncology Group 0132. Ann Surg Oncol 2012;19(4):1074–80.

55. Andtbacka RH, Ng CS, Scaife CL, et al. Surgical resection of gastrointestinal stromal tumors after treatment with imatinib. Ann Surg Oncol 2007;14(1):14–24.
56. Fiore M, Palassini E, Fumagalli E, et al. Preoperative imatinib mesylate for unresectable or locally advanced primary gastrointestinal stromal tumors (GIST). Eur J Surg Oncol 2009;35(7):739–45.
57. Agaimy A, Wünsch PH, Hofstaedter F, et al. Minute gastric sclerosing stromal tumors (GIST tumorlets) are common in adults and frequently show c-KIT mutations. Am J Surg Pathol 2007;31(1):113–20.
58. Kawanowa K, Sakuma Y, Sakurai S, et al. High incidence of microscopic gastrointestinal stromal tumors in the stomach. Hum Pathol 2006;37(12):1527–35.
59. Otani Y, Kitajima M. Laparoscopic surgery for GIST: too soon to decide. Gastric Cancer 2005;8(3):135–6.
60. Otani Y, Furukawa T, Yoshida M, et al. Operative indications for relatively small (2–5 cm) gastrointestinal stromal tumor of the stomach based on analysis of 60 operated cases. Surgery 2006;139(4):484–92.
61. Novitsky YW, Kercher KW, Sing RF, et al. Long-term outcomes of laparoscopic resection of gastric gastrointestinal stromal tumors. Ann Surg 2006;243(6): 738–45.
62. Dematteo RP, Ballman KV, Antonescu CR, et al. Adjuvant imatinib mesylate after resection of localised, primary gastrointestinal stromal tumour: a randomised, double-blind, placebo-controlled trial. Lancet 2009;373(9669):1097–104.
63. Joensuu H, Eriksson M, Sundby Hall K, et al. One vs three years of adjuvant imatinib for operable gastrointestinal stromal tumor: a randomized trial. J Am Med Assoc 2012;307(12):1265–72.

Liposarcomas

Joern Henze, MD, Sebastian Bauer, MD*

KEYWORDS

- Liposarcoma • Treatment • Grading • Tumor • Therapy

KEY POINTS

- Liposarcoma (LPS) is a heterogeneous disease with distinct subentities presenting with differential clinical behavior.
- From a clinical perspective, *grading* of liposarcomas is of greatest importance for decision making in localized tumors, as it greatly determines prognosis and aggressiveness of local treatment.
- Patients suspected of LPS should be managed by a multidisciplinary team with expertise in treating sarcomas.
- For the treatment of locally advanced liposarcomas, several neoadjuvant or definitive treatment modalities can be used to achieve local tumor control.
- Although important oncogenic events in well-differentiated and dedifferentiated LPS (MDM2/CDK4 amplifications) have been known for many years, targeted approaches have been hampered by the lack of drugs for clinical use. Recently, a multitude of compounds targeting CDK4 and MDM2 have entered clinical development and may soon change the landscape of systemic treatment for LPS.

INTRODUCTION

Liposarcomas (LPSs) represent one of the most common soft tissue sarcoma subtypes. In the National Cancer Institute's Surveillance, Epidemiology, and End Results study, LPSs account for approximately 12.8% of all sarcomas.[1,2] LPSs represent 24% of all extremity and 45% of all retroperitoneal soft tissue sarcomas[3] and the annual incidence is estimated to be 2.5 per 1 million inhabitants in population-based studies.[4]

LPS is defined as a malignant mesenchymal neoplasm that is composed of lipogenic tissue with a varying degree of cellular atypia, possibly including nonlipogenic sarcoma cells.

Funding sources: Dr S. Bauer: Deutsche Krebshilfe, Life-Raft-Group, Novartis.
Conflict of Interest: Dr S. Bauer: Research support: Novartis; Speakers Honoraria: Novartis, Pfizer, Pharmamar, GSK, Bayer. Dr J. Henze: nil.
Department of Medical Oncology, Sarcoma Center, West German Cancer Center, University Hospital Essen, University of Duisburg-Essen, Hufelandstrasse 55, Essen 45239, Germany
* Corresponding author.
E-mail address: sebastian.bauer@uk-essen.de

Hematol Oncol Clin N Am 27 (2013) 939–955
http://dx.doi.org/10.1016/j.hoc.2013.07.010
0889-8588/13/$ – see front matter © 2013 Elsevier Inc. All rights reserved.

However, LPS is a heterogeneous disease with distinct subentities presenting with differential clinical behavior. LPS can be subdivided into 4 important histologic subtypes:

- well-differentiated LPS (WDLPS)/atypical lipomatous tumor (ALT; 40%–45% of all LPS)
- dedifferentiated LPS (DDLPS) (5% respectively of all LPS)
- myxoid LPS (MLPS)/round-cell LPS (RCLPS) (30%–35% of all LPS)
- pleomorphic LPS (PLPS) (<15% of all LPS)[5–7]

From a conceptual standpoint, WDLPS and DDLPS should be grouped together, as DDLPS usually arises from WDLPS. Exact classification of the LPS subtypes is crucial for decision making in patients, as the aggressiveness of local and systemic treatment modalities may vary substantially (**Table 1**).

Pathology and Molecular Pathology

In differentiated LPS, the lipogenic origin can typically be seen with lipoblasts paired with atypical stromal cells in the context of mature fat. With increasing dedifferentiation, LPSs develop greater similarity to other pleomorphic high-grade sarcomas, such as undifferentiated pleomorphic sarcomas, and may not even display adipocytic components. Benign lipomas, in contrast, consist only of mature adipocytes and usually occur subcutaneously, whereas LPSs are generally deep seated. Given this anatomic difference and the underlying biology, LPS and lipoma are classified as 2 distinct entities with an independent evolution.

From a clinical perspective, *grading* of LPSs is of greatest importance for decision making in localized tumors, as it greatly determines prognosis and aggressiveness of

Table 1
Overview of LPS subtypes

Subtype	Pathology	Molecular Characteristics/ "Actionable" Targets	MRI/CT Appearance
ALT/WDLPS	Low grade, positive IHC for MDM2, CDK4, p16	MDM2 and CDK4 amplifications	Large encapsulated lipomatous mass (high signal intensity both in T1-weighted and T2-weighted MRI) with thick internal septations; Signal loss on fat-saturated T1-weighted images, and focal nodules (>1 cm is suggestive of a DDLPS)
DDLPS	High grade, positive IHC for MDM2, CDK4, p16	MDM2 and CDK4 amplifications	
MLPS and RCLPS	Low grade (percentage of round cells important for grading)	*FUS-CHOP* fusion gene, PI3K mutations (~20%)	Pathognomonically low signal intensity in T1-weighted and marked signal intensity in T2-weighted MRI
PLPS	High grade, pleomorphic, cellular sarcoma	Complex structural rearrangements	Nonspecific soft tissue mass, often including areas of necrosis and hemorrhage

Abbreviations: ALT, atypical lipomatous tumor; CT, computed tomography; DDLPS, dedifferentiated liposarcoma; IHC, immunohistochemistry; LPS, liposarcoma; MLPS, myxoid liposarcoma; MRI, magnetic resonance imaging; PI3K, phosphatidylinositol 3-kinase; PLPS, pleomorphic liposarcoma; RCLPS, round-cell liposarcoma; WDLPS, well-differentiated liposarcoma.

local treatment. WDLPS and pure MLPS are considered low grade. These tumors have very little to no metastatic potential and their prognosis is mostly favorable: 11% of all patients with WDLPS and MLPS die of their disease.[8,9] DDLPS, RCLPS, and PLPS usually are classified as high-grade tumors with a disease-related mortality of 28% for DDLPS, 21% for myxoid-round cell, and 35% to 50% for PLPS.[9-12] Histologic subtype plays a prominent role in MLPS, as these are highly sensitive to radiotherapy and often substantially shrink to neoadjuvant treatment.

WDLPS/DDLPS

The most common subtype of LPS is WDLPS. According to the most recent World Health Organization classification, ALT has replaced the term of WDLPS, as these tumors show no potential for metastases unless they undergo dedifferentiation. Biologically, ALT and WDLPS are the same, but tumors are named differently for patient reassurance: ALT should be used for resectable well-differentiated LPSs of the extremities, as local relapse is usually manageable and the term is more reflective of the benign course of disease.[13] In contrast, WDLPSs in the retroperitoneum or mediastinum are biologically the same as ALT, but wide margins are difficult to achieve, and patients are more likely to die of local relapse. Karyotypically, WDLPSs are characterized by giant marker and ring chromosomes.[14] This neochromosome contains an amplification of genes regularly based on chromosome 12q13-15. This set of genes includes oncogenes, such as MDM2 and CDK4.[15] Nearly all WDLPSs and DDLPSs overexpress MDM2 and CDK4,[16] making it the most important marker to differentiate from lipomas or other high-grade sarcomas. DDLPSs have been defined as "ALT that shows progression in a tumor with variable histologic grade."[7] Both, MDM2 and CDK4 have recently been identified as relevant therapeutic targets in LPS. Biologically, WDLPS and DDLPS represent a continuum, they share the same underlying genetic alterations and clinical features are similar. However, DDLPSs tend to grow more aggressively and are mostly found in the retroperitoneum.[10]

MLPS/RCLPS

The second most common subtype is MLPS/RCLPS (20% of all LPSs), which more often occurs in younger patients. MLPS is even the most common LPS in children and adolescents. High histologic grade is often defined as greater than 5% round-cell component and low grade is usually associated with a metastatic risk of less than 10%.[9,17] As MLPS progresses, more round-cell components can be found, either as isolated nodules or transitional areas with mixed cell types. Genetically, MLPS/RCLPS is characterized by a reciprocal translocation of chromosomes 12 and 16;t(12;16)(q13; p11), which can be found in approximately 95% of all cases.[18,19] This translocation leads to the fusion of the CHOP gene with the TLS (Translocated in Liposarcoma; also called FUS) gene and consecutively to the generation of a FUS-CHOP hybrid protein.[18,20] The CHOP gene encodes for a transcription factor that is involved in adipocyte differentiation and growth arrest.[21] TLS is an RNA-binding protein involved in RNA processing that interacts with steroid, thyroid hormone, and retinoid receptors.[22] This fusion gene encodes for 3 different transcripts (Types I–III); type II is the one most commonly found in MLPS/RCLPS.[23] Kuroda and colleagues[23] demonstrated that the introduction of the FUS-CHOP fusion gene into preadipocytes caused oncogenic transformation and inhibited adipocytic conversion. Thus, the FUS-CHOP fusion gene is believed to act as an aberrant transcriptional regulator that interferes with adipocyte differentiation, thereby stimulating adipocytic proliferation and tumor initiation.

PLPS

PLPS is defined as a pleomorphic high-grade sarcoma that contains lipoblasts but no areas of WDLPS or any other line of differentiation.[24] Immunohistochemistry may help in the differential diagnosis with other pleomorphic high-grade sarcomas. Approximately 30% to 50% of all PLPSs may stain positive for S-100; the nonlipogenic areas may stain positive for smooth muscle actin (45%–49%), CD34 (40%), and desmin (13%–19%)[11,12]; and a subset of PLPS may stain positive for epithelial markers (epithelial membrane antigen [EMA], 26%; keratin-6, 21%).[11,12] Genetically, PLPSs usually have high chromosome counts and complex structural rearrangements.[25] Unlike WDLPS/DDLPS and MLPS/RCLPS, no consistent oncogenic event can be found.[26]

Approximately 5% of all LPSs cannot easily be categorized into the previously mentioned categories. Sometimes more than one growth pattern may be observed; in this case, these tumors may be classified as LPS of mixed type.

Clinical Appearance

LPS usually presents as a painless enlarging mass. Men and women are equally affected, most patients are diagnosed in the sixth decade.[27] Depending on growth rate and site of the primary, LPS can attain a very large size and still remain asymptomatic. WDLPS is a locally aggressive, nonmetastasizing tumor that grows slowly and is rarely symptomatic. Retroperitoneal WDLPSs do not have metastatic potential; however, they can progress to high-grade DDLPS and have a high tendency to recur, with then an unfavorable prognosis. Progression to DDLPS occurs more frequently in retroperitoneal than in extremity WDLPS (17% vs 6%)[8] and more often in recurrent disease; 20% of first-time retroperitoneal recurrences compared with 44% of second time local recurrences progress.[28]

MLPSs occur mainly in the deep soft tissues of the extremities with a predilection within the musculature of the thigh. Retroperitoneal MLPSs are rare, and patients are generally younger than patients with WDLPS/DDLPS.[17] These tumors frequently recur, and 1 in 3 patients develops distant metastases and dies of disease. These metastases often occur in unusual sites, such as soft tissues rather than in the lungs.[17] Notably, rate of osseous metastasis (17%) is as high as the rate of pulmonary metastases (14%).[29]

PLPSs are high-grade LPSs that tend to occur in the lower extremities (47%); other sites, such as the upper limb (18%), trunk (14%), or retroperitoneum (7%), are rare.[11,12] Compared with other LPS subtypes, they behave more aggressively. They grow quicker, recur locally in 30% to 50%, have a 30% to 50% metastasis rate, and an overall tumor-associated mortality of 35% to 50%.[11,12] In contrast to WDLPS and MLPS, the preferred site of metastasis is the lung.[11,12] When compared with other high-grade, pleomorphic sarcomas, however, PLPS shows a comparatively prolonged clinical course.[6,30]

Diagnosis/Imaging

Patients suspected of LPS should be managed by a multidisciplinary team with expertise in treating sarcomas. As LPSs often present as heterogeneous masses with both well-differentiated and dedifferentiated areas, magnetic resonance imaging (MRI) or computed tomography (CT) scans should be done *before* biopsy. WDLPS usually exhibits as a large encapsulated lipomatous mass with thick internal septations and may include focal nodules.[31] A nodular focus of nonlipogenic tissue larger than 1 cm inside a WDLPS is suggestive of a DDLPS.[31] Therefore, a biopsy should be directed at the nonlipogenic focus. Open biopsies should be preferred over needle biopsies, when feasible, to maximize the chance to detect dedifferentiated areas, as these are of greatest importance for treatment decisions.

Owing to their high water content, MLPSs often pathognomonically present with low signal intensity on T1-weighted and marked signal intensity on T2-weighted MRI. The tumors are usually large, well-defined, and multilobulated intermuscular lesions, with inclusions of adipose tissue.[31] Staging should be completed in all patients diagnosed with LPSs using chest CT, abdominal CT, and a bone scan at baseline. As low-grade LPSs, especially at the extremities, very rarely metastasize, chest radiographs can substitute for CT scans during follow-up.

As MLPSs frequently metastasize to the spine, whole-spine MRI should be routinely performed to screen for spinal metastasis. Even though local therapy for metastatic disease in this setting is mostly palliative, some long-term survivors have been seen after wide resection of solitary lesions.[29]

Prognostic Factors

Most prognostic data on LPSs are based on retrospective analyses from large sarcoma centers; population-based studies are available from Scandinavia (**Table 2**).[8–12,17,24,27,30,32–35] Even though patient groups varied considerably between the different studies, histology/grade and site were the most important factors.

Low-grade LPSs of the extremities or trunk have a 95% disease-specific survival (DSS), compared with 70% DSS of high-grade LPSs of the same location.[32] Low-grade LPS of the retroperitoneum had an 87% DSS, whereas high-grade tumors had only 50% DSS.[32] Other reported prognostic factors included margins and treatment at large sarcoma centers.[27,33]

For WDLPS, Weiss and Rao[8] were able to show that almost all (91%) retroperitoneal tumors recurred, compared with 43% of those with extremity site. For DDLPS, the risk of metastatic disease was similar regardless of site of primary, but the DSS was considerably worse for the latter (89% vs 66%).[10]

In MLPS and RCLPS, several groups have identified a round-cell component (5%–25%) and presence of necrosis as prognostic factors. In the analyses of Kilpatrick and colleagues,[9] tumors with a round-cell component of more than 25% metastasized in 58% and had a 10-year DSS of 40% compared with a metastatic risk of 26% and 10-year DSS of 66% in those with a round-cell component of less than 25%.

For PLPS, Hornick and colleagues[12] reported age older than 60 years, central location, tumor size, and mitotic rate as predictors for an adverse outcome.

Table 2
Prognosis depending on LPS subtype

Subtype	Recurrence, %	Metastasis, %	OS, %	DSS, %	Prognosis Factors
WDLPS	13–46 (extremity) 91 (retroperitoneal)	Very low	76–93	86	Location; margin
DDLPS	18–57	13–47	54–64	66–89	Location; mitotic count
MLPS/RCLPS	7–28	10–58	40–75	69–100	Age; RC-component
PLPS	16–45	32–44	0–63	50	Mostly none

Abbreviations: DDLPS, dedifferentiated liposarcoma; DSS, disease-specific survival; LPS, liposarcoma; MLPS, myxoid liposarcoma; OS, overall survival; PLPS, pleomorphic liposarcoma; RCLPS, round-cell liposarcoma; WDLPS, well-differentiated liposarcoma.
Data from Refs.[8–12,17,24,27,30,33–35]

Therapeutic Strategies in LPS

Treatment of localized disease

Like other well-differentiated sarcomas, low-grade LPSs are treated by surgery alone when negative margins can be achieved. As ALTs of the extremities very rarely metastasize, re-resection can be omitted in selected patients with positive margins when this procedure would be associated with increased morbidity.[13] However, in these patients, a regular, reliable follow-up must be ensured.

A wide resection is the standard of care for LPSs with intermediate to high grade, and most investigators recommend a resection margin of at least 10 mm of adjacent normal fat or muscle tissue.[36,37] In case of close or positive margins, re-resection should be considered whenever feasible. For high-grade LPSs that are located close or adjacent to a neurovascular bundle, it may be necessary to sacrifice important structures so as to achieve wide margins.[3] Alternatively, neoadjuvant or adjuvant treatment using radiotherapy and/or isolated limb perfusion (extremities only) may allow smaller margins (<10 mm). Amputation does not improve survival compared with resection followed by radiotherapy, but can be necessary in patients with chronic infections, severe pain, or lymphedema that results in severe functional impairment.[38,39] Adjuvant radiotherapy in soft tissue sarcoma of the extremities has been shown to effectively prolong relapse-free survival (RFS), but not overall survival (OS).[40]

Neoadjuvant radiotherapy allows smaller radiation fields with equal local disease control. Although short-term wound complications are more common, late effects of radiotherapy are substantially less frequent.[41]

The role of chemotherapy (CTX) in soft tissue sarcoma remains a matter of dispute and cannot be unequivocally recommended. A limited number of mostly small randomized trials are available for the group of all sarcomas, and no subtype-specific trials have been performed for LPSs. In 1997, the sarcoma meta-analysis collaboration (SMAC) published a meta-analysis of 14 adjuvant trials showing a 10% absolute benefit in RFS, and a 4% improved OS after 10 years, which was not statistically significant.[42] Most trials did not incorporate ifosfamide or used inadequate doses and some trials also included low-risk sarcomas, hence limiting the value of the analysis from today's perspective. Only 10% LPSs were included. An updated meta-analysis published in 2008 incorporated 4 new ifosfamide-containing combination studies, which amounted to an 11% absolute benefit in OS for combination regimen.[43] The strongest evidence in this meta-analysis was based on the Italian Sarcoma Group trial that had focused on patients with stage III, G2-3, and extremity sarcomas, and who were treated with high doses of ifosfamide and epirubicin.[44] The trial, albeit small, resulted in a 19% absolute benefit in OS after 4 years. This trial was recently contrasted with the results from the European Organisation for Research and Treatment of Cancer (EORTC) Soft Tissue and Bone Sarcoma Group trial of adjuvant CTX using doxorubicin and ifosfamide in soft tissue sarcoma, which did not improve OS (66.5% vs 67.8% after 5 years).[45] Unfortunately, this trial had used rather low doses of ifosfamide and also included intra-abdominal and stage II sarcomas. Again, no LPS-specific data have been extracted from these trials.

The largest analyses on the role of adjuvant CTX in LPS (n = 246) was published in 2004 by Eilber and colleagues,[46] who retrospectively analyzed all primary resectable high-grade extremity LPSs treated at the University of California Los Angeles and Memorial Sloan-Kettering Cancer Center (MSKCC) from 1975 to 2003. They compared the impact of a doxorubicin-based regimen used from 1975 to 1990 and an ifosfamide-based regimen used from 1990 to 2003 with patients who did not receive adjuvant CTX in the same period of time. In their analysis, ifosfamide-containing treatment was associated with improved OS (92% vs 65% after 5 years), whereas doxorubicin treatment was not. Subgroup analyses showed that tumors larger than 10 cm benefited the most from CTX.[46]

For patients with retroperitoneal LPS, local recurrence rates of more than 80% are reported and because of their location, tumors tend to grow large and often infiltrate adjacent structures at the time of diagnosis.[28] Wide resection is the only curative treatment approach and complete resection is associated with significantly longer DSS than incomplete resection (73% vs 43% at 3 years).[28] A median survival for completely resected tumors of 103 months has been described compared with 18 months after incomplete resection.[47] Aggressive surgery generally aims at en bloc resections of the tumor and adjacent organs that are infiltrated by the tumor. Frontline aggressive surgery that is performed in high-volume centers is safe and associated with better outcome compared with less-aggressive strategies.[48,49] Very few data are available on the role of CTX in retroperitoneal LPS.[46] Additive radiotherapy can be used in incompletely resected tumors, but usually postoperative radiotherapy is limited by the size of the fields and intestinal toxicity. As tumors may serve as their own spacers to reduce radiation to the intestine, neoadjuvant radiotherapy strategies are currently being investigated in retroperitoneal sarcomas (EORTC 62092).

Treatment of locally advanced or recurrent disease For the treatment of locally advanced LPSs, several neoadjuvant or definitive treatment modalities can be used to achieve local tumor control, including radiotherapy with and without CTX or hyperthermic isolated limb perfusion.

For isolated limb perfusion, the circulation of the extremity is isolated from the body circulation and perfused with a hyperthermic solution of melphalan and tumor necrosis factor (TNF)-α using a heart-lung machine. This prevents TNF-α from entering the systemic circulation, which may cause severe toxicity, such as capillary leak syndrome. Effectiveness in extremity soft tissue sarcoma has been shown in large multicenter studies with response rates of 75% to 85% and limb salvage in more than 85% of patients.[50–52] Perfusion may allow function-sparing surgery, as frequently tumor margins are completely devitalized, allowing nerve- and vessel-sparing resection.[53] Subtype-specific data are scarce, but some evidence suggests that LPS may respond less frequently than other subtypes, such as undifferentiated sarcomas, leiomyosarcoma, or clear-cell sarcoma.[54]

In patients for whom no acceptable surgical option is available, definitive radiotherapy represents a treatment option, with 5-year local control rates of 30% to 45% and 5-year OS of 25% to 35%.[55,56]

Systemic CTX may improve the response rate when combined with radiotherapy, but few data are available on the different LPS subtypes; however, combinations of doxorubicin ± ifosfamide are used in combination with radiotherapy.[57–60] In MLPS, trabectedin treatment has yielded remissions rates of 24%.[61]

In retroperitoneal recurrences, surgery represents the only viable treatment modality; however, surgical approaches cause 3% to 6% mortality and considerable morbidity. A watch-and-wait strategy can be safely applied in asymptomatic recurrences of WDLPS; symptomatic or progressive LPS should, however, be evaluated for surgical treatment. Lewis and colleagues[47] proclaimed that once retroperitoneal soft tissue sarcoma recurs, the outcome of the patient is dictated by tumor biology rather than treatment variables, such as resection margins. Park and colleagues[62] analyzed 105 patients with recurrence of retroperitoneal LPS and were able to show that only patients with a growth rate of less than 0.9 cm per month gain a survival benefit from aggressive resection. They proposed the "1 cm per month rule," by which tumors with faster growth rate will not benefit from surgery. Therefore, these patients should be offered systemic treatment, potentially followed by surgery in case of response.[62] As incomplete resection does not prolong survival, it should be restricted to patients with existing or immanent tumor-related symptoms.

In patients in whom local treatments cannot be offered because of decreased performance status or extent of disease, CTX should be offered in analogy to patients with metastatic disease.

Treatment of Metastatic Disease

In patients with low-grade, slow-growing tumors, surgery may allow disease control over many years, especially in patients with intra-abdominal tumor spread. Complete resection of metastases restricted to the lung has been associated with prolonged disease-free intervals in sarcomas in general.[63–66] Notably, histology of LPS was associated with an unfavorable outcome in a large series of patients who underwent metastasectomy.[63–66]

In patients with fast-growing, high-grade tumors, systemic CTX remains the mainstay of treatment. Approved drugs for LPS are doxorubicin, ifosfamide, dacarbacin (DTIC), and trabectedin (EMA) with gemcitabine ± docetaxel being frequently used in clinical practice. In general, sequential monotherapy represents the standard approach in LPS and doxorubicin the standard first-line therapy for this subtype.

Most clinical trials published on soft tissue sarcomas report on LPSs as a whole group regardless of the fact that response rates may vary considerably between different LPS subgroups. Few large retrospective studies have addressed this lack of detail (**Table 3**).

Myxoid LPSs are considered most responsive to CTX, with remission rates of up to 50%, followed by PLPS (33%) and DDLPS (12%–25%), as nicely summarized by Jones and others.[67,68] In a large retrospective analysis of palliative CTX in 208 patients with WD/DDLPS, Italiano[68] reported an response rate (RR) of 12% and a progression-free survival (PFS) and OS of 4.6 and 15.2 months, respectively. In this context, LPS seem to be less responsive to ifosfamide than other sarcoma subtypes.[67,69,70]

Ifosfamide-containing CTX combinations have resulted in improved response rates in non-LPS sarcomas. Interestingly, data from a meta-analysis of several EORTC soft tissue sarcoma trials suggested that patients with LPS benefited less from ifosfamide combinations compared with doxorubicin alone ($P = .0324$). Response rates for doxorubicin were 32% compared with 21% for the ifosfamide-containing regimen. Whether this finding is true for all LPS subtypes has not been shown in this context. Promising data have been retrospectively collected for the combination of doxorubicin (75 mg/m^2) and DTIC (2×400 mg/m^2). Reichardt and colleagues achieved 5% complete response, 35% partial response, and 50% disease stabilizations with a median PFS of 9 months in 22 patients with LPSs.[71]

Trabectedin has been studied mostly in pretreated leiomyosarcoma and LPSs, and although objective remissions in these sarcomas are rare (6% for the overall study populations), prolonged disease stabilizations are commonly observed with PFS rates of 52% at 3 months and 36% at 6 months.[72] Given a favorable toxicity profile, trabectedin represents an important treatment option and patients may derive clinical benefit despite heavy pretreatment and advanced age.[73,74] Of note, MLPSs exhibit an exquisite sensitivity toward trabectedin, with a response rate of 51% even in pretreated patients,[75] which may justify the use of trabectedin even in first-line therapy when a clinical situation requires tumor shrinkage.

Table 3
Overview on large chemotherapy studies depending on LPS subtype

Subtype	Study	No. of Cases	Drug	RR, %	PFS, mo	Med. OS, mo
LPS (subtype not reported)	Nielsen et al,[70] 2000	13	Ifosfamide	8		
	Le Cesne et al,[79] 2000	19	Doxorubicin/ Ifosfamide	26		
	Demetri et al,[72] 2009 (both LMS and LPS)	270	Trabectedin	2–6	2.3-3.3 (6-mo PFS: 28%–36%)	11.8–13.9
WDLPS	Italiano et al,[68] 2012	37	Various chemotherapeutic drugs	13	8.7	33.5
DDLPS	Italiano et al,[68] 2012	171	Various chemotherapeutic drugs	12	4.0	13.9
MLPS/RCLPS	Grosso et al,[75] 2007	51	Trabectedin	51	14.0	
	Katz et al,[80] 2012	37	Doxorubicin/ Ifosfamide	43	23.0	31.1
PLPS	Italiano et al,[81] 2012	39	Various chemotherapeutic drugs	37	4.3	14.0

Abbreviations: DDLPS, dedifferentiated liposarcoma; LMS, leiomyosarcoma; LPS, liposarcoma; MLPS, myxoid liposarcoma; Med. OS, medium overall survival; PFS, progression-free survival; PLPS, pleomorphic liposarcoma; RCLPS, round-cell liposarcoma; RR, response rate; WDLPS, well-differentiated liposarcoma.
Data from Refs.[67,72,75,79–81]

Very few data are available on the LPS-specific benefit of gemcitabine-containing therapies. Maki and colleagues[76] also showed a subgroup analysis for LPS, and found objective remissions in 2 of 3 patients with pleomorphic LPS. Prolonged (>24 weeks) disease stabilizations were seen in only 2 of 12 patients with WD/DDLPS.

Pazopanib, a vascular endothelial growth factor receptor/multi–tyrosine kinase inhibitor, has been extensively studied in soft tissue sarcomas. A phase II study including 19 patients with LPSs suggested a limited value in this subtype, which led to the exclusion of patients with LPS from the Pazopanib for Metastatic Soft-Tissue Sarcoma phase III trial.[77,78] A subset of patients still exhibited disease stabilization exceeding 3 months, which prompted a trial by the Spanish and German Sarcoma Groups that currently investigate the role of pazopanib in a larger group of LPSs (**Table 3**).

Outlook on Molecular Therapeutic Approaches

Although important oncogenic events in WDLPS and DDLPS, such as MDM2 and CDK4 amplifications, have been known for many years, targeted approaches have been hampered by the lack of drugs for clinical use. This situation is rapidly changing. A multitude of compounds targeting CDK4 and MDM2 have entered early clinical development, which may soon change the landscape of systemic treatment for patients with LPS.

MDM2 is a major physiologic antagonist of the tumor suppressor p53, and MDM2 serves as an E3 ubiquitin ligase that promotes p53 proteasomal degradation and furthermore interferes with p53 transcriptional activity.[82] The p53 transcription factor is an important cell cycle regulator that plays a key role in the cellular defense against neoplastic transformation.[83] Functional inactivation of p53 is a common finding in many human tumors and is caused by either direct inactivation of p53 by mutations or indirect inactivation by loss of upstream regulator p14^ARF or overexpression of the murine double-minute 2 cellular oncoprotein,[82] the major physiologic antagonist of p53. MDM2 inhibitors, such as nutlin-3, bind MDM2 in the p53 binding pocket and inhibit interaction with p53. This inhibition is followed by upregulation of p53 and induction of apoptosis, but only in the absence of inactivating p53 mutations.[84–86] LPSs represent the ideal disease model for MDM2 inhibitors, as strong MDM2 amplification is a universal finding in WDLPS and DDLPS and p53 mutations are rare. In preclinical models, LPSs exhibit an exquisite sensitivity to MDM2 inhibitors.[84] Currently, RG7112 and CGM097 are in clinical evaluation for various malignancies, including LPS.[87–89] Ray-Coquard and colleagues[90] recently reported a groundbreaking study in WD/DDLPS evaluating neoadjuvant RG7112. Patients with localized and resectable LPS (n = 20) were treated for 10 days in a 28-day cycle for up to 3 cycles of therapy preceding curative surgery. One patient developed a partial remission and 14 patients had stable disease with strong evidence of target inhibition as measured by p53 and p21 levels in resected tumors. Although the formulation and schedule used in this trial were still associated with substantial toxicity, especially hematological toxicity, Ray-Coquard and colleagues'[90] findings nonetheless proved the concept of this approach. These findings were also supported by a partial remission in 1 of 5 patients with LPS treated with RG7112 in a phase I dose-escalation study.[89] Further studies will be necessary to identify the optimal schedule and/or compound. In addition, MDM2 inhibitors may work best in combination with other cytotoxic/targeted drugs, such as CDK4 inhibitors, and combination studies are currently ongoing.[88]

The rationale for the use of CDK4 inhibitors in LPSs is equally compelling, as high amplifications can be invariably found in most patients with WD/DDLPS. CDK4 is involved in the regulation of the cell cycle, by phosphorylating Retinoblastoma-protein, CDK4 enables G1-S transition.[91] A phase II trial at MSKCC recently reported results of a study on CDK4/CDK6 inhibitor PD0332991 in LPS.[92,93] Treatment with the CDK4/6 inhibitor was associated with a median PFS of 4.5 months and a 12-week PFS of 66%.[92] As with the MDM2 inhibitors, targeted interference with cell-cycle proteins was associated with substantial hematological toxicity, suggesting a narrow therapeutic window.

For many years, peroxisome proliferator-activated receptor gamma (PPAR-γ) has been known to induce terminal differentiation in LPS cell lines.[94] Promising clinical observations in patients with MLPS and PLPS who were treated with traglitazone, a PPAR-γ agonist,[95] prompted clinical trials that surprisingly failed to prove a clinical benefit except for an anecdotal remission in a patient with LPS in a phase I trial.[96,97] Further molecular studies will be needed to identify patients who may benefit from this approach. Of note, a recent preclinical study has demonstrated an additive effect of PPAR-γ agonist with trabectedin in a mouse model of myxoid round-cell LPS, which may serve as a rationale for the use of PPAR-γ in an LPS subtype.[98]

Last, different groups have reported additional "actionable" pathways that may play a role in the pathogenesis of LPS.[99–101] Notably, myxoid round-cell LPS harbors up to 19% phosphatidylinositol 3-kinase (PI3K) mutations,[99,102] which serve as a strong rationale to explore inhibitors that target the PI3K/AKT/mammalian target of rapamycin pathway in these tumors.

REFERENCES

1. Mack TM. Sarcomas and other malignancies of soft tissue, retroperitoneum, peritoneum, pleura, heart, mediastinum, and spleen. Cancer 1995;75(1):211–44.
2. Gadgeel SM, Harlan LC, Zeruto CA, et al. Patterns of care in a population-based sample of soft tissue sarcoma patients in the United States. Cancer 2009; 115(12):2744–54. http://dx.doi.org/10.1002/cncr.24307.
3. Crago AM, Singer S. Clinical and molecular approaches to well differentiated and dedifferentiated liposarcoma. Curr Opin Oncol 2011;23(4):373–8. http://dx.doi.org/10.1097/CCO.0b013e32834796e6.
4. Kindblom LG, Angervall L, Svendsen P. Liposarcoma: a clinicopathologic, radiographic and prognostic study. Acta Pathol Microbiol Scand Suppl 1975;(253): 1–71.
5. Evans HL. Liposarcoma: a study of 55 cases with reassessment of its classification. Am J Surg Pathol 1979;3(6):507–23.
6. Fletcher CD, Unni KK, Mertens F, editors. World Health Organization classification of tumours Pathology and genetics of tumours of soft tissue and bone. Lyon: IARC Press; 2013.
7. Fletcher CD, Bridge JA, Hogendoorn PC, et al. WHO classification of tumours of soft tissue and bone. 4th edition; 2013. p. 468.
8. Weiss SW, Rao VK. Well-differentiated liposarcoma (atypical lipoma) of deep soft tissue of the extremities, retroperitoneum, and miscellaneous sites. Am J Surg Pathol 1992;16(11):1051–8.
9. Kilpatrick SE, Doyon J, Choong PF, et al. The clinicopathologic spectrum of myxoid and round cell liposarcoma. Cancer 1996;77(8):1450–8.
10. Henricks WH, Chu YC, Goldblum JR, et al. Dedifferentiated liposarcoma: a clinicopathological analysis of 155 cases with a proposal for an expanded definition of dedifferentiation. Am J Surg Pathol 1997;21(3):271–81.
11. Gebhard S, Coindre JM, Michels JJ, et al. Pleomorphic liposarcoma: clinicopathologic, immunohistochemical, and follow-up analysis of 63 cases: a study from the French Federation of Cancer Centers Sarcoma Group. Am J Surg Pathol 2002;26(5):601–16.
12. Hornick JL, Bosenberg MW, Mentzel T, et al. Pleomorphic liposarcoma. Am J Surg Pathol 2004;28(10):1257–67. http://dx.doi.org/10.1097/01.pas.0000135524. 73447.4a.
13. Canter RJ, Qin LX, Ferrone CR, et al. Why do patients with low-grade soft tissue sarcoma die? Ann Surg Oncol 2008;15(12):3550–60. http://dx.doi.org/10.1245/s10434-008-0163-0.
14. Fletcher CD, Akerman M, Dal Cin P, et al. Correlation between clinicopathological features and karyotype in lipomatous tumors. A report of 178 cases from the Chromosomes and Morphology (CHAMP) Collaborative Study Group. Am J Pathol 1996;148(2):623–30.
15. Pedeutour F, Forus A, Coindre JM, et al. Structure of the supernumerary ring and giant rod chromosomes in adipose tissue tumors. Genes Chromosomes Cancer 1999;24(1):30–41.
16. Binh M, Sastre-Garau X, Guillou L, et al. MDM2 and CDK4 immunostainings are useful adjuncts in diagnosing well-differentiated and dedifferentiated liposarcoma subtypes: a comparative analysis of 559 soft tissue neoplasms. Am J Surg Pathol 2005;29(10):1340–7.
17. Antonescu CR, Tschernyavsky SJ, Decuseara R, et al. Prognostic impact of P53 status, TLS-CHOP fusion transcript structure, and histological grade in myxoid

liposarcoma: a molecular and clinicopathologic study of 82 cases. Clin Cancer Res 2001;7:3977–87.

18. Aman P, Ron D, Mandahl N, et al. Rearrangement of the transcription factor gene CHOP in myxoid liposarcomas with t(12;16)(q13;p11). Genes chromosomes cancer 1992;5(4):278–85.

19. Knight JC, Renwick PJ, Cin PD, et al. Translocation t(12;16)(q13;p11) in myxoid liposarcoma and round cell liposarcoma: molecular and cytogenetic analysis. Cancer Res 1995;55:24–7.

20. Rabbitts TH, Forster A, Larson R, et al. Fusion of the dominant negative transcription regulator CHOP with a novel gene FUS by translocation t(12;16) in malignant liposarcoma. Nat Genet 1993;4(2):175–80.

21. Ron D, Habener JF. CHOP, a novel developmentally regulated nuclear protein that dimerizes with transcription factors C/EBP and LAP and functions as a dominant-negative inhibitor of gene transcription. Genes Dev 1992;6(3):439–53.

22. Powers CA, Mathur M, Raaka BM, et al. Is a high-affinity interactor for steroid, thyroid hormone, and retinoid receptors. Mol Endocrinol 1998;4–18.

23. Kuroda M, Ishida T, Takanashi M, et al. Oncogenic transformation and inhibition of adipocytic conversion of preadipocytes by TLS/FUS-CHOP type II chimeric protein. Am J Pathol 1997;151(3):735–44.

24. Downes KA, Goldblum JR, Montgomery EA, et al. Pleomorphic liposarcoma: a clinicopathologic analysis of 19 cases. Mod Pathol 2001;14(3):179–84.

25. Mertens F, Fletcher CD, Dal Cin P, et al. Cytogenetic analysis of 46 pleomorphic soft tissue sarcomas and correlation with morphologic and clinical features: a report of the CHAMP Study Group. Chromosomes and MorPhology. Genes Chromosomes Cancer 1998;22(1):16–25.

26. Schneider-Stock R, Walter H, Radig K, et al. MDM2 amplification and loss of heterozygosity at Rb and p53 genes: no simultaneous alterations in the oncogenesis of liposarcomas. J Cancer Res Clin Oncol 1998;124:532–40.

27. Engström K, Bergh P, Gustafson P, et al. Liposarcoma: outcome based on the Scandinavian Sarcoma Group register. Cancer 2008;113(7):1649–56. http://dx.doi.org/10.1002/cncr.23784.

28. Singer S, Antonescu CR, Riedel E, et al. Histologic subtype and margin of resection predict pattern of recurrence and survival for retroperitoneal liposarcoma. Ann Surg 2003;238(3):358–70. http://dx.doi.org/10.1097/01.sla.0000086542.11899.38 [discussion: 370–1].

29. Schwab JH, Boland PJ, Antonescu C, et al. Spinal metastases from myxoid liposarcoma warrant screening with magnetic resonance imaging. Cancer 2007;110(8):1815–22. http://dx.doi.org/10.1002/cncr.22992.

30. McCormick D, Mentzel T, Beham A, et al. Dedifferentiated liposarcoma: clinicopathologic analysis of 32 cases suggesting a better prognostic subgroup among pleomorphic sarcomas. Am J Surg Pathol 1994;18(12):1213–23.

31. Murphy MD, Arcara LK, Fanburg-Smith J. Imaging of musculoskeletal liposarcoma with radiologic-pathologic correlation. Radiographics 2005;25:1371–95.

32. Linehan DC, Lewis JJ, Leung D, et al. Influence of biologic factors and anatomic site in completely resected liposarcoma. J Clin Oncol 2000;18(8):1637–43.

33. Kim HS, Lee J, Yi SY, et al. Liposarcoma: exploration of clinical prognostic factors for risk based stratification of therapy. BMC Cancer 2009;9:205. http://dx.doi.org/10.1186/1471-2407-9-205.

34. Lucas DR, Nascimento AG, Sanjay BK, et al. Well-differentiated liposarcoma. The Mayo Clinic experience with 58 cases. Am J Clin Pathol 1994;102(5):677–83.

35. Moreau LC, Turcotte R, Ferguson P, et al. Myxoid\round cell liposarcoma (MRCLS) revisited: an analysis of 418 primarily managed cases. Ann Surg Oncol 2012;19(4):1081–8. http://dx.doi.org/10.1245/s10434-011-2127-z.

36. McKee MD, Liu DF, Brooks JJ, et al. The prognostic significance of margin width for extremity and trunk sarcoma. J Surg Oncol 2004;85(2):68–76. http://dx.doi.org/10.1002/jso.20009.

37. Liu CY, Yen CC, Chen WM, et al. Soft tissue sarcoma of extremities: the prognostic significance of adequate surgical margins in primary operation and reoperation after recurrence. Ann Surg Oncol 2010;17(8):2102–11. http://dx.doi.org/10.1245/s10434-010-0997-0.

38. Rosenberg SA, Tepper J, Glatstein E, et al. The treatment of soft-tissue sarcomas of the extremities: prospective randomized evaluation of (1) limb-sparing surgery plus radiation therapy compared with amputation and (2) the role of adjuvant chemotherapy. Ann Surg 1982;196(3):305–14.

39. Ghert MA, Abudu A, Driver N, et al. The indications for and the prognostic significance of amputation as the primary surgical procedure for localized soft tissue sarcoma of the extremity 2005;12(1):10–7. http://dx.doi.org/10.1245/ASO.2005.03.097.

40. Yang JC, Chang AE, Baker AR, et al. Randomized prospective study of the benefit of adjuvant radiation therapy in the treatment of soft tissue sarcomas of the extremity. J Clin Oncol 1998;16(1):197–203.

41. O'Sullivan B, Davis AM, Turcotte R, et al. Preoperative versus postoperative radiotherapy in soft-tissue sarcoma of the limbs: a randomised trial. Lancet 2002;359(9325):2235–41. http://dx.doi.org/10.1016/S0140-6736(02)09292-9.

42. Tierney JF, Stewart LA, Parmar MK. Adjuvant chemotherapy for localised resectable soft-tissue sarcoma of adults: meta-analysis of individual data. Lancet 1997;350:1647–54.

43. Pervaiz N, Colterjohn N, Farrokhyar F, et al. A systematic meta-analysis of randomized controlled trials of adjuvant chemotherapy for localized resectable soft-tissue sarcoma. Cancer 2008;113(3):573–81. http://dx.doi.org/10.1002/cncr.23592.

44. Frustaci BS, Gherlinzoni F, De Paoli A, et al. Adjuvant chemotherapy for adult soft tissue sarcomas of the extremities and girdles: results of the Italian randomized cooperative trial. J Clin Oncol 2001;19(5):1238–47.

45. Woll PJ, Reichardt P, Le Cesne A, et al. Adjuvant chemotherapy with doxorubicin, ifosfamide, and lenograstim for resected soft-tissue sarcoma (EORTC 62931): a multicentre randomised controlled trial. Lancet Oncol 2012; 2045(EORTC 62931):1–10. http://dx.doi.org/10.1016/S1470-2045(12)70346-7.

46. Eilber FC, Eilber FR, Eckardt J, et al. The impact of chemotherapy on the survival of patients with high-grade primary extremity liposarcoma. Ann Surg 2004;240(4):686–97. http://dx.doi.org/10.1097/01.sla.0000141710.74073.0d.

47. Lewis JJ, Leung D, Woodruff JM, et al. Retroperitoneal soft-tissue sarcoma: analysis of 500 patients treated and followed at a single institution. Ann Surg 1998;228(3):355–65.

48. Gronchi A, Lo Vullo S, Fiore M, et al. Aggressive surgical policies in a retrospectively reviewed single-institution case series of retroperitoneal soft tissue sarcoma patients. J Clin Oncol 2009;27(1):24–30. http://dx.doi.org/10.1200/JCO.2008.17.8871.

49. Bonvalot S, Miceli R, Berselli M, et al. Aggressive surgery in retroperitoneal soft tissue sarcoma carried out at high-volume centers is safe and is associated with

improved local control. Ann Surg Oncol 2010;17(6):1507–14. http://dx.doi.org/
10.1245/s10434-010-1057-5.

50. Lienard D, Ewalenko P, Delmotte JJ, et al. High-dose recombinant tumor necrosis factor alpha in combination with interferon gamma and melphalan in isolation
perfusion of the limbs for melanoma and sarcoma. J Clin Oncol 1992;10(1):
52–60.

51. Eggermont AM, Schraffordt Koops H, Klausner JM, et al. Isolated limb perfusion
with tumor necrosis factor and melphalan for limb salvage in 186 patients with
locally advanced soft tissue extremity sarcomas. The Cumulative Multicenter
European Experience. Ann Surg 1996;224(6):756–64.

52. Grunhagen DJ, De Wilt JH, Graveland WJ, et al. Outcome and prognostic factor
analysis of 217 consecutive isolated limb perfusions with tumor necrosis factor-
alpha and melphalan for limb-threatening soft tissue sarcoma. Cancer 2006;
106(8):1776–84. http://dx.doi.org/10.1002/cncr.21802.

53. Grabellus F, Kraft C, Sheu SY, et al. Evaluation of 47 soft tissue sarcoma resection specimens after isolated limb perfusion with TNF-alpha and melphalan: histologically characterized improved margins correlate with absence of
recurrences. Ann Surg Oncol 2009;16(3):676–86. http://dx.doi.org/10.1245/
s10434-008-0277-4.

54. Grabellus F, Kraft C, Sheu-Grabellus S-Y, et al. Tumor vascularization and histopathologic regression of soft tissue sarcomas treated with isolated limb perfusion with TNF-α and melphalan. J Surg Oncol 2011;103(5):371–9. http://dx.
doi.org/10.1002/jso.21724.

55. Tepper JE, Suit HD. Radiation therapy alone for sarcoma of soft tissue. Cancer
1985;56:475–9.

56. Kepka L, DeLaney TF, Suit HD, et al. Results of radiation therapy for unresected
soft-tissue sarcomas. Int J Radiat Oncol Biol Phys 2005;63(3):852–9. http://dx.
doi.org/10.1016/j.ijrobp.2005.03.004.

57. Gortzak E, Azzarelli A, Buesa J, et al. A randomised phase II study on neoadjuvant chemotherapy for "high-risk" adult soft-tissue sarcoma. Eur J Cancer
2001;37(9):1096–103.

58. DeLaney TF, Spiro IJ, Suit HD, et al. Neoadjuvant chemotherapy and radiotherapy for large extremity soft-tissue sarcomas. Int J Radiat Oncol Biol Phys
2003;56(4):1117–27. http://dx.doi.org/10.1016/S0360-3016(03)00186-X.

59. Kraybill WG, Harris J, Spiro IJ, et al. Phase II study of neoadjuvant chemotherapy and radiation therapy in the management of high-risk, high-grade,
soft tissue sarcomas of the extremities and body wall: Radiation Therapy
Oncology Group Trial 9514. J Clin Oncol 2006;24(4):619–25. http://dx.doi.org/
10.1200/JCO.2005.02.5577.

60. Kraybill WG, Harris J, Spiro IJ, et al. Long-term results of a phase 2 study of neoadjuvant chemotherapy and radiotherapy in the management of high-risk, high-
grade, soft tissue sarcomas of the extremities and body wall: Radiation Therapy
Oncology Group Trial 9514. Cancer 2010;116(19):4613–21. http://dx.doi.org/10.
1002/cncr.25350.

61. Gronchi A, Bui BN, Bonvalot S, et al. Phase II clinical trial of neoadjuvant trabectedin in patients with advanced localized myxoid liposarcoma. Ann Oncol 2012;
23(3):771–6. http://dx.doi.org/10.1093/annonc/mdr265.

62. Park JO, Qin LX, Prete FP, et al. Predicting outcome by growth rate of locally
recurrent retroperitoneal liposarcoma. Ann Surg 2009;250(6):977–82. http://dx.
doi.org/10.1097/SLA.0b013e3181b2468b.

63. Van Geel AN, Pastorino U, Jauch K, et al. Surgical treatment of lung metastases: The European Organization for Research and Treatment of Cancer-Soft Tissue and Bone Sarcoma Group Study of 255 Patients. Cancer 1995;77(4): 675–82.
64. Billingsley KG, Burt ME, Jara E, et al. Pulmonary metastases from soft tissue sarcoma analysis of patterns of disease and postmetastasis survival. Ann Surg 1999;229(5):602–12.
65. Rehders A, Hosch SB, Scheunemann P, et al. Benefit of surgical treatment of lung metastasis in soft tissue sarcoma. Arch Surg 2007;142(1):70–5. http://dx.doi.org/10.1001/archsurg.142.1.70 [discussion: 76].
66. Blackmon SH, Shah N, Roth JA, et al. Resection of pulmonary and extrapulmonary sarcomatous metastases is associated with long-term survival. Ann Thorac Surg 2009;88(3):877–84. http://dx.doi.org/10.1016/j.athoracsur.2009. 04.144 [discussion: 884–5].
67. Jones RL, Fisher C, Al-Muderis O, et al. Differential sensitivity of liposarcoma subtypes to chemotherapy. Eur J Cancer 2005;41(18):2853–60. http://dx.doi.org/10.1016/j.ejca.2005.07.023.
68. Italiano A, Toulmonde M, Cioffi A, et al. Advanced well-differentiated/dedifferentiated liposarcomas: role of chemotherapy and survival. Ann Oncol 2012;23(6):1601–7. http://dx.doi.org/10.1093/annonc/mdr485.
69. Patel SR, Vadhan-Raj S, Papadopolous N, et al. High-dose ifosfamide in bone and soft tissue sarcomas: results of phase II and pilot studies—dose-response and schedule dependence. J Clin Oncol 1997;15:2378–84.
70. Nielsen OS, Judson I, Van Hoesel Q, et al. Effect of high-dose ifosfamide in advanced soft tissue sarcomas. A multicentre phase II study of the EORTC Soft Tissue and Bone Sarcoma Group. Eur J Cancer 2000;36(1):61–7.
71. Bitz U, Pink D, Busemann C, et al. Doxorubicin (Doxo) and dacarbacin (DTIC) as first-line therapy for patients (pts) with locally advanced or metastatic leiomyosarcoma (LMS) and liposarcoma (LPS). J Clin Oncol 2011;29:(suppl; abstr 10094).
72. Demetri GD, Chawla SP, Von Mehren M, et al. Efficacy and safety of trabectedin in patients with advanced or metastatic liposarcoma or leiomyosarcoma after failure of prior anthracyclines and ifosfamide: results of a randomized phase II study of two different schedules. J Clin Oncol 2009;27(25):4188–96. http://dx.doi.org/10.1200/JCO.2008.21.0088.
73. Samuels BL, Chawla S, Patel S, et al. Clinical outcomes and safety with trabectedin therapy in patients with advanced soft tissue sarcomas following failure of prior chemotherapy: results of a worldwide expanded access program study. Ann Oncol 2013;24(6):1703–9. http://dx.doi.org/10.1093/annonc/mds659.
74. Hoiczyk M, Grabellus F, Podleska L, et al. Trabectedin in metastatic soft tissue sarcomas: role of pretreatment and age. Ann Oncol 2013;43:23–8. http://dx.doi.org/10.3892/ijo.2013.1928.
75. Grosso F, Jones RL, Demetri GD, et al. Efficacy of trabectedin (ecteinascidin-743) in advanced pretreated myxoid liposarcomas: a retrospective study. Lancet Oncol 2007;8:595–602. http://dx.doi.org/10.1016/S1470-2045(07)70175-4.
76. Maki RG, Wathen JK, Patel SR, et al. Randomized phase II study of gemcitabine and docetaxel compared with gemcitabine alone in patients with metastatic soft tissue sarcomas: results of sarcoma alliance for research through collaboration study 002 [corrected]. J Clin Oncol 2007;25(19):2755–63. http://dx.doi.org/10.1200/JCO.2006.10.4117.

77. Sleijfer S, Ray-Coquard I, Papai Z, et al. Pazopanib, a multikinase angiogenesis inhibitor, in patients with relapsed or refractory advanced soft tissue sarcoma: a phase II study from the European Organisation for Research and Treatment of Cancer—Soft Tissue and Bone Sarcoma Group (EORTC study 620. J Clin Oncol 2009;27(19):3126–32. http://dx.doi.org/10.1200/JCO.2008.21.3223.

78. Van der Graaf WT, Blay JY, Chawla SP, et al. Pazopanib for Metastatic Soft-Tissue Sarcoma (PALETTE): a randomised, double-blind, placebo-controlled phase 3 trial. Lancet 2012;379(9829):1879–86. http://dx.doi.org/10.1016/S0140-6736(12)60651-5.

79. Le Cesne A, Judson I, Crowther D, et al. Randomized phase III study comparing conventional-dose doxorubicin plus ifosfamide versus high-dose doxorubicin plus ifosfamide plus recombinant human granulocyte-macrophage colony-stimulating factor in advanced soft tissue sarcomas: a trial of the European Organization for Research and Treatment of Cancer/Soft Tissue and Bone Sarcoma Group. J Clin Oncol 2000;18(14):2676–84.

80. Katz D, Boonsirikamchai P, Choi H, et al. Efficacy of first-line doxorubicin and ifosfamide in myxoid liposarcoma. Clin Sarcoma Res 2012;2(1):2. http://dx.doi.org/10.1186/2045-3329-2-2.

81. Italiano A, Garbay D, Cioffi A, et al. Advanced pleomorphic liposarcomas: clinical outcome and impact of chemotherapy. Ann Oncol 2012;23(8):2205–6. http://dx.doi.org/10.1093/annonc/mds221.

82. Michael D, Oren M. The p53-Mdm2 module and the ubiquitin system. Semin Cancer Biol 2003;13(1):49–58. http://dx.doi.org/10.1016/S1044-579X(02)00099-8.

83. Oren M, Damalas A, Gottlieb T, et al. Regulation of p53: intricate loops and delicate balances. Ann N Y Acad Sci 2002;973:374–83.

84. Singer S, Socci ND, Ambrosini G, et al. Gene expression profiling of liposarcoma identifies distinct biological types/subtypes and potential therapeutic targets in well-differentiated and dedifferentiated liposarcoma. Cancer research 2007;67(14):6626–36. http://dx.doi.org/10.1158/0008-5472.CAN-07-0584.

85. Vassilev L, Vu B, Graves B, et al. In vivo activation of the p53 pathway by small-molecule antagonists of MDM2. Science 2004;303:844. http://dx.doi.org/10.1126/science.1092472.

86. Henze J, Mühlenberg T, Simon S, et al. p53 modulation as a therapeutic strategy in gastrointestinal stromal tumors. PLoS One 2012;7(5):e37776. http://dx.doi.org/10.1371/journal.pone.0037776.

87. Stühmer T, Arts J, King P, et al. A first-in-class HDM2-inhibitor (JNJ-26854165) in phase I development shows potent activity against multiple myeloma (MM) cells in vitro and ex vivo. J Clin Oncol 2008;26(suppl; abstr 14694):1–2.

88. Ray-Coquard IL, Blay J, Italiano A, et al. Neoadjuvant MDM2 antagonist RG7112 for well-differentiated and dedifferentiated liposarcomas (WD/DD LPS): a pharmacodynamic (PD) biomarker study. J Clin Oncol 2011;29(suppl; abstr 10007b):2–4.

89. Kurzrock R, Blay J, Nguyen BB, et al. A phase I study of MDM2 antagonist RG7112 in patients (pts) with relapsed/refractory solid tumors. J Clin Oncol 2012;30:(suppl; abstr e136000).

90. Ray-Coquard I, Blay JY, Italiano A, et al. Effect of the MDM2 antagonist RG7112 on the P53 pathway in patients with MDM2-amplified, well-differentiated or dedifferentiated liposarcoma: an exploratory proof-of-mechanism study. Lancet Oncol 2012;13(11):1133–40. http://dx.doi.org/10.1016/S1470-2045(12)70474-6.

91. Ortega S, Malumbres M, Barbacid M. Cyclin D-dependent kinases, INK4 inhibitors and cancer. Biochim Biophys Acta 2002;1602(1):73–87.

92. Dickson MA, Keohan ML, Tap WD, et al. Phase II trial of the CDK4 inhibitor PD0332991 in CDK4-amplified well-differentiated or dedifferentiated liposarcoma. J Clin Oncol 2012;30:(suppl; abstr 10002).
93. Dickson MA, Tap WD, Keohan ML, et al. Phase II trial of the CDK4 inhibitor PD0332991 in patients with advanced CDK4-amplified well-differentiated or dedifferentiated liposarcoma. J Clin Oncol 2013;31(16):2024–8. http://dx.doi.org/10.1200/JCO.2012.46.5476.
94. Tontonoz P, Singer S, Forman BM, et al. Terminal differentiation of human liposarcoma cells induced by ligands for peroxisome proliferator-activated receptor gamma and the retinoid X receptor. Proc Natl Acad Sci U S A 1997;94(1):237–41.
95. Demetri GD, Fletcher CD, Mueller E, et al. Induction of solid tumor differentiation by the peroxisome proliferator-activated receptor-gamma ligand troglitazone in patients with liposarcoma. Proc Natl Acad Sci U S A 1999;96(7):3951–6.
96. Debrock G, Vanhentenrijk V, Sciot R, et al. A phase II trial with rosiglitazone in liposarcoma patients. Br J Cancer 2003;89(8):1409–12. http://dx.doi.org/10.1038/sj.bjc.6601306.
97. Pishvaian MJ, Cotarla I, Wagner AJ, et al. Final reporting of a phase I clinical trial of the oral PPAR-gamma agonist, CS-7017, in patients with advanced malignancies. J Clin Oncol 2010;28(15s):(suppl; abstr 2526).
98. Charytonowicz E, Terry M, Coakley K, et al. PPARγ agonists enhance ET-743–induced adipogenic differentiation in a transgenic mouse model of myxoid round cell liposarcoma. J Clin Invest 2012;122(3):886–98. http://dx.doi.org/10.1172/JCI60015DS1.
99. Barretina J, Taylor BS, Banerji S, et al. Subtype-specific genomic alterations define new targets for soft-tissue sarcoma therapy. Nat Genet 2010;42(8):715–21. http://dx.doi.org/10.1038/ng.619.
100. Peng T, Zhang P, Liu J, et al. An experimental model for the study of well-differentiated and dedifferentiated liposarcoma; deregulation of targetable tyrosine kinase receptors. Lab Invest 2011;91(3):392–403. http://dx.doi.org/10.1038/labinvest.2010.185.
101. Gutierrez A, Snyder EL, Marino-Enriquez A, et al. Aberrant AKT activation drives well-differentiated liposarcoma. Proc Natl Acad Sci U S A 2011;108(39):16386–91. http://dx.doi.org/10.1073/pnas.1106127108/-/DCSupplemental. Available at. www.pnas.org/cgi/doi/10.1073/pnas.1106127108.
102. Demicco EG, Torres KE, Ghadimi MP, et al. Involvement of the PI3K/Akt pathway in myxoid/round cell liposarcoma. Mod Pathol 2012;25(2):212–21. http://dx.doi.org/10.1038/modpathol.2011.148.

Leiomyosarcoma

César Serrano, MD[a,b], Suzanne George, MD[b,*]

KEYWORDS

- Leiomyosarcoma • Chemotherapy • Targeted therapy • Prognostic factors
- Uterine leiomyosarcoma

KEY POINTS

- Leiomyosarcoma is a malignant mesenchymal tumor that derives from the smooth muscle lineage.
- The underlying genetic mechanisms remain unclear, and complex and unbalanced karyotypic defects are the only shared features observed across the different leiomyosarcoma subtypes.
- Cell-cycle perturbations, mainly through RB1 defects, and phosphatidylinositol 3 kinase/Akt pathway activation caused by *PTEN* genomic deletion are the two most consistent drivers commonly observed in sarcomas, including leiomyosarcoma.
- Patients with unresectable metastatic leiomyosarcoma are considered incurable and the treatment intention for systemic disease is always palliative.
- Unlike other soft tissue sarcomas, leiomyosarcomas are particularly sensitive to the combination of gemcitabine-docetaxel, which is currently regarded as a standard of care in this population.
- Chemotherapy treatment with trabectedin has shown exquisite activity in leiomyosarcoma, mainly in the form of long disease stabilization.
- Pazopanib is an oral multikinase inhibitor recently approved for the treatment of soft tissue sarcomas in leiomyosarcoma.

EPIDEMIOLOGY

Leiomyosarcoma is one of the most frequent soft tissue sarcomas, with an estimated incidence ranging between 10% and 20% of all newly diagnosed soft tissue sarcomas. Population-based data on the incidence of leiomyosarcoma were investigated in a study from the Surveillance, Epidemiology, and End Results (SEER) program, covering

Funding Sources: Spanish Society of Medical Oncology (SEOM) Translational Award (C. Serrano); Driscoll Family Leiomyosarcoma Research Fund (S. George).
Conflict of Interest: Nil.
[a] Fletcher Laboratory, Department of Pathology, Brigham and Women's Hospital, 75 Francis Street, Thorn 528, Boston, MA 02115, USA; [b] Center for Sarcoma and Bone Oncology, Dana-Farber Cancer Institute, 450 Brookline Avenue, Boston, MA 02215, USA
* Corresponding author.
E-mail address: sgeorge2@partners.org

Hematol Oncol Clin N Am 27 (2013) 957–974
http://dx.doi.org/10.1016/j.hoc.2013.07.002
0889-8588/13/$ – see front matter © 2013 Elsevier Inc. All rights reserved.

a total of 35,359 soft tissue sarcomas diagnosed during 2005 to 2009. Leiomyosarcoma comprised a significant percentage of soft tissues and abdominal-pelvic sarcomas, only outnumbered by liposarcomas, and is the predominant sarcoma arising from large blood vessels.[1] Aside from these locations, it is less common in the extremities, accounting for perhaps 10% to 15% of limb sarcomas, with a preference for the thigh.[2] In addition, leiomyosarcomas of the uterus, with an estimated incidence of 0.64 cases per 100,000 women, are among the most common uterine sarcomas and likely account for the single largest site-specific group of leiomyosarcomas.[3]

As in soft tissue sarcomas in general, overall incidence of leiomyosarcoma increases with age, and peaks at the seventh decade. By contrast, uterine leiomyosarcoma occurs from the third decade into old age, but is most common in the perimenopausal age group, in the fifth decade.[4] The sex incidence depends on tumor location, with most patients with retroperitoneal and inferior vena cava leiomyosarcoma being women,[5] whereas there is a mild male predominance in noncutaneous soft tissue sites[2] and cutaneous leiomyosarcoma.[6]

Causes and Predisposing Factors

There are few clear causal or predisposing factors identified for this disease. Several exogenous agents have been studied, but only Epstein-Barr virus (EBV) infection, in the setting of severe immunosuppression, has been associated with leiomyosarcomas among patients with acquired immunodeficiency syndrome (AIDS) and after kidney, cardiac, and liver transplantation. Most of EBV-related leiomyosarcomas occur in children and young adults, and develop in organs not traditionally considered preferred sites for leiomyosarcoma.[7] Other traditional risk factors for sarcomas, such as radiotherapy, rarely lead to the development of leiomyosarcomas.[8] In addition, the role for estrogenic stimulation remains unclear.[9] Patients with hereditary retinoblastoma have a cumulative risk of 13.1% for developing any soft tissue sarcoma as a secondary malignancy,[10] including leiomyosarcoma, which further agrees with the relevance of RB1 loss in sporadic leiomyosarcoma (discussed later). In contrast, although clearly reported, leiomyosarcoma is an uncommon subtype of sarcoma among patients with Li-Fraumeni syndrome.[11]

There is no solid evidence showing that leiomyoma (the benign counterpart of leiomyosarcomas) can undergo malignant transformation, and it is currently widely accepted that leiomyosarcomas are tumors that arise de novo.[9]

PATHOLOGY AND TUMOR BIOLOGY
Histopathology

Leiomyosarcoma is a malignant mesenchymal tumor composed of cells showing distinct features of the smooth muscle lineage. The typical histologic pattern of leiomyosarcomas of any origin is that of intersecting, sharply marginated fascicles of spindle cells with abundant eosinophilic cytoplasm and elongated and hyperchromatic nuclei (**Fig. 1**). Large leiomyosarcomas frequently contain coagulative tumor necrosis regions. Focal pleomorphism is common, and some cases show extensive pleomorphism, resembling any undifferentiated soft tissue sarcoma.[12] Most leiomyosarcomas are reactive for alpha smooth muscle actin, desmin, and h-caldesmon on immunohistochemistry, although none of these markers are specific for smooth muscle differentiation.

Tumor Biology

From a molecular genetics standpoint, sarcomas are conceptually classified in 2 broad categories[13]: the first category comprises sarcomas with near-diploid

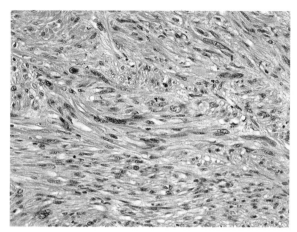

Fig. 1. Representative hematoxylin and eosin stain (40×) of a leiomyosarcoma. (*Courtesy of Dr Jason Hornick, Boston, MA.*)

karyotypes and simple but essential genetic alterations, such as translocations or activating mutations. The second category includes tumors with complex and unbalanced karyotypes, which are characteristic from tumors with severe genome instability, thus resulting in multiple genomic aberrations, and leiomyosarcomas are in this second category (**Fig. 2**).

Standard karyotyping and fluorescence in situ hybridization techniques have shown that the cytogenetic and molecular changes in leiomyosarcomas are complex and there are no consistent, recurrent aberrations shown at the chromosomal level.[14] DNA copy number changes also depict a complex landscape in all leiomyosarcomas, and likewise some other cancer types, and the extent of gains/losses and cytogenetic changes seems to be associated with tumor evolution and worse survival.[15,16] The most consistent changes detected across several studies are losses in chromosomes 10q11 to 21.2 and 13q14.3 to q21.1, and gains at 17p11 to p12. Regions deleted in 10q and 13q harbor 2 important tumor suppressor genes: *RB1* and *PTEN*, respectively.

The underlying genetic mechanisms of sarcomas with complex karyotypic defects, such as leiomyosarcomas, although poorly understood, frequently include disturbances in key cell-cycle genes.[17] The aforementioned 13q loss specifically targets the tumor suppressor *RB1* gene, and entails lack of regulation of the cell cycle at the G1-S checkpoint, thus leading to uncontrolled cell division. Analysis of components of the RB1-cyclin D1 pathway (RB1, CDKN2A, CCND1, CCND3) in leiomyosarcomas revealed alterations in up to 90% of patients[17,18] and association with poorer prognosis (reviewed by Yang and colleagues[19] in 2009). Therefore, loss of RB1 function may be an important driver for proliferation in at least a subset of leiomyosarcoma. In contrast, molecular studies focused on p53/MDM2 abnormalities in leiomyosarcoma have observed a lower rate of p53 mutations and amplification of MDM2 compared with other sarcoma types.[17,20]

From a gene expression standpoint, gene expression profiling studies using expression microarrays have identified 3 reproducible molecular subtypes that are distributed similarly over leiomyosarcomas of gynecologic and nongynecologic origins.[21] Group I comprises approximately 25% of all leiomyosarcomas, is highly enriched for genes related to muscle contraction and the actin cytoskeleton, tends to be of

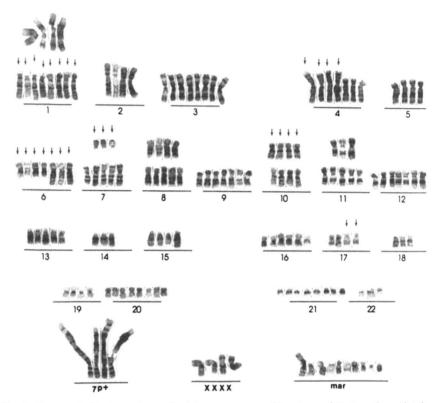

Fig. 2. Representative karyotype of a leiomyosarcoma. (*Courtesy of* Dr Jonathan Fletcher, Boston, MA.)

the conventional leiomyosarcoma histologic subtype, and shows improved outcome compared with leiomyosarcoma groups II and III,[21,22] which in turn overlaps to a greater extent with undifferentiated pleomorphic sarcomas. These results agree with previous data showing that some leiomyosarcomas cluster with undifferentiated pleomorphic sarcomas and liposarcomas in microarray studies performed in pooled sarcoma subtypes.[23] Profiling studies have also contributed to the identification of new targets, such as Aurora-A and Aurora-B kinases, which are consistently overexpressed in uterine leiomyosarcoma,[24] and in vitro and in vivo targeting of Aurora-A kinase induces cell-cycle arrest and apoptosis.[25]

Several pathways and signal intermediates have been investigated in leiomyosarcoma, and the relevance of phosphatidylinositol 3 kinase (PI3K)/AKT pathway activation has been consistently shown throughout several studies. Genomic deletion of chromosome 10q targets the *PTEN* tumor suppressor gene and leads to hyperactivation of PI3K/AKT, which is a common finding in leiomyosarcoma. Mice with genetic inactivation of *PTEN* in the smooth cell muscle lineage accordingly develop a rapid onset of abdominal leiomyosarcomas with constitutive mammalian target of rapamycin (mTOR) activation.[26] Although approximately half of leiomyosarcomas express insulinlike growth factor (IGF)-1R and IGF-II, the relevance of the IGFR/AKT pathway in the proliferation and survival of leiomyosarcoma is yet to be elucidated.

PRINCIPLES OF GENERAL MANAGEMENT
Diagnosis

Clinical presentation of leiomyosarcomas, as of other soft tissue sarcomas, is often associated with nonspecific symptoms caused by displacement of structures, rather than invasion, in specific anatomic locations of the primary tumor and its metastasis. Pretreatment biopsy is mandatory, but further pathologic evaluation with the primary tumor is typically performed following complete resection.

Imaging approaches include magnetic resonance imaging (MRI) in soft tissue tumors, and contrast-enhanced computed tomography (CT) scan for retroperitoneal lesions. Chest and abdominal CT scan is required in the initial work-up, because hematogenous spread is a frequent event in leiomyosarcomas, and lung and liver are two common sites of metastasis.

Prognostic Factors

In leiomyosarcoma, as in soft tissue sarcomas, histologic grade, tumor size, and tumor depth are the three major clinicopathologic factors that establish the risk profile, and all are included in the American Joint Committee on Cancer (AJCC) staging system for soft tissue sarcomas.[27,28] However, relationship between AJCC staging and prognosis of leiomyosarcoma arising from the gastrointestinal tract or uterus is not clear.[29] Perhaps the major limitation of the AJCC staging system is that it does not include histology and anatomic site, and both have been shown to affect prognosis. Pisters and colleagues[28] reported the risk factors associated with soft tissue sarcoma in a series of 1,041 cases. Among several risk factors, patients with leiomyosarcoma were at higher risk for distant recurrence and decreased disease-specific survival than other histotypes, which corroborates the intrinsic aggressive behavior of leiomyosarcoma.

Grade and location are two independent prognosis factors of similar importance to stage.[28] Histologic grading is an independent indicator of the degree of malignancy, probability of distant metastasis, and disease-specific survival,[27,28,30] and, accordingly, leiomyosarcoma is a subtype of soft tissue sarcoma with substantial intrinsic aggressiveness: approximately 90% of leiomyosarcoma are reported to be moderate to high grade.[27] Regarding location, soft tissue sarcomas from extremities have better overall survival than those arising in the retroperitoneum.[30] Atypical intradermal smooth muscle neoplasm (formerly called cutaneous leiomyosarcoma) constitutes a distinctive entity with excellent prognosis, because it arises in the dermis, and does not develop metastasis.[9,31] Tumor size and bone or neurovascular involvement are two other risk factors, together with grade, that have been significantly associated with poor outcome specifically in leiomyosarcoma.[27]

Surgery

Surgical resection is the cornerstone treatment of all patients with localized soft tissue sarcomas, and subsequently for leiomyosarcomas. The standard surgical procedure involves a complete excision with wide negative margins (R0 resection), which offers the best chance of cure, with or without adjuvant treatment.

Leiomyosarcomas are commonly found in the retroperitoneum, and surgical R0 resection in retroperitoneal leiomyosarcoma is often hampered by the large tumor size, coupled with the anatomic constrains. Thus, in clinical practice, many resections are grossly complete but with microscopically positive margins,[32] which is essential because the ability to perform a complete surgical resection at the time of initial presentation is the most important prognostic factor for survival.[33]

In addition, surgery may benefit certain metastatic patients, particularly pulmonary metastasectomy in patients with a low number of metastases appearing late after primary resection.[34]

Radiotherapy

The therapeutic role of radiotherapy in soft tissue sarcomas has been shown to improve local control with preservation of the function, decrease in local recurrence rate, but not to improve overall survival.[35] Thus, preoperative or postoperative radiotherapy are considered to be the standard of care for nearly all intermediate-grade or high-grade leiomyosarcomas of the limbs and trunk. The radiotherapy approach in soft tissue sarcomas is discussed in detail elsewhere.[36,37]

Radiation therapy has shown benefit in the treatment of soft tissue sarcoma of the extremity and trunk, but there are no randomized data addressing this question in retroperitoneal sarcomas and hence there is institutional variation on its use in this setting. The largest retrospective series investigated the role of preoperative radiation therapy in 33 retroperitoneal sarcomas, 12 of which were leiomyosarcomas. In this series, leiomyosarcomas, unlike liposarcomas, had a lower 3-year local recurrence rate (18.8%) and a higher 3-year distance recurrence rate (35.4%).[38]

SYSTEMIC TREATMENT OF LEIOMYOSARCOMAS

The most life-threatening aspect of sarcomas in general, and leiomyosarcomas in particular, is their propensity for hematogenous dissemination,[39] and therefore systemic control is desired.

The role of postoperative chemotherapy remains unproven, and is not further discussed here because it is not the focus of this article. Most trials evaluating adjuvant chemotherapy in sarcoma evaluate patients with high-risk soft tissue sarcomas and including many histologic subtypes, making it difficult to discern a subtype-specific recommendation. The largest such trial was recently reported by the European Organisation for Research and Treatment of Cancer (EORTC) and did not show an overall survival benefit with adjuvant chemotherapy.

Almost all patients with unresectable metastatic leiomyosarcoma are considered incurable; hence, in almost all cases, the treatment intention for systemic disease is palliative, with the goal of decreasing tumor bulk, diminishing symptoms, improving quality of life, and prolonging survival. It is widely recognized that different histologic subtypes have variable patterns of chemosensitivity, and leiomyosarcomas show moderate sensitivity to chemotherapy (reviewed by Grimer and colleagues[37] in 2010), although uterine leiomyosarcoma seems to be more responsive to many chemotherapy agents, in contrast with visceral leiomyosarcomas. Systemic treatment of uterine leiomyosarcoma is described separately below.

Anthracyclines

Single-agent doxorubicin is a standard systemic treatment of soft tissue sarcomas, and subsequently for leiomyosarcomas as well. Doxorubicin, as a single agent, has reported response rates varying between 10% and 25% (reviewed by Krikelis and Judson[40] in 2010), although leiomyosarcoma seems to be less responsive than other sarcoma subtypes, such as synovial sarcoma and liposarcoma. A review of 2185 patients with sarcoma treated with doxorubicin showed that leiomyosarcomas had a nonsignificant lower response rate (11%) compared with other sarcoma subtypes.[39] An updated study on 488 metastatic patients, 85% of whom received doxorubicin as first-line treatment and including 171 leiomyosarcomas, also concluded that synovial sarcoma and liposarcoma were independent favorable predictive factors of response and longer survival compared with leiomyosarcomas.[41]

Various doxorubicin-based combination regimens have been tested in the hopes of achieving superior response rates and overall survival, and higher response rates (of approximately 45%) have been consistently shown in several randomized clinical trials and pooled analyses with combination regimens compared with single-agent doxorubicin.[40,42] However, none of these studies have been able to show whether the observed increased activity leads to a statistically significant advantage in overall survival. In addition, more toxic effects were observed with the combination regimens. Therefore, the higher response rates suggest that doxorubicin/ifosfamide might be justified in selected patients and if tumor shrinkage is critical.

In addition, alternative anthracyclines might be used to minimize secondary effects, such as epirubicin and liposomal anthracyclines. Epirubicin is less cardiotoxic and provides outcomes that are comparable with doxorubicin. Liposomal doxorubicin has a better toxicity profile, although whether it is as efficacious as unencapsulated doxorubicin is still unproved in large trials.

Ifosfamide

Single-agent ifosfamide seems to have similar antitumor activity to doxorubicin in soft tissue sarcomas, but entails a worse toxicity profile,[43] and thus may be regarded as a second-line regimen. Treatment with ifosfamide among patients who previously failed a doxorubicin-based regimen achieves approximate response rates of 25%,[40] with an observed dose-response relationship.[44]

Sleijfer and colleagues[45] undertook a retrospective analysis on prognostic and predictive factors for outcome to first-line single-agent ifosfamide and ifosfamide-containing regimens in 1337 advanced or metastatic patients with soft tissue sarcoma. The median progression-free and overall survivals were 19 and 54 weeks respectively. There was a nonsignificant trend in leiomyosarcomas toward a lower response rate and a lower median progression-free survival compared with synovial sarcomas, liposarcomas, and other sarcoma histologies (not including gastrointestinal stromal tumors).

Gemcitabine and Gemcitabine-based Regimens

Gemcitabine is a nucleoside metabolite that has shown efficacy in a variety of solid tumors, and several phase II clinical trials have shown a response rate of approximately 10% in previously treated soft tissue sarcomas, including leiomyosarcomas.[46–51]

Several other agents have been tested in soft tissue sarcomas, and none, as single therapy, has achieved response rates greater than 20%. The activity of docetaxel[52,53] and vinorelbine[54] as single agents is almost nill. Dacarbazine and temozolomide seem to have modest antitumor effects, with some predilection for leiomyosarcomas, and data from a phase II clinical trial showed an overall response rate of 15.5%.[55] The combination of gemcitabine with any of these aforementioned drugs seems to yield significant synergistic activity, and a gemcitabine/docetaxel doublet has been shown to be highly active in patients with unresectable leiomyosarcomas or in those with leiomyosarcoma that has progressed to prior doxorubicin-based therapy.

Activity for fixed-dose rate gemcitabine plus docetaxel was initially reported in a prospective phase II study that recruited patients with advanced leiomyosarcoma of uterine (n = 29) or other (n = 5) primary sites progressing to prior treatment. Complete response was observed in 3 patients and partial response in 15, for an overall response rate of 53%. Among 16 patients previously treated with doxorubicin with or without ifosfamide, objective responses were observed in 8 patients (50%). Among the 5 patients with nonuterine primary leiomyosarcoma, partial responses were observed in 2 patients (40%), stable disease in 2, and progression of disease in 1. The median progression-free survival was 5.6 months.[56] The activity of the combination and the activity in leiomyosarcoma were later confirmed in 2 independent series of soft tissue sarcomas.[57,58]

It was unknown whether adding docetaxel produces synergy in the combination, or whether most of the treatment effect arises from the fixed dose rate of gemcitabine. Two multicenter phase II randomized clinical trials addressed this question. The SARC002 study showed that the combination was associated with superior response rate (16% vs 8%), median progression-free survival (6.2 vs 3.0 months), and overall survival (17.9 vs 11.5 months) compared with gemcitabine alone in patients with advanced soft tissue sarcoma who had received a median of 1 line of treatment.[59] This study also confirmed the higher sensitivity of leiomyosarcoma to this regimen. By contrast, results from the French clinical trial differed from previous data and only confirmed the benefit of the combination in uterine leiomyosarcomas, but not in those of nonuterine origin, in which the combination seemed to be detrimental.[60] The French study, unlike the SARC02 trial, included only patients with leiomyosarcomas after progressing to a first line of systemic treatment, and the dose of gemcitabine in the control arm was slightly higher. Whether these nuances might explain the differences observed between the current conflicting data remains unknown.

Two other gemcitabine-based combinations have shown benefit in soft tissue sarcomas, and exquisite efficacy in leiomyosarcomas. García del Muro and colleagues[61] explored the feasibility and activity of fixed-dose-rate gemcitabine plus dacarbazine in a phase II randomized clinical trial. The combination was superior to single-agent dacarbazine, and histology showed that leiomyosarcomas of any origin benefited significantly from the doublet, achieving a median progression-free survival and an overall survival of 4.9 and 18.3 months respectively (2.1 and 7.8 months respectively in nonleiomyosarcoma subtypes). The combination of gemcitabine and vinorelbine similarly achieved greater benefit in leiomyosarcomas, although the complete benefit rate was lower, and the trial did not have a control arm.[62] **Table 1** summarizes gemcitabine-based phase II clinical trials.

Table 1
Phase II clinical trials with gemcitabine-based regimens. Data regarding patients with leiomyosarcoma refer to those treated only with the combinations

Regimen	Prior Lines in mts Disease	N (Total)	N (LMS)	Uterine/ Extrauterine	CR/PR (%)	mPFS (mo)
Gem-Doc[55]	0–2	29	29	29/5	53	5.6
Gem-Doc[56]	0–5	35	12	2/10	58	NA
Gem-Doc[58]	0–3	122	29	NA	17	NA
Gem-Doc[59]	0–1	46	46	24/22	9	3.4–4.7
Gem-DTIC[60]	≥1	57	16	NA	19	4.9
Gem-VNR[61]	0–1	40	19	NA	16	NA

Abbreviations: CR, complete response; Doc, docetaxel; DTIC, dacarbazine; Gem, gemcitabine; LMS, leiomyosarcoma; mPFS, median progression-free survival; mts, metastatic; NA, not available; PR, partial response; VNR, vinorelbine.

Trabectedin

Trabectedin (also known as ecteinascidin, or ET-743) is a unique, novel, marine-derived chemotherapy agent. This agent forms covalent bonds with the DNA minor groove, distorting DNA and blocking the transcription activation of several genes regulated by the minor groove.

Several phase II trials have tested single-agent trabectedin as second-line treatment and in heavily pretreated metastatic or unresectable soft tissue sarcomas, and leiomyosarcomas of any origin have been found to have a particularly sensitive histology,[63-66] mainly in the form of disease stabilization, rather than major objective responses. The efficacy of trabectedin in leiomyosarcomas has been extensively confirmed in the recently published expanded access program.[67] Data from 431 leiomyosarcomas of any origin revealed an overall response rate of 7.5%, whereas all sarcomas grouped together achieved 5.9%. Likewise, L-sarcomas (leiomyosarcomas and liposarcomas) obtained a higher clinical benefit rate (54%) and median overall survival (16.2 months) than non–L-sarcomas (38% and 8.4 months, respectively).

A higher response rate (17.1%) was found in a phase II, single-arm clinical trial conducted in 36 chemotherapy-naive patients with sarcoma. The median duration of response was 16.5 months, and approximately three-fourths of enrolled patients were still alive at 1 year. Two out of the 15 patients with leiomyosarcoma recruited achieved partial responses.[68] These results led to the design of a randomized, multicenter, phase III clinical trial that is to evaluate the effectiveness of trabectedin versus standard doxorubicin-based chemotherapy as first-line treatment of patients with advanced translocation-related sarcomas.

Trabectedin was approved by the European Medicines Agency (EMEA) in 2007, and is currently available in Europe and some other countries, but not yet in the United States, Australia, or Brazil. A phase III randomized trial comparing trabectedin with dacarbacine in patients with advanced leiomyosarcoma and liposarcomas is currently underway in the United States.

Targeted Therapies

Antiangiogenic inhibitors

Antiangiogenic inhibitors have traditionally shown modest activity in soft tissue sarcoma, especially in terms of objective response rate. The addition of bevacizumab to doxorubicin did not improve the response rates seen with single-agent therapy and caused increased cardiac toxicity.[69] Sunitinib and sorafenib, two multitargeted tyrosine kinase inhibitors, only show some benefit in a small subset of sarcomas, but not in leiomyosarcomas.[70,71]

In contrast, pazopanib, an oral tyrosine kinase inhibitor that also shows potent inhibition of vascular endothelial growth factor and platelet-derived growth factor receptors, was active in leiomyosarcoma and synovial sarcoma cohorts in a single-arm phase II trial.[72] A subsequent randomized, placebo-controlled, multicenter phase III clinical trial further confirmed initial data, and resulted in a significant increase in progression-free survival compared with placebo (4.6 months vs 1.6 months, respectively). As expected, the overall response rate was low (6%), but up to 67% of the patients achieved disease stabilization as best response.[73] Based on these results, pazopanib obtained US Food and Drug Administration approval for the treatment of patients with metastatic soft tissue sarcomas who have received prior chemotherapy.

mTOR inhibitors

Despite the strong rationale behind mTOR inhibition in leiomyosarcoma preclinical models,[26] temsirolimus and ridaforolimus have both failed to show significant benefit in soft tissue sarcomas. An initial single-arm phase II study of ridaforolimus in 216 patients with sarcoma previously treated with chemotherapy yielded a low response rate (1.9%),[74] but a clinical benefit rate including prolonged stabilization (16 weeks or greater) of approximately 30%. However, a subsequent placebo-controlled, phase III trial, which compared ridaforolimus with placebo as maintenance therapy after initial chemotherapy in advanced sarcomas, reported a statistically significant, but unlikely to be relevant, short median progression-free survival advantage (3.1 weeks) in those patients who received ridoforalimus.[75] Temsirolimus, only tested in a phase II, single-arm, clinical trial, also had poor activity.[76]

Therefore, clinical evidence has failed to show benefit of mTOR inhibitors in patients with sarcoma in general, and specifically in leiomyosarcomas. It is possible that the adaptive capabilities of oncogenic signaling networks, such as enhanced signaling through IGF-1R and other growth factors, hamper the antiproliferative effect of these compounds in the clinical setting.[77] Based on this evidence, 2 clinical trials investigated whether the combination of an mTOR inhibitor with an IGF-1R inhibitor provides greater benefit in patients with sarcoma. Interesting activity could be observed in a subset of patients (mainly bone sarcomas), although the combination did not yield significant activity in leiomyosarcomas, beyond stabilization in a minor proportion of patients.[78,79]

UTERINE LEIOMYOSARCOMA

Uterine sarcomas are rare and constitute approximately 3% of all uterine neoplasms, with leiomyosarcoma being the most common mesenchymal malignancy of the uterus.[80] Uterine leiomyosarcoma is associated with poor outcome, because rates of local and distant failure are usually high (45%–80%), and median overall survival of 2 years once disease is disseminated.[81]

There are no distinctive symptoms or pathognomonic features on any imaging technique, therefore the diagnosis is made by histologic examination of the tumor specimen. Diagnosis of uterine leiomyosarcoma must include at least 2 of the following 3 criteria: diffuse nuclear atypia, increased mitotic rate, and coagulative necrosis.[82] Differential diagnosis with benign or borderline entities is occasionally challenging, because there is a continuum from benign forms to borderline disease to high-grade leiomyosarcoma, which sometimes makes it challenging to establish a univocal diagnosis. Standard surgical management for nonmetastatic disease is total abdominal hysterectomy with bilateral salpingo-oophorectomy, although in premenopausal women a simple hysterectomy without oophorectomy can be considered. Lymph node invasion is uncommon and lymphadenectomy is not shown to be useful in the absence of macroscopic involvement.[36,83] To date, no adjuvant treatment strategies have shown a survival benefit, and therefore adjuvant radiotherapy and chemotherapy are not recommended routinely.

Regarding adjuvant radiotherapy, a phase III clinical trial randomized surgically resected uterine sarcomas of stages I and II to either observation or pelvic radiation (51 Gy in 28 fractions over 5 weeks). 103 patients with leiomyosarcoma were recruited. Radiation therapy was shown to reduce significantly the local relapse rate, but without any impact on disease-free survival and overall survival.[84]

Adjuvant chemotherapy is being explored in uterine leiomyosarcoma because of its propensity for early hematogenous spread, leading to a high risk of systemic relapse.[85] Nonetheless, the role of adjuvant chemotherapy remains unclear. Adjuvant doxorubicin was compared with placebo in a phase II clinical trial that pooled 156 patients with different uterine sarcomas.[86] In the subgroup of patients with leiomyosarcoma (n = 48), the recurrence rate was 61% in the control arm compared with 44% among patients assigned to doxorubicin. The combination of fixed-dose gemcitabine plus docetaxel was studied in a single-arm, phase II study in 25 patients with uterine leiomyosarcomas, International Federation of Gynecology and Obstetrics (FIGO) stages I to IV. After 4 cycles of treatment, 45% of patients remained progression free at 2 years, with a median progression-free survival of 13 months.[87] A more recent phase II trial evaluated adjuvant gemcitabine plus docetaxel for 4 cycles, followed by doxorubicin for 4 cycles in patients with resected high-risk uterine leiomyosarcoma. After a median follow-up of 3 years, disease-free survival seems similar to that of historical controls who did not receive chemotherapy.[88] These results have led to the development of an ongoing phase III clinical trial that randomizes patients with FIGO stage I uterine leiomyosarcoma to observation or 4 cycles of docetaxel plus gemcitabine followed by 4 cycles of doxorubicin.

In advanced-stage or recurrent disease, treatment is palliative only. Current options comprise classic treatments such as doxorubicin or ifosfamide, which yield responses rates around 20%.[89,90] In recent years, 3 prospective phase II trials have led to the recommendation of the combination of fixed-dose-rate gemcitabine and docetaxel as first-line or second-line treatment of uterine leiomyosarcomas.[56,87,91] Response rate and median progression-free survival were 35.8% and 4.4 months, respectively, in the first-line treatment, and 27% and 5.4 months in the second-line treatment, respectively.

Trabectedin has shown comparable efficacy in leiomyosarcomas of different origins, including uterine leiomyosarcomas, with outcomes similar to those obtained with well-established agents such as doxorubicin, ifosfamide, and gemcitabine.[92] A later single-arm phase II clinical trial specifically assessed the efficacy of trabectedin in 20 chemonaive patients with uterine leiomyosarcoma. Two patients (10%) achieved a partial response, and 10 achieved disease stabilization (50%). Median progression-free survival and median overall survival were 5.8 months and greater than 26 months respectively.[93]

Other agents have been reported to show activity in uterine leiomyosarcomas and include single-agent gemcitabine,[94] temozolomide,[95] liposomal doxorubicin,[96] and etoposide.[97]

In addition, anecdotal case reports and 1 retrospective series have reported some benefit of antihormone therapies in patients with metastatic uterine leiomyosarcomas (reviewed by Amant and colleagues[3] in 2009). However, it is possible that there was some bias toward patients with a more favorable outcome, and so the effects observed might be caused by the particular tumor biology rather than a therapeutic effect of hormone therapy. Expression of estrogen and progesterone receptors is present in some high-grade uterine leiomyosarcomas, the relationship between expression and response to hormonal manipulation remains unclear.[98]

INFERIOR VENA CAVA LEIOMYOSARCOMAS

Leiomyosarcoma of the inferior vena cava (IVC) is an uncommon clinical entity that accounts for only about 0.5% of all adult soft tissue sarcomas.[99] Given its rarity, current knowledge is based on case reports and experience from single institutions. Leiomyosarcoma of IVC peaks in the sixth decade of life, and is predominantly observed in women, with a female/male ratio of about 3:1. The most common presenting symptom across several series is abdominal or flank pain. Other presenting signs and symptoms include abdominal distention, lower extremity edema, Budd-Chiari syndrome, and deep vein thrombosis.

Complete surgical resection constitutes the only curative procedure for localized primary tumor, which may also involve en bloc resection of adjacent organs. Complete macroscopic resection is the treatment with the greatest impact on survival and, accordingly, Hollenbeck and colleagues[99] claimed a 3-year overall survival rate of 76% for patients with IVC leiomyosarcoma managed in this manner, but a 0% survival for patients with incompletely excised tumors. Nonetheless, adequate surgery with negative margins remains a challenge because of the location of the tumor and the occasional involvement of vital structures such as right atrium or hepatic vessels.[100]

In addition, leiomyosarcomas of the IVC usually develop early relapse despite aggressive multimodality therapy, and often metastasize to liver and lungs. Single institutions, registries, and comprehensive literature reviews document a poor 5-year survival of between 33% and 68% for surgically treated patients with IVC leiomyosarcoma, with greater chances of superior survival for patients who undergo curative resections without documented macroscopic residual disease.[100,101]

REFERENCES

1. Howlader N, Noone AM, Krapcho M, et al, editors. SEER Cancer Statistics Review. Bethesda, MD: National Cancer Institute; 1975–2010. Available at: http://seer.cancer.gov/csr/1975_2010/. Accessed April, 2013.
2. Gustafson P. Soft tissue sarcoma. Epidemiology and prognosis in 508 patients. Acta Orthop Scand Suppl 1994;259:1–31.
3. Amant F, Coosemans A, Dbiec-Rychter M, et al. Clinical management of uterine sarcomas. Lancet Oncol 2009;10:1188–98.
4. Miettinen M. Smooth muscle tumors. In: Miettinen M, editor. Modern soft tissue pathology. 1st edition. New York: Cambridge University Press; 2010. p. 460–90.
5. Hashimoto H, Tsuneyoshi M, Enjoji M. Malignant smooth muscle tumors of the retroperitoneum and mesentery: a clinicopathologic analysis of 44 cases. J Surg Oncol 1985;28:177–86.
6. Fields JP, Helwig EB. Leiomyosarcoma of the skin and subcutaneous tissue. Cancer 1981;47:156–69.
7. McClain KL, Leach CT, Jenson HB, et al. Association of Epstein-Barr virus with leiomyosarcomas in children with AIDS. N Engl J Med 1995;332:12–8.
8. Robinson E, Neugut AI, Wylie P. Clinical aspects of postirradiation sarcomas. J Natl Cancer Inst 1988;80:233–40.
9. Weiss SW, Goldblum JR. Chapter 18. Leiomyosarcoma. In: Enzinger & Weiss's soft tissue tumors. 5th edition. Mosby, Elsevier; 2008. p. 545–64.
10. Kleinerman RA, Tucker MA, Abramson DH, et al. Risk of soft tissue sarcomas by individual subtype in survivors of hereditary retinoblastoma. J Natl Cancer Inst 2007;99:24–31.
11. Ognjanovic S, Olivier M, Bergemann TL, et al. Sarcomas in TP53 germline mutation carriers: a review of the IARC TP53 database. Cancer 2012;118:1387–96.
12. Chen E, O'Connell F, Fletcher CD. Dedifferentiated leiomyosarcoma: clinicopathological analysis of 18 cases. Histopathology 2011;59:1135–43.
13. Helman LJ, Meltzer P. Mechanisms of sarcoma development. Nat Rev Cancer 2003;3:685–94.
14. Wang R, Lu YJ, Fisher C, et al. Characterization of chromosome aberrations associated with soft-tissue leiomyosarcomas by twenty-four-color karyotyping and comparative genomic hybridization analysis. Genes Chromosomes Cancer 2001;31:54–64.

15. El-Rifai W, Sarlomo-Rikala M, Knuutila S, et al. DNA copy number changes in development and progression in leiomyosarcomas of soft tissues. Am J Pathol 1998;153:985–90.
16. Gibault L, Perot G, Chibon F, et al. New insights in sarcoma oncogenesis: a comprehensive analysis of a large series of 160 soft tissue sarcomas with complex genomics. J Pathol 2011;223:64–71.
17. Dei Tos AP, Maestro R, Doglioni C, et al. Tumor suppressor genes and related molecules in leiomyosarcoma. Am J Pathol 1996;148:1037–45.
18. Meza-Zepeda LA, Kresse SH, Barragan-Polania AH, et al. Array comparative genomic hybridization reveals distinct DNA copy number differences between gastrointestinal stromal tumors and leiomyosarcomas. Cancer Res 2006;66: 8984–93.
19. Yang J, Du X, Chen K, et al. Genetic aberrations in soft tissue leiomyosarcoma. Cancer Lett 2009;275:1–8.
20. Cordon-Cardo C, Latres E, Drobnjak M, et al. Molecular abnormalities of mdm2 and p53 genes in adult soft tissue sarcomas. Cancer Res 1994;54:794–9.
21. Beck AH, Lee CH, Witten DM, et al. Discovery of molecular subtypes in leiomyosarcoma through integrative molecular profiling. Oncogene 2010;29:845–54.
22. Mills AM, Beck AH, Montgomery KD, et al. Expression of subtype-specific group 1 leiomyosarcoma markers in a wide variety of sarcomas by gene expression analysis and immunohistochemistry. Am J Surg Pathol 2011;35:583–9.
23. Nielsen TO, West RB, Linn SC, et al. Molecular characterisation of soft tissue tumours: a gene expression study. Lancet 2002;359:1301–7.
24. Shan W, Akinfenwa PY, Savannah KB, et al. A small-molecule inhibitor targeting the mitotic spindle checkpoint impairs the growth of uterine leiomyosarcoma. Clin Cancer Res 2012;18:3352–65.
25. Brewer Savannah KJ, Demicco EG, Lusby K, et al. Dual targeting of mTOR and aurora-A kinase for the treatment of uterine leiomyosarcoma. Clin Cancer Res 2012;18:4633–45.
26. Hernando E, Charytonowicz E, Dudas ME, et al. The AKT-mTOR pathway plays a critical role in the development of leiomyosarcomas. Nat Med 2007;13:748–53.
27. Coindre JM, Terrier P, Guillou L, et al. Predictive value of grade for metastasis development in the main histologic types of adult soft tissue sarcomas: a study of 1240 patients from the French Federation of Cancer Centers Sarcoma Group. Cancer 2001;91:1914–26.
28. Pisters PW, Leung DH, Woodruff J, et al. Analysis of prognostic factors in 1,041 patients with localized soft tissue sarcomas of the extremities. J Clin Oncol 1996;14:1679–89.
29. Pautier P, Genestie C, Rey A, et al. Analysis of clinicopathologic prognostic factors for 157 uterine sarcomas and evaluation of a grading score validated for soft tissue sarcoma. Cancer 2000;88:1425–31.
30. Zagars GK, Ballo MT, Pisters PW, et al. Prognostic factors for patients with localized soft-tissue sarcoma treated with conservation surgery and radiation therapy: an analysis of 1225 patients. Cancer 2003;97:2530–43.
31. Kraft S, Fletcher CD. Atypical intradermal smooth muscle neoplasms: clinicopathologic analysis of 84 cases and a reappraisal of cutaneous "leiomyosarcoma". Am J Surg Pathol 2011;35:599–607.
32. Pierie JP, Betensky RA, Choudry U, et al. Outcomes in a series of 103 retroperitoneal sarcomas. Eur J Surg Oncol 2006;32:1235–41.
33. Anaya DA, Lev DC, Pollock RE. The role of surgical margin status in retroperitoneal sarcoma. J Surg Oncol 2008;98:607–10.

34. Temple LK, Brennan MF. The role of pulmonary metastasectomy in soft tissue sarcoma. Semin Thorac Cardiovasc Surg 2002;14:35–44.

35. Yang JC, Chang AE, Baker AR, et al. Randomized prospective study of the benefit of adjuvant radiation therapy in the treatment of soft tissue sarcomas of the extremity. J Clin Oncol 1998;16:197–203.

36. Demetri GD, Antonia S, Benjamin RS, et al. Soft tissue sarcoma. J Natl Compr Canc Netw 2010;8:630–74.

37. Grimer R, Judson I, Peake D, et al. Guidelines for the management of soft tissue sarcomas. Sarcoma 2010;2010:506182.

38. McBride SM, Raut CP, Lapidus M, et al. Locoregional recurrence after preoperative radiation therapy for retroperitoneal sarcoma: adverse impact of multifocal disease and potential implications of dose escalation. Ann Surg Oncol 2013; 20(7):2140–7.

39. van GM, van Oosterom AT, Oosterhuis JW, et al. Prognostic factors for the outcome of chemotherapy in advanced soft tissue sarcoma: an analysis of 2,185 patients treated with anthracycline-containing first-line regimens–a European Organization for Research and Treatment of Cancer Soft Tissue and Bone Sarcoma Group Study. J Clin Oncol 1999;17:150–7.

40. Krikelis D, Judson I. Role of chemotherapy in the management of soft tissue sarcomas. Expert Rev Anticancer Ther 2010;10:249–60.

41. Karavasilis V, Seddon BM, Ashley S, et al. Significant clinical benefit of first-line palliative chemotherapy in advanced soft-tissue sarcoma: retrospective analysis and identification of prognostic factors in 488 patients. Cancer 2008;112:1585–91.

42. van der Graaf WTA, Judson I, Verweij J, et al. Results of a randomized phase III trial (EORTC 62012) of single agent doxorubicin versus doxorubicin plus ifosfamide as first line chemotherapy for patients with advanced or metastatic soft tissue sarcoma: A survival study by the EORTC Soft Tissue and Bone Sarcoma Group. 2012 ESMO Congress. Abstract LBA7. Presented October 1, 2012.

43. Rahal AS, Cioffi A, Rahal C, et al. High-dose ifosfamide (HDI) in metastatic synovial sarcoma: the Institut Gustave Roussy experience. J Clin Oncol 2012; 30(suppl):[abstract 10044].

44. Le CA, Antoine E, Spielmann M, et al. High-dose ifosfamide: circumvention of resistance to standard-dose ifosfamide in advanced soft tissue sarcomas. J Clin Oncol 1995;13:1600–8.

45. Sleijfer S, Ouali M, van GM, et al. Prognostic and predictive factors for outcome to first-line ifosfamide-containing chemotherapy for adult patients with advanced soft tissue sarcomas: an exploratory, retrospective analysis on large series from the European Organization for Research and Treatment of Cancer-Soft Tissue and Bone Sarcoma Group (EORTC-STBSG). Eur J Cancer 2010;46:72–83.

46. Patel SR, Gandhi V, Jenkins J, et al. Phase II clinical investigation of gemcitabine in advanced soft tissue sarcomas and window evaluation of dose rate on gemcitabine triphosphate accumulation. J Clin Oncol 2001;19:3483–9.

47. Merimsky O, Meller I, Flusser G, et al. Gemcitabine in soft tissue or bone sarcoma resistant to standard chemotherapy: a phase II study. Cancer Chemother Pharmacol 2000;45:177–81.

48. Okuno S, Ryan LM, Edmonson JH, et al. Phase II trial of gemcitabine in patients with advanced sarcomas (E1797): a trial of the Eastern Cooperative Oncology Group. Cancer 2003;97:1969–73.

49. Svancarova L, Blay JY, Judson IR, et al. Gemcitabine in advanced adult soft-tissue sarcomas. A phase II study of the EORTC Soft Tissue and Bone Sarcoma Group. Eur J Cancer 2002;38:556–9.

50. Ferraresi V, Ciccarese M, Cercato MC, et al. Gemcitabine at fixed dose-rate in patients with advanced soft-tissue sarcomas: a mono-institutional phase II study. Cancer Chemother Pharmacol 2008;63:149–55.
51. Spath-Schwalbe E, Genvresse I, Koschuth A, et al. Phase II trial of gemcitabine in patients with pretreated advanced soft tissue sarcomas. Anticancer Drugs 2000;11:325–9.
52. van Hoesel QG, Verweij J, Catimel G, et al. Phase II study with docetaxel (Taxotere) in advanced soft tissue sarcomas of the adult. EORTC Soft Tissue and Bone Sarcoma Group. Ann Oncol 1994;5:539–42.
53. Verweij J, Lee SM, Ruka W, et al. Randomized phase II study of docetaxel versus doxorubicin in first- and second-line chemotherapy for locally advanced or metastatic soft tissue sarcomas in adults: a study of the European Organization for Research and Treatment of Cancer Soft Tissue and Bone Sarcoma Group. J Clin Oncol 2000;18:2081–6.
54. Anderson SE, Keohan ML, D'Adamo DR, et al. A retrospective analysis of vinorelbine chemotherapy for patients with previously treated soft-tissue sarcomas. Sarcoma 2006;2006:15947.
55. Garcia del Muro X, Lopez-Pousa A, Martin J, et al. A phase II trial of temozolomide as a 6-week, continuous, oral schedule in patients with advanced soft tissue sarcoma: a study by the Spanish Group for Research on Sarcomas. Cancer 2005;104:1706–12.
56. Hensley ML, Maki R, Venkatraman E, et al. Gemcitabine and docetaxel in patients with unresectable leiomyosarcoma: results of a phase II trial. J Clin Oncol 2002;20:2824–31.
57. Leu KM, Ostruszka LJ, Shewach D, et al. Laboratory and clinical evidence of synergistic cytotoxicity of sequential treatment with gemcitabine followed by docetaxel in the treatment of sarcoma. J Clin Oncol 2004;22:1706–12.
58. Bay JO, Ray-Coquard I, Fayette J, et al. Docetaxel and gemcitabine combination in 133 advanced soft-tissue sarcomas: a retrospective analysis. Int J Cancer 2006;119:706–11.
59. Maki RG, Wathen JK, Patel SR, et al. Randomized phase II study of gemcitabine and docetaxel compared with gemcitabine alone in patients with metastatic soft tissue sarcomas: results of sarcoma alliance for research through collaboration study 002 [corrected]. J Clin Oncol 2007;25:2755–63.
60. Pautier P, Floquet A, Penel N, et al. Randomized multicenter and stratified phase II study of gemcitabine alone versus gemcitabine and docetaxel in patients with metastatic or relapsed leiomyosarcomas: a Federation Nationale des Centres de Lutte Contre le Cancer (FNCLCC) French Sarcoma Group Study (TAXOGEM study). Oncologist 2012;17:1213–20.
61. Garcia-Del-Muro X, Lopez-Pousa A, Maurel J, et al. Randomized phase II study comparing gemcitabine plus dacarbazine versus dacarbazine alone in patients with previously treated soft tissue sarcoma: a Spanish Group for Research on Sarcomas study. J Clin Oncol 2011;29:2528–33.
62. Dileo P, Morgan JA, Zahrieh D, et al. Gemcitabine and vinorelbine combination chemotherapy for patients with advanced soft tissue sarcomas: results of a phase II trial. Cancer 2007;109:1863–9.
63. Garcia-Carbonero R, Supko JG, Manola J, et al. Phase II and pharmacokinetic study of ecteinascidin 743 in patients with progressive sarcomas of soft tissues refractory to chemotherapy. J Clin Oncol 2004;22:1480–90.
64. Le CA, Blay JY, Judson I, et al. Phase II study of ET-743 in advanced soft tissue sarcomas: a European Organisation for the Research and Treatment of Cancer

(EORTC) soft tissue and bone sarcoma group trial. J Clin Oncol 2005;23: 576–84.

65. Yovine A, Riofrio M, Blay JY, et al. Phase II study of ecteinascidin-743 in advanced pretreated soft tissue sarcoma patients. J Clin Oncol 2004;22: 890–9.

66. Demetri GD, Chawla SP, von MM, et al. Efficacy and safety of trabectedin in patients with advanced or metastatic liposarcoma or leiomyosarcoma after failure of prior anthracyclines and ifosfamide: results of a randomized phase II study of two different schedules. J Clin Oncol 2009;27:4188–96.

67. Samuels BL, Chawla S, Patel S, et al. Clinical outcomes and safety with trabectedin therapy in patients with advanced soft tissue sarcomas following failure of prior chemotherapy: results of a worldwide expanded access program study. Ann Oncol 2013;24(6):1703–9.

68. Garcia-Carbonero R, Supko JG, Maki RG, et al. Ecteinascidin-743 (ET-743) for chemotherapy-naive patients with advanced soft tissue sarcomas: multicenter phase II and pharmacokinetic study. J Clin Oncol 2005;23:5484–92.

69. D'Adamo DR, Anderson SE, Albritton K, et al. Phase II study of doxorubicin and bevacizumab for patients with metastatic soft-tissue sarcomas. J Clin Oncol 2005;23:7135–42.

70. George S, Merriam P, Maki RG, et al. Multicenter phase II trial of sunitinib in the treatment of nongastrointestinal stromal tumor sarcomas. J Clin Oncol 2009;27: 3154–60.

71. Maki RG, D'Adamo DR, Keohan ML, et al. Phase II study of sorafenib in patients with metastatic or recurrent sarcomas. J Clin Oncol 2009;27:3133–40.

72. Sleijfer S, Ray-Coquard I, Papai Z, et al. Pazopanib, a multikinase angiogenesis inhibitor, in patients with relapsed or refractory advanced soft tissue sarcoma: a phase II study from the European Organisation for Research and Treatment of Cancer-Soft Tissue and Bone Sarcoma Group (EORTC study 62043). J Clin Oncol 2009;27:3126–32.

73. van der Graaf WT, Blay JY, Chawla SP, et al. Pazopanib for metastatic soft-tissue sarcoma (PALETTE): a randomised, double-blind, placebo-controlled phase 3 trial. Lancet 2012;379:1879–86.

74. Chawla SP, Staddon AP, Baker LH, et al. Phase II study of the mammalian target of rapamycin inhibitor ridaforolimus in patients with advanced bone and soft tissue sarcomas. J Clin Oncol 2012;30:78–84.

75. Chawla SP, Blessing J, Ray-Coquard I, et al. Results of the phase III, placebo-controlled trial (SUCCEED) evaluating the mTOR inhibitor ridaforolimus (R) as maintenance therapy in advanced sarcoma patients (pts) following clinical benefit from prior standard cytotoxic chemotherapy (CT). J Clin Oncol 2011; 29:606s [abstract 10005].

76. Okuno S, Bailey H, Mahoney MR, et al. A phase 2 study of temsirolimus (CCI-779) in patients with soft tissue sarcomas: a study of the Mayo phase 2 consortium (P2C). Cancer 2011;117:3468–75.

77. O'Reilly KE, Rojo F, She QB, et al. mTOR inhibition induces upstream receptor tyrosine kinase signaling and activates Akt. Cancer Res 2006;66:1500–8.

78. Quek R, Wang Q, Morgan JA, et al. Combination mTOR and IGF-1R inhibition: phase I trial of everolimus and figitumumab in patients with advanced sarcomas and other solid tumors. Clin Cancer Res 2011;17:871–9.

79. Schwartz GK, Tap WD, Qin LX, et al. Cixutumumab and temsirolimus for patients with bone and soft-tissue sarcoma: a multicentre, open-label, phase 2 trial. Lancet Oncol 2013;14:371–82.

80. Harlow BL, Weiss NS, Lofton S. The epidemiology of sarcomas of the uterus. J Natl Cancer Inst 1986;76:399–402.
81. Raut CP, Nucci MR, Wang Q, et al. Predictive value of FIGO and AJCC staging systems in patients with uterine leiomyosarcoma. Eur J Cancer 2009;45: 2818–24.
82. Bell SW, Kempson RL, Hendrickson MR. Problematic uterine smooth muscle neoplasms. A clinicopathologic study of 213 cases. Am J Surg Pathol 1994; 18:535–58.
83. ESMO/European Sarcoma Network Working Group. Soft tissue and visceral sarcomas: ESMO Clinical Practice Guidelines for diagnosis, treatment and follow-up. Ann Oncol 2012;23(Suppl 7):vii92–9.
84. Reed NS, Mangioni C, Malmstrom H, et al. Phase III randomised study to evaluate the role of adjuvant pelvic radiotherapy in the treatment of uterine sarcomas stages I and II: an European Organisation for Research and Treatment of Cancer Gynaeco-logical Cancer Group study (protocol 55874). Eur J Cancer 2008;44:808–18.
85. Rose PG, Piver MS, Tsukada Y, et al. Patterns of metastasis in uterine sarcoma. An autopsy study. Cancer 1989;63:935–8.
86. Omura GA, Blessing JA, Major F, et al. A randomized clinical trial of adjuvant adriamycin in uterine sarcomas: a Gynecologic Oncology Group Study. J Clin Oncol 1985;3:1240–5.
87. Hensley ML, Ishill N, Soslow R, et al. Adjuvant gemcitabine plus docetaxel for completely resected stages I-IV high grade uterine leiomyosarcoma: results of a prospective study. Gynecol Oncol 2009;112:563–7.
88. Hensley ML, Wathen JK, Maki RG, et al. Adjuvant therapy for high-grade, uterus-limited leiomyosarcoma: results of a phase 2 trial (SARC 005). Cancer 2013;119:1555–61.
89. Omura GA, Major FJ, Blessing JA, et al. A randomized study of adriamycin with and without dimethyl triazenoimidazole carboxamide in advanced uterine sarcomas. Cancer 1983;52:626–32.
90. Sutton GP, Blessing JA, Barrett RJ, et al. Phase II trial of ifosfamide and mesna in leiomyosarcoma of the uterus: a Gynecologic Oncology Group study. Am J Obstet Gynecol 1992;166:556–9.
91. Hensley ML, Blessing JA, Mannel R, et al. Fixed-dose rate gemcitabine plus do-cetaxel as first-line therapy for metastatic uterine leiomyosarcoma: a Gyneco-logic Oncology Group phase II trial. Gynecol Oncol 2008;109:329–34.
92. Ray-Coquard I. An increasing role for trabectedin in gynecological cancers: efficacy in uterine sarcomas. Int J Gynecol Cancer 2011;21(Suppl 1):S3–5.
93. Monk BJ, Blessing JA, Street DG, et al. A phase II evaluation of trabectedin in the treatment of advanced, persistent, or recurrent uterine leiomyosarcoma: a gynecologic oncology group study. Gynecol Oncol 2012;124:48–52.
94. Look KY, Sandler A, Blessing JA, et al. Phase II trial of gemcitabine as second-line chemotherapy of uterine leiomyosarcoma: a Gynecologic Oncology Group (GOG) study. Gynecol Oncol 2004;92:644–7.
95. Anderson S, Aghajanian C. Temozolomide in uterine leiomyosarcomas. Gynecol Oncol 2005;98:99–103.
96. Sutton G, Blessing J, Hanjani P, et al. Phase II evaluation of liposomal doxoru-bicin (Doxil) in recurrent or advanced leiomyosarcoma of the uterus: a Gyneco-logic Oncology Group study. Gynecol Oncol 2005;96:749–52.
97. Slayton RE, Blessing JA, Angel C, et al. Phase II trial of etoposide in the man-agement of advanced and recurrent leiomyosarcoma of the uterus: a Gyneco-logic Oncology Group study. Cancer Treat Rep 1987;71:1303–4.

98. Leitao MM Jr, Hensley ML, Barakat RR, et al. Immunohistochemical expression of estrogen and progesterone receptors and outcomes in patients with newly diagnosed uterine leiomyosarcoma. Gynecol Oncol 2012;124:558–62.

99. Hollenbeck ST, Grobmyer SR, Kent KC, et al. Surgical treatment and outcomes of patients with primary inferior vena cava leiomyosarcoma. J Am Coll Surg 2003;197:575–9.

100. Ito H, Hornick JL, Bertagnolli MM, et al. Leiomyosarcoma of the inferior vena cava: survival after aggressive management. Ann Surg Oncol 2007;14:3534–41.

101. Laskin WB, Fanburg-Smith JC, Burke AP, et al. Leiomyosarcoma of the inferior vena cava: clinicopathologic study of 40 cases. Am J Surg Pathol 2010;34: 873–81.

Angiosarcomas and Other Sarcomas of Endothelial Origin

Angela Cioffi, MD[a,b], Sonia Reichert, MD[a],
Cristina R. Antonescu, MD[c], Robert G. Maki, MD, PhD, FACP[a,b,d],*

KEYWORDS

- Angiosarcoma • Epithelioid hemangioendothelioma • Vascular sarcoma
- Kaposi sarcoma • VEGF • KDR • FLT4 • Translocation • Organ transplant

KEY POINTS

- Vascular sarcomas are rare and collectively affect fewer than 600 people a year in the United States (incidence approximately 2/million).
- Because angiosarcomas, hemangioendotheliomas, and other vascular tumors have unique embryonal derivation, it is not surprising that they have a unique sensitivity pattern to chemotherapy agents.
- Surgery, when possible, remains the primary treatment for angiosarcomas.
- Adjuvant radiation for primary disease seems prudent for at least some angiosarcoma, given the high local-regional recurrence rate of these tumors. Angiosarcomas also have a high rate of metastasis, but it is not clear that adjuvant chemotherapy improves survival.
- Epithelioid hemangioendothelioma is a unique form of sarcoma often presenting as multifocal disease. Most patients can do well with observation alone, although a fraction of patients have more aggressive disease and have difficulties in both local control and metastatic disease.

Continued

Disclosures: R.G. Maki receives clinical research support from Morphotek/Eisai, Ziopharm, and Imclone/Lilly. He has also consulted for Eisai, Morphotek/Eisai, Imclone/Lilly, Taiho, Glaxo-SmithKline, Merck, Champions Biotechnology, and Pfizer. He has received speaker's fees from Novartis. He is an unpaid consultant for the Sarcoma Foundation of America, SARC: Sarcoma Alliance for Research through Collaboration, n-of-one, and 23 & me. C.R. Antonescu, A. Cioffi, and S. Reichert report no conflicts.
Research Support: NCI P01-CA47179, P50-CA14014 (C.R. Antonescu); Hyundai Hope on Wheels (R.G. Maki).
a Department of Medicine, Mount Sinai School of Medicine, 1 Gustave L. Levy Place, Box 1128, New York, NY 10029-6574, USA; b Department of Pediatrics, Mount Sinai School of Medicine, 1 Gustave L. Levy Place, Box 1128, New York, NY 10029-6574, USA; c Department of Pathology, Memorial Sloan-Kettering Cancer Center, 1275 York Avenue, New York, NY 10065, USA; d Tisch Cancer Institute, Mount Sinai School of Medicine, 1 Gustave L. Levy Place, Box 1128, New York, NY 10029-6574, USA
* Corresponding author.
E-mail address: bobmakimd@gmail.com

Hematol Oncol Clin N Am 27 (2013) 975–988
http://dx.doi.org/10.1016/j.hoc.2013.07.005
0889-8588/13/$ – see front matter © 2013 Elsevier Inc. All rights reserved.

hemonc.theclinics.com

Continued

- Anthracyclines, alkylating agents such as ifosfamide, are active against at least some vascular sarcomas. Angiosarcomas demonstrate a unique sensitivity to taxanes, and gemcitabine, vinorelbine, and vascular endothelial growth factor (VEGF) or vascular endothelial growth factor receptors (VEGFR) antagonists all have at least some activity against these tumors.
- New targets to consider for therapy include angiopoietin antagonists as well as inhibitors notch or ephrin signaling pathways.

INTRODUCTION

Of the 14,000 cases of sarcoma diagnosed in the United States annually, sarcomas arising from endothelium and other elements of blood vessels constitute ~2% to 3%, and thus it is likely that fewer than 600 people in the United States are affected each year.[1] This fact is surprising, given the common nature of the benign counterpart of these tumors, hemangiomas, arteriovenous malformations, and other lesions in the population.

In this review, examined are some of the unique characteristics and therapeutic options for patients with tumors that arise from endothelium or its precursors, highlighting the potential of new agents for these tumors. Given the activity of anti-angiogenic therapy in both vascular sarcomas and other cancers, new agents will have an impact on both vascular sarcomas and more common cancers.

SCOPE OF THE DIAGNOSES DISCUSSED

The World Health Organization (WHO) fascicle for soft tissue sarcomas was updated in 2013. The terminology for soft tissue vascular sarcomas is largely unchanged from the prior 2002 version. For bone vascular tumors, changes are anticipated to make terminology for both groups of vascular tumors more consistent. Technically, leiomyosarcoma could be considered vascular sarcomas, because they frequently arise from branches of veins, presumably from smooth muscle cells of blood vessels or their precursors, but they are not discussed here. For space considerations, also not addressed are other tumors that arise from other cellular structures associated with blood vessels (eg, solitary fibrous tumor or intimal sarcoma, each of which has unique biology and sensitivity to systemic therapeutics as well). Finally, there are also vascular components of other tumors such as angiomyolipoma, but these are also not discussed in this review.

DEMOGRAPHICS

Kaposi sarcoma (KS) is an AIDS (acquired immune deficiency syndrome)-defining diagnosis and happily has been observed less frequently, with the advent of newer generations of anti-retroviral therapy for people with human immunodeficiency virus (HIV) infections. KS also arises in approximately 1 in 200 patients with organ transplants due to immunosuppressive drugs. KS is also seen in an endemic form in patients from the Mediterranean basin and endemically in Africa and the Mideast as well. In the United States, what was a rare cancer became common with the advent of AIDS, with a peak incidence of 10 to 20/1000 HIV-positive patients per year in the United States, but an ~80% decrease with the broad use of multitargeted anti-retroviral therapy.[2] Nonetheless, KS remains more common than other vascular sarcomas.

Angiosarcoma may arise in any part of the body but is more common in soft tissue than in bone. The peak age of incidence seems to be the 7th decade, and men are affected more than women.[1] The head and neck area is probably the most common site of diagnosis, and the most common site of radiation-induced angiosarcoma development is the breast. With an increasing incidence of breast cancer, an increase in angiosarcoma of the breast has also been observed with a cumulative incidence of 0.9 per 1000 breast cancer cases over 15 years.[3] The median latency is 4 to 8 years after treatment.

In addition, it is worth noting that after rhabdomyosarcoma, angiosarcoma is likely the second most common sarcoma to arise from germ cell tumors.[4,5] In all, angiosarcoma and epithelioid hemangioendothelioma (EHE) represent under 2% to 3% of all sarcoma diagnoses.

Epithelioid hemangioendothelioma (EHE) is substantially less common than angiosarcoma, but given the more indolent nature of the tumor, there is a relatively larger prevalent population. It occurs in a younger population, with a peak incidence in the 4th to 5th decade.[6] Women seem to be affected more commonly than men. In a survey of EHE patients from an EHE support group, overall survival was 73% at 5 years.[7]

ANGIOGENESIS VERSUS VASCULOGENESIS AND THE GROWTH OF ENDOTHELIAL TUMORS

There is significant confusion in the literature regarding the terms vasculogenesis and angiogenesis. Vasculogenesis typically has been a term applied to de novo blood vessel formation during embryonic development. Conversely, classically, angiogenesis was described to be the formation of new capillaries by sprouting or splitting of preexisting vessels. In common oncological parlance today, angiogenesis is used to describe the growth of any new blood vessel of any size. It has been proposed that capillarogenesis is a more accurate term to describe the "universal formation of new capillaries, during development and in the adult, without any implications regarding possible underlying mechanisms, processes, or the cells that give rise to this outcome" and distinguishable from the growth and maturation of these smallest of vessels into larger ones.[8]

Clearly, KS, angiosarcomas, and hemangioendotheliomas fall into the categories of tumors of endothelial cells or their precursors. Clinicians see both nodular masses and superficial spreading versions of endothelial tumors (**Fig. 1**). Pathologists have described some microscopic features of cutaneous angiosarcomas as having areas that are more solid (which one can hypothesize as being local aggressiveness of the tumor) as well as a characteristic dissecting pattern among existing collagen bundles, which could be construed as an aberrant version of capillarogenesis. These features seem to correlate with the gross pictures of tumor growth. The dissecting features may also account for the very common marginal recurrence of these tumors after primary resection. The authors further hypothesize that the multifocal pattern of these tumors, seen in particular in some versions of EHE, may arise from an unusual pattern of self-seeding as described by Comen and colleagues and Kim and colleagues.[9,10]

Like angiosarcoma, KS is described as evolving between a patch stage, a plaque stage, and frankly nodular disease, again harkening to the pattern of growth seen in other endothelial tumors in which aberrant capillarogenesis is involved.

CAUSE OF SARCOMAS OF ENDOTHELIAL ORIGIN

The most common cause of angiosarcoma seems to be therapeutic radiation, which was a well-recognized cause of hepatic angiosarcoma in the era when the

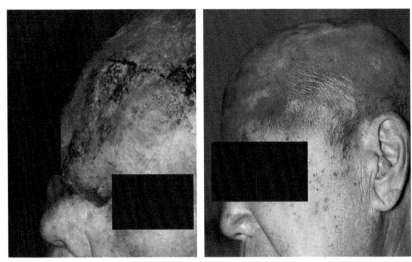

Fig. 1. Nodular (*left,* most notable on the bridge of the nose) and spreading (*right*) patterns of spread of cutaneous angiosarcoma of the head and neck.

thorium-containing contrast agent Thorotrast was used.[11] Presently, the breast is the most common anatomic site affected by radiation-induced angiosarcoma, raising the question of the use of lumpectomy and radiation for ductal carcinoma in situ, a noninvasive form of breast cancer in which this recommendation is often made in lieu of wide surgical resection.[3,12]

Angiosarcomas also arise after exposure to vinyl chloride, although they remain rare tumors even in an exposed population.[13,14] Angiosarcomas are also observed after lymphedema from any cause, be it surgical, filarial, or congenital, and carries the term Stewart-Treves syndrome from the pathologists who first described it.[15]

Whether arising in its epidemic HIV-associated form or endemic form, KS is caused by human herpesvirus-8 (HHV8), a γ-2 herpesvirus also termed Kaposi sarcoma herpesvirus. HHV8 functions at least in part through stimulation of chemokines, a viral version of interleukin-6, and anti-apoptotic proteins for its growth and transmission.[16–19] The role of microRNA networks in its propagation as well as change from latent to lytic state is under scrutiny.[20]

GENETIC CHANGES IN ENDOTHELIAL-BASED SARCOMAS

Specific sarcomas of endothelial derivation are described in **Table 1**, along with genetic alterations observed for each subtype. The specifics of HHV8 biology are beyond the scope of this review, but point to specific genes that may be important in the conversion of an endothelial cell to a sarcoma cell, for example, cyclin D homologues and a G-protein-coupled receptor.[21] Also not discussed here are the very interesting findings with respect to genetic knockout mice and vascular development; arteriovenous malformations arise in several of these mice and understanding of these pathways could affect therapy for patients with vascular sarcomas.[22–24]

Angiosarcomas are largely aneuploid tumors, which for at least some of them makes sense, given their association with therapeutic irradiation. Because there are only rare cases of angiosarcomas that seem to arise from a benign lesion such as a hemangioma,[25] the pathway leading to the 2 types of vascular lesions seems distinct, although clearly a genetic examination of such rare compound lesions would be of

Table 1
Genetics of sarcomas of apparent endothelial cell origin

Histology	Characteristic Genetic Changes/etiology
Kaposi sarcoma	HHV-8/Kaposi sarcoma herpesvirus
Angiosarcoma	MYC amplification (in radiation-induced angiosarcoma more than primary angiosarcoma) KDR/VEGFR2 mutations, FLT4/VEGFR3 amplifications (frequency well under 50%)
Epithelioid hemangioendothelioma	t(1;3) (p36.3;q25) WWTR1-CAMTA1 (more common) t(X;11) (p11.23;q22.1) YAP1-TFE3
Pseudomyogenic hemangioendothelioma	t(7;19) (q22;q13); frequency unknown

Data from Refs.[19,20,26–28,30–34,41,77,82–84]

great interest to understand angiosarcomagenesis. ERG (ETS [E twenty six]-related gene) is overexpressed in most angiosarcomas as well as other benign and malignant vascular tumors and seems to be a consistent endothelial lineage marker.[26] MYC amplification seems to be more common in secondary than primary angiosarcomas.[27–29] miR17-92 seems to be up-regulated with MYC in radiation-induced angiosarcomas as well, with concurrent downregulation of anti-angiogenic gene THBS1.[27] KDR mutation and FLT4 amplification have been observed in a fraction of angiosarcomas.[28,30] There does not sem to be a correlation between mutation status and outcome with vascular endothelial growth factors (VEGFs).

EHE has been found to be associated with the t(1;3) (p36.3;q25) WWTR1-CAMTA1 translocation,[31,32] and less commonly t(X;11) (p11.23;q22.1) YAP1-TFE3.[33] WWTR1, also called TAZ, is a gene involved in 14-3-3 transcriptional factor activation and signaling in the hippo pathway that is normally highly expressed in endothelial cells. CAMTA1 is part of a family of calmodulin-binding transcription activators, normally found only in brain. YAP1 is another gene in the hippo pathway, thus closely EHE to hippo signaling in all cases examined to date. These fusions are not directly targetable with present day therapeutics but may reveal downstream targets. Of note, the multiple lesions examined from a single patient all seem to have the same translocation, providing evidence that this is a matter of tumor metastasis or self-seeding at an early stage of development.[34]

PATHOLOGIC ABNORMALITY OF ENDOTHELIAL TUMORS

All angiosarcomas are presently considered high-grade neoplasms, regardless of degree of vascular differentiation or cytology, save primary breast angiosarcomas, where the Rosen 3-tier grading scheme is used. The concept angiosarcoma grading was challenged in one analysis of what was largely consultation material. In this study of 49 patients Rosen grade was not prognostic, in keeping with outcomes from other primary sites of disease.[35]

As noted above, angiosarcomas demonstrate a dissecting pattern of blood vessel formation and bear the endothelial markers characteristic of this cell lineage. There are variations of the histology based on anatomic site, with cutaneous lesions demonstrating dissecting and solid patterns of growth, and some tumors of visceral origin more commonly displaying epithelioid features. In comparison to benign lesions, areas with multilayered endothelial growth are characteristic of angiosarcoma, and there is at least some evidence of cytologic atypia. Mitotic rate is variable, but greater than that seen for hemangiomas.

Immunohistochemical markers for angiosarcoma include CD31, ERG, and CD34, among others. Although FLT4/vascular endothelial growth factor receptor3 was proposed as a lymphatic-specific marker based on in situ hybridization in developing mice,[36] a significant number of angiosarcomas express one or more lymphatic markers, without direct correlation with FLT4 gene amplification.[28] It is hoped that work on the association of ephrin B2 and EphB4 expression in arterial versus venous development will shed some light on this fundamental issue regarding the nature of these tumors.[37–40]

EHE are characterized by endothelial cells arranged in single files, nest, or more solid growth, and distinct lack of vessel formation that is characteristic of angiosarcomas. Intracytoplasmic vacuoles are often seen, and some of these may have red blood cells in them as well. Like angiosarcomas, EHE are positive for CD31, CD34, and ERG, and often are keratin positive.

KS usually shows a greater number of spindle-shaped cells than angiosarcoma and also forms vascular channels containing red blood cells, like angiosarcoma. Lymphoplasmacytic infiltrates may be observed. Eosinophilic hyaline inclusions can be observed in more advanced lesions. Although CD31 and CD34 immunohistochemicals are also common in KS, HHV8 latent nuclear antigen-1 is only positive in KS and not in the other diagnoses.

The 2013 WHO classification adds the unifying entity pseudomyogenic hemangioendothelioma, which has also been called epithelioid sarcoma-like hemangioendothelioma.[41–43] It will be included in the "rarely metastasizing" category of the WHO soft tissue sarcoma classification. Like EHE, it can be multifocal, and at least some cases are associated with a t(7;19) (q22;q13) translocation, distinct from other forms of hemangioendothelioma described above. There are presently no data regarding chemotherapy sensitivity of this unique vascular sarcoma subtype.

PRIMARY THERAPY
Kaposi Sarcoma

For KS, observation alone, in particular in someone with improving CD4 counts after the institution of anti-retroviral therapy, seems prudent except for those patients with obvious symptoms. For transplant-related KS patients cautious decrease or withdrawal of immunosuppressive therapy is often effective, but this benefit comes at the risk of allograft rejection.[44,45] The switch of the immunosuppressive regimen from calcineurin inhibitors to target rapamycin inhibitor sirolimus has been reported to induce significant regression of KS lesions.[45,46]

KS lesions are usually not isolated, and thus "primary therapy" takes on a different tone. Intralesional chemotherapy such as vinblastine can be used for symptomatic isolated lesions,[47,48] as can topical retinoids. Radiation therapy is usually used as primary therapy disease that is symptomatic and too extensive to treat with more localized treatments.

Angiosarcoma and EHE

When feasible, primary treatment of angiosarcoma or EHE is surgical. However, for the relatively common site of head and neck it is not uncommon to encounter unresectable disease that covers too large an area of the scalp to treat surgically, in which case electron beam radiation sometimes can be used for local control. In the situation of radiation-induced angiosarcoma of the breast, the local recurrence risk of these lesions highlights the need for resection of irradiated parenchyma and skin as primary therapy to attempt to improve the local control rate.[3,49]

For primary therapy of EHE or angiosarcoma involving the liver, embolization can be useful, taking advantage of the differences between tumor and normal tissue tolerance for hypoxia. Shamefully, there remain no comparative data on chemoembolization versus bland embolization, despite thousands of patients with a variety of diagnoses being treated with either modality.

After primary therapy for angiosarcoma (or potentially EHE in the correct anatomic location), general principles regarding adjuvant therapy in sarcoma apply, with some caveats. If an angiosarcoma was caused by radiation, it is oftentimes not possible to administer adjuvant radiation. In some cases a way to boost local doses of radiation can be considered, such as brachytherapy, but these are considered on a case-by-case basis.

In terms of adjuvant chemotherapy, the low response rate to chemotherapy in EHE makes it a relatively unattractive prospect. In addition, the small number of people with localized disease with EHE at presentation makes this clinical situation uncommon.

As for adjuvant chemotherapy for angiosarcoma, meta-analysis data indicate that patients with unselected sarcomas have a survival benefit from ifosfamide-based chemotherapy.[50] However, for the few positive individual studies over the last few decades of adjuvant therapy in soft tissue sarcomas, there are multiple negative individual studies, including the largest such randomized study,[51] making the recommendation of adjuvant anthracycline-ifosfamide a difficult decision. As with all clinical decision-making in which there are conflicting data, decisions should be made on a patient-by-patient basis.

TREATMENT OF RECURRENT DISEASE BY DIAGNOSIS
Kaposi Sarcoma

As noted below for angiosarcoma, anthracyclines and taxanes both demonstrate significant activity in KS. Chemotherapy is generally used for more extensive skin disease, edema, visceral disease, and disease not responding to local therapy. PEGylated liposomal doxorubicin (PLD; Doxil/Caelyx) showed a greater response rate and less toxicity than a combination of vincristine, doxorubicin, and bleomycin in 2 studies, and thus is a good standard of care.[52,53] Liposomal daunorubicin was also shown similar to a combination of vincristine, doxorubicin, and bleomycin in terms of response rate and median survival and is another potential option.[54] In a small study (n = 60), PLD was more active than liposomal daunorubicin, giving further support for its use.[55]

Taxanes also have activity in KS. There are concerns about the interaction of antiretroviral agents and cytochrome p450 metabolism, so care should be taken in their use. In one poorly accruing randomized study (n = 73 evaluable), clinical outcomes were similar with PLD 20 mg/m^2 IV every 3 weeks versus paclitaxel at a dose of 100 mg/m^2 IV every 2 weeks.[56] For patients for whom PLD is not a good option, paclitaxel or other agents such as docetaxel[57] or the yet to be tested nab-paclitaxel may be reasonable second-line options for treatment.

Other agents with some activity in KS include vinorelbine,[58] bevacizumab,[59] or sirolimus[60] (at very low doses due to pharmacokinetic interactions). However, given the lack of data on newer agents, clinical trials are advisable in advanced disease.

Angiosarcoma

Angiosarcoma is one of the few sarcoma diagnoses with a significant response rate to taxanes,[61] as had been noted previously with KS. In a similar fashion, PLD was shown to have activity in angiosarcoma,[62] with less toxicity than that of standard doxorubicin.

A single-center review demonstrated that anthracyclines had slightly greater activity than taxanes.[63] However, prospective studies in angiosarcoma patients have been few and far between. There are no prospective studies of anthracyclines treating angiosarcoma specifically, although there are data from studies involving multiple sarcoma histologies that anthracyclines and/or ifosfamide have activity in angiosarcoma patients (eg, the phase II study of mitomycin-doxorubicin-cisplatin showing 3 of 4 angiosarcoma patients with responses).[64]

Paclitaxel was studied in France in 30 patients, using 80 mg/m^2 IV on days 1, 8, and 15 of a 28-day cycle. The aggressiveness of advanced disease was highlighted by the median time to progression of 4 months and median overall survival of 8 months. For other cytotoxic agents, after small numbers of patients with angiosarcoma in all-sarcoma phase II studies, Stacchiotti and colleagues[65] examined the experience with gemcitabine in a traditional 1000 mg/m^2 schedule days 1, 8, and 15 every 28 days in 25 angiosarcoma patients across several centers in Italy, showing a median progression-free survival (PFS) of 7 months and median overall survival of 17 months. Radiation-induced angiosarcomas seemed to fare as well to therapy as those that arose spontaneously. There are anecdotal data that the combination of gemcitabine-docetaxel is active in angiosarcoma, but it is not clear if it is any more active than, for example, sequential therapy with the 2 agents. Given the relatively short PFS for people on systemic therapy in general, this seems a difficult proposition to prove.

As part of a multi-arm phase II study, Maki and colleagues[66] showed 5 of 37 angiosarcoma patients with Response Evaluation Criteria in Solid Tumors (RECIST) responses to oral daily sorafenib. Median PFS was 3.8 months, and overall survival was 14.9 months for the angiosarcoma patients. These data were quite different from the French experience with sorafenib, in which 26 patients with superficial tumors and 15 with visceral angiosarcomas were enrolled. The median PFS times for cutaneous and visceral disease were 1.8 months and 3.8 months, respectively, and median overall survival times were 12.0 months and 9.0 months, respectively.[67] The reasons for the differences between the 2 studies remain unclear. Differences between specific kinase inhibitors were also highlighted by the SARC001 study, in which there were only 2 patients of 16 treated who did not progress within 16 weeks of starting therapy.[68] Bevacizumab has also been examined prospectively and was shown to have a 15% response rate in 30 evaluable patients with angiosarcoma (n = 23) or EHE (n = 7) in a phase II study.[69] Median PFS was 12 weeks, whereas median overall survival was 52.7 weeks in the angiosarcoma population.

Epithelioid Hemangioendothelioma

The rarity of EHE has led to little prospective evaluation of this diagnosis in clinical trials. The Agulnik study is the only one to prospectively capture these patients properly, showing median PFS and overall survival of 7 patients of 39.1 and 142.6 weeks, respectively.[69] These data highlight the much more indolent nature of this diagnosis in some patients, with liver or other organ failure in a significant proportion of patients. The authors have observed anecdotal responses to single agents, but no consistent pattern of activity, of PLD, doxorubicin, ifosfamide, vinorelbine, sorafenib, pazopanib, or other agents. For example, a patient on oral cyclophosphamide and prednisolone achieved a complete response,[70] but the authors have been unable to replicate this finding on a consistent basis. In treating a large number of patients with a variety of agents, Stacchiotti and colleagues[71] have found activity of sirolimus in EHE, making this an interesting agent to consider even as first-line therapy, given the lack of consistent responses with other agents. Sirolimus is also an obvious choice of immunosuppressant in patients who have liver transplant for liver-predominant EHE.

For EHE involving the liver, even in the setting of metastasis-proven disease in other organs such as lung, liver transplant is an option for continued survival in the setting of a failing liver if the disease is indolent enough over time. Of course, this means the use of anti-rejection drugs and attendant complications thereafter, but in the proper clinical setting, such a procedure can be life-extending. An evaluation by a liver transplant team during a patient's course is advisable; however, transplant should not be considered as primary therapy for EHE of the liver, because a substantial proportion of patients can have indolent disease that evolves only slowly over a decade or more; the 5-year survival rate in one small series was 67%.[72] Furthermore, recurrence of EHE is common in the transplanted liver.[73,74] It would be a waste to discard a patient's liver that is still even somewhat functional by rushing to liver transplant. The success rate of liver transplant in the literature does not take into account the long survival of patients with primary disease.

EMERGING THERAPEUTIC OPTIONS

Local therapy also may be improving for patients with angiosarcoma or EHE in an end organ. Yttrium 90 is an electron emitter with a 64-hour half-life and has been used in primary hepatocellular carcinoma with some success. Selective internal radiotherapy with Yttrium 90 microspheres is a way to deliver radiation therapy in a measured way to the liver and is a possible consideration for EHE or angiosarcoma metastatic to liver or other end organ, although there are no prospective data available.

A variety of developments in biology may have an impact on angiogenesis in cancer and thus also have an impact on treatment of endothelial tumors such as angiosarcoma. Advances in the developmental biology of blood vessel formation point out new pathways that may be worth pursuing as therapies for KS, angiosarcoma, or EHE.

The finding of the importance of ephrin signaling and the notch pathway in the development of vasculature gives hope that inhibitors of these pathways will be useful.[75–77] Dasatinib is an inhibitor of at least one of the very complex family of ephrins/Eph signaling pathways and has not been examined in detail in angiosarcoma, for example. Unfortunately, γ-secretase inhibitors, which represent one mechanism to block notch signaling, essentially have been abandoned as of 2013 for study in solid tumors. Agents that attack other important steps in angiogenesis are under study as well, such as inhibitors of angiopoietin signaling via receptor TIE2.[78] Given the differences in mechanism of action compared with small molecule tyrosine kinase inhibitors, antibodies to VEGF or platelet-derived growth factor receptors could provide activity alone or in combination with these other agents, trying to mimic the concept of early aggressive blockade of a tyrosine kinase signaling pathways (eg, HER2 in breast cancer, BRAF and MEK in melanoma) to achieve better tumor control.[79–81] Looking for general principles that will apply to more than one type of cancer is one strategy to insure patients with common and rare diseases alike may benefit from new therapeutic strategies.

PERSPECTIVE

Elegant basic science studies of vertebrate development have led to a greater appreciation of the differences between arteries, veins, and lymphatics. These data inform thinking regarding the yin and yang of therapeutic angiogenesis in cardiac disease versus anti-angiogenic therapy in cancer. Given only modest benefit of existing agents in metastatic endothelial tumors such as KS, EHE, and angiosarcoma, these developmental and other mechanistic pathways, such as signaling downstream from ERG or MYC, aim to help guide future generations of studies of this diverse group of sarcomas. Because proportions of patients respond to therapy directed at the VEGF axis, there are clearly differences in the VEGF dependence of this family of tumors. Perhaps by reconstructing downstream signaling pathways in patient material, it will be bests to discern circumstances in which receptor or downstream signaling inhibitors will benefit patients most.

REFERENCES

1. Brennan MF, Antonescu CR, Maki RG. Management of soft tissue sarcoma. New York: Springer; 2013.
2. Semeere AS, Busakhala N, Martin JN. Impact of antiretroviral therapy on the incidence of Kaposi's sarcoma in resource-rich and resource-limited settings. Curr Opin Oncol 2012;24(5):522–30.
3. Seinen JM, Styring E, Verstappen V, et al. Radiation-associated angiosarcoma after breast cancer: high recurrence rate and poor survival despite surgical treatment with R0 resection. Ann Surg Oncol 2012;19(8):2700–6.
4. Contreras AL, Punar M, Tamboli P, et al. Mediastinal germ cell tumors with an angiosarcomatous component: a report of 12 cases. Hum Pathol 2010;41(6):832–7.
5. Malagon HD, Valdez AM, Moran CA, et al. Germ cell tumors with sarcomatous components: a clinicopathologic and immunohistochemical study of 46 cases. Am J Surg Pathol 2007;31(9):1356–62.
6. Miettinen M, editor. Modern soft tissue pathology: tumors and non-neoplastic conditions. 1st edition. Cambridge (UK): Cambridge University Press; 2010.
7. Lau K, Massad M, Pollak C, et al. Clinical patterns and outcome in epithelioid hemangioendothelioma with or without pulmonary involvement: insights from an internet registry in the study of a rare cancer. Chest 2011;140(5):1312–8.
8. Kovacic JC, Moore J, Herbert A, et al. Endothelial progenitor cells, angioblasts, and angiogenesis–old terms reconsidered from a current perspective. Trends Cardiovasc Med 2008;18(2):45–51.
9. Comen E, Norton L, Massague J. Clinical implications of cancer self-seeding. Nat Rev Clin Oncol 2011;8(6):369–77.
10. Kim MY, Oskarsson T, Acharyya S, et al. Tumor self-seeding by circulating cancer cells. Cell 2009;139(7):1315–26.
11. Lipshutz GS, Brennan TV, Warren RS. Thorotrast-induced liver neoplasia: a collective review. J Am Coll Surg 2002;195(5):713–8.
12. Buchholz TA, Theriault RL, Niland JC, et al. The use of radiation as a component of breast conservation therapy in National Comprehensive Cancer Network Centers. J Clin Oncol 2006;24(3):361–9.
13. Marion MJ, Boivin-Angele S. Vinyl chloride-specific mutations in humans and animals. IARC Sci Publ 1999;150:315–24.
14. Elliott P, Kleinschmidt I. Angiosarcoma of the liver in Great Britain in proximity to vinyl chloride sites. Occup Environ Med 1997;54(1):14–8.
15. Stewart FW, Treves N. Lymphangiosarcoma in postmastectomy lymphedema; a report of six cases in elephantiasis chirurgica. Cancer 1948;1(1):64–81.
16. Giraldo G, Beth E, Coeur P, et al. Kaposi's sarcoma: a new model in the search for viruses associated with human malignancies. J Natl Cancer Inst 1972;49(6): 1495–507.
17. Cai Q, Verma SC, Lu J, et al. Molecular biology of Kaposi's sarcoma-associated herpesvirus and related oncogenesis. In: Maramorosch K, Shatkin AJ, Murphy FA, editors. Advances in virus research, vol. 78. London UK: Academic Press; 2010. p. 87–142.

18. Chang Y, Cesarman E, Pessin MS, et al. Identification of herpesvirus-like DNA sequences in AIDS-associated Kaposi's sarcoma. Science 1994;266(5192): 1865–9.
19. Russo JJ, Bohenzky RA, Chien MC, et al. Nucleotide sequence of the Kaposi sarcoma-associated herpesvirus (HHV8). Proc Natl Acad Sci U S A 1996; 93(25):14862–7.
20. Dahlke C, Maul K, Christalla T, et al. A microRNA encoded by Kaposi sarcoma-associated herpesvirus promotes b-cell expansion in vivo. PLoS One 2012; 7(11):e49435.
21. Cesarman E, Nador RG, Bai F, et al. Kaposi's sarcoma-associated herpesvirus contains G protein-coupled receptor and cyclin D homologs which are expressed in Kaposi's sarcoma and malignant lymphoma. J Virol 1996;70(11):8218–23.
22. Mahmoud M, Allinson KR, Zhai Z, et al. Pathogenesis of arteriovenous malformations in the absence of endoglin. Circ Res 2010;106(8):1425–33.
23. Krebs LT, Starling C, Chervonsky AV, et al. Notch1 activation in mice causes arteriovenous malformations phenocopied by ephrinB2 and EphB4 mutants. Genesis 2010;48(3):146–50.
24. Urness LD, Sorensen LK, Li DY. Arteriovenous malformations in mice lacking activin receptor-like kinase-1. Nat Genet 2000;26(3):328–31.
25. Rossi S, Fletcher CD. Angiosarcoma arising in hemangioma/vascular malformation: report of four cases and review of the literature. Am J Surg Pathol 2002; 26(10):1319–29.
26. McKay KM, Doyle LA, Lazar AJ, et al. Expression of ERG, an Ets family transcription factor, distinguishes cutaneous angiosarcoma from histological mimics. Histopathology 2012;61(5):989–91.
27. Italiano A, Thomas R, Breen M, et al. The miR-17-92 cluster and its target THBS1 are differentially expressed in angiosarcomas dependent on MYC amplification. Genes Chromosomes Cancer 2012;51(6):569–78.
28. Guo T, Zhang L, Chang NE, et al. Consistent MYC and FLT4 gene amplification in radiation-induced angiosarcoma but not in other radiation-associated atypical vascular lesions. Genes Chromosomes Cancer 2011;50(1):25–33.
29. Manner J, Radlwimmer B, Hohenberger P, et al. MYC high level gene amplification is a distinctive feature of angiosarcomas after irradiation or chronic lymphedema. Am J Pathol 2010;176(1):34–9.
30. Antonescu CR, Yoshida A, Guo T, et al. KDR activating mutations in human angiosarcomas are sensitive to specific kinase inhibitors. Cancer Res 2009; 69(18):7175–9.
31. Tanas MR, Sboner A, Oliveira AM, et al. Identification of a disease-defining gene fusion in epithelioid hemangioendothelioma. Sci Transl Med 2011;3(98):98ra82.
32. Errani C, Zhang L, Sung YS, et al. A novel WWTR1-CAMTA1 gene fusion is a consistent abnormality in epithelioid hemangioendothelioma of different anatomic sites. Genes Chromosomes Cancer 2011;50(8):644–53.
33. Antonescu CR, Le Loarer F, Mosquera JM, et al. Novel YAP1-TFE3 fusion defines a distinct subset of epithelioid hemangioendothelioma. Genes Chromosomes Cancer 2013;52(8):775–84.
34. Errani C, Sung YS, Zhang L, et al. Monoclonality of multifocal epithelioid hemangioendothelioma of the liver by analysis of WWTR1-CAMTA1 breakpoints. Cancer Genet 2012;205(1–2):12–7.
35. Nascimento AF, Raut CP, Fletcher CD. Primary angiosarcoma of the breast: clinicopathologic analysis of 49 cases, suggesting that grade is not prognostic. Am J Surg Pathol 2008;32(12):1896–904.

36. Kaipainen A, Korhonen J, Mustonen T, et al. Expression of the fms-like tyrosine kinase 4 gene becomes restricted to lymphatic endothelium during development. Proc Natl Acad Sci U S A 1995;92(8):3566–70.

37. Wang Y, Nakayama M, Pitulescu ME, et al. Ephrin-B2 controls VEGF-induced angiogenesis and lymphangiogenesis. Nature 2010;465(7297):483–6.

38. Wang HU, Chen ZF, Anderson DJ. Molecular distinction and angiogenic interaction between embryonic arteries and veins revealed by ephrin-B2 and its receptor Eph-B4. Cell 1998;93(5):741–53.

39. Shin D, Garcia-Cardena G, Hayashi S, et al. Expression of ephrinB2 identifies a stable genetic difference between arterial and venous vascular smooth muscle as well as endothelial cells, and marks subsets of microvessels at sites of adult neovascularization. Dev Biol 2001;230(2):139–50.

40. Gerety SS, Wang HU, Chen ZF, et al. Symmetrical mutant phenotypes of the receptor EphB4 and its specific transmembrane ligand ephrin-B2 in cardiovascular development. Mol Cell 1999;4(3):403–14.

41. Trombetta D, Magnusson L, von Steyern FV, et al. Translocation t(7;19)(q22;q13)-a recurrent chromosome aberration in pseudomyogenic hemangioendothelioma? Cancer Genet 2011;204(4):211–5.

42. Hornick JL, Fletcher CD. Pseudomyogenic hemangioendothelioma: a distinctive, often multicentric tumor with indolent behavior. Am J Surg Pathol 2011; 35(2):190–201.

43. Billings SD, Folpe AL, Weiss SW. Epithelioid sarcoma-like hemangioendothelioma. Am J Surg Pathol 2003;27(1):48–57.

44. Riva G, Luppi M, Barozzi P, et al. How I treat HHV8/KSHV-related diseases in posttransplant patients. Blood 2012;120(20):4150–9.

45. Stallone G, Schena A, Infante B, et al. Sirolimus for Kaposi's sarcoma in renal-transplant recipients. N Engl J Med 2005;352(13):1317–23.

46. Monaco AP. The role of mTOR inhibitors in the management of posttransplant malignancy. Transplantation 2009;87(2):157–63.

47. Epstein JB. Treatment of oral Kaposi sarcoma with intralesional vinblastine. Cancer 1993;71(5):1722–5.

48. Tucker SB, Winkelmann RK. Treatment of Kaposi sarcoma with vinblastine. Arch Dermatol 1976;112(7):958–61.

49. Morgan EA, Kozono DE, Wang Q, et al. Cutaneous radiation-associated angiosarcoma of the breast: poor prognosis in a rare secondary malignancy. Ann Surg Oncol 2012;19(12):3801–8.

50. Pervaiz N, Colterjohn N, Farrokhyar F, et al. A systematic meta-analysis of randomized controlled trials of adjuvant chemotherapy for localized resectable soft-tissue sarcoma. Cancer 2008;113(3):573–81.

51. Woll PJ, Reichardt P, Le Cesne A, et al. Adjuvant chemotherapy with doxorubicin, ifosfamide, and lenograstim for resected soft-tissue sarcoma (EORTC 62931): a multicentre randomised controlled trial. Lancet Oncol 2012;13(10): 1045–54.

52. Northfelt DW, Dezube BJ, Thommes JA, et al. Pegylated-liposomal doxorubicin versus doxorubicin, bleomycin, and vincristine in the treatment of AIDS-related Kaposi's sarcoma: results of a randomized phase III clinical trial. J Clin Oncol 1998;16(7):2445–51.

53. Stewart S, Jablonowski H, Goebel FD, et al. Randomized comparative trial of pegylated liposomal doxorubicin versus bleomycin and vincristine in the treatment of AIDS-related Kaposi's sarcoma. International Pegylated Liposomal Doxorubicin Study Group. J Clin Oncol 1998;16(2):683–91.

54. Gill PS, Wernz J, Scadden DT, et al. Randomized phase III trial of liposomal daunorubicin versus doxorubicin, bleomycin, and vincristine in AIDS-related Kaposi's sarcoma. J Clin Oncol 1996;14(8):2353–64.

55. Cooley T, Henry D, Tonda M, et al. A randomized, double-blind study of pegylated liposomal doxorubicin for the treatment of AIDS-related Kaposi's sarcoma. Oncologist 2007;12(1):114–23.

56. Cianfrocca M, Lee S, Von Roenn J, et al. Randomized trial of paclitaxel versus pegylated liposomal doxorubicin for advanced human immunodeficiency virus-associated Kaposi sarcoma: evidence of symptom palliation from chemotherapy. Cancer 2010;116(16):3969–77.

57. Lim ST, Tupule A, Espina BM, et al. Weekly docetaxel is safe and effective in the treatment of advanced-stage acquired immunodeficiency syndrome-related Kaposi sarcoma. Cancer 2005;103(2):417–21.

58. Nasti G, Errante D, Talamini R, et al. Vinorelbine is an effective and safe drug for AIDS-related Kaposi's sarcoma: results of a phase II study. J Clin Oncol 2000; 18(7):1550–7.

59. Uldrick TS, Wyvill KM, Kumar P, et al. Phase II study of bevacizumab in patients with HIV-associated Kaposi's sarcoma receiving antiretroviral therapy. J Clin Oncol 2012;30(13):1476–83.

60. Krown SE, Roy D, Lee JY, et al. Rapamycin with antiretroviral therapy in AIDS-associated Kaposi sarcoma: an AIDS Malignancy Consortium study. J Acquir Immune Defic Syndr 2012;59(5):447–54.

61. Fata F, O'Reilly E, Ilson D, et al. Paclitaxel in the treatment of patients with angiosarcoma of the scalp or face. Cancer 1999;86(10):2034–7.

62. Skubitz KM, Haddad PA. Paclitaxel and pegylated-liposomal doxorubicin are both active in angiosarcoma. Cancer 2005;104(2):361–6.

63. Fury MG, Antonescu CR, Van Zee KJ, et al. A 14-year retrospective review of angiosarcoma: clinical characteristics, prognostic factors, and treatment outcomes with surgery and chemotherapy. Cancer J 2005;11(3):241–7.

64. Edmonson JH, Long HJ, Richardson RL, et al. Phase II study of a combination of mitomycin, doxorubicin and cisplatin in advanced sarcomas. Cancer Chemother Pharmacol 1985;15(2):181–2.

65. Stacchiotti S, Palassini E, Sanfilippo R, et al. Gemcitabine in advanced angiosarcoma: a retrospective case series analysis from the Italian Rare Cancer Network. Ann Oncol 2012;23(2):501–8.

66. Maki RG, D'Adamo DR, Keohan ML, et al. Phase II study of sorafenib in patients with metastatic or recurrent sarcomas. J Clin Oncol 2009;27(19):3133–40.

67. Ray-Coquard I, Italiano A, Bompas E, et al. Sorafenib for patients with advanced angiosarcoma: a phase II Trial from the French Sarcoma Group (GSF/GETO). Oncologist 2012;17(2):260–6.

68. Chugh R, Wathen JK, Maki RG, et al. Phase II multicenter trial of imatinib in 10 histologic subtypes of sarcoma using a bayesian hierarchical statistical model. J Clin Oncol 2009;27(19):3148–53.

69. Agulnik M, Yarber JL, Okuno SH, et al. An open-label, multicenter, phase II study of bevacizumab for the treatment of angiosarcoma and epithelioid hemangioendotheliomas. Ann Oncol 2013;24(1):257–63.

70. Mir O, Domont J, Cioffi A, et al. Feasibility of metronomic oral cyclophosphamide plus prednisolone in elderly patients with inoperable or metastatic soft tissue sarcoma. Eur J Cancer 2011;47(4):515–9.

71. Stacchiotti S, Palassini E, Libertini M, et al. Sirolimus in advanced hemangioendothelioma. J Clin Oncol 2013;31(Suppl):[abstract: 10565].

72. Weitz J, Klimstra DS, Cymes K, et al. Management of primary liver sarcomas. Cancer 2007;109(7):1391–6.
73. Bonaccorsi-Riani E, Lerut JP. Liver transplantation and vascular tumours. Transpl Int 2010;23(7):686–91.
74. Nudo CG, Yoshida EM, Bain VG, et al. Liver transplantation for hepatic epithelioid hemangioendothelioma: the Canadian multicentre experience. Can J Gastroenterol 2008;22(10):821–4.
75. Herbert SP, Huisken J, Kim TN, et al. Arterial-venous segregation by selective cell sprouting: an alternative mode of blood vessel formation. Science 2009; 326(5950):294–8.
76. Kim YH, Hu H, Guevara-Gallardo S, et al. Artery and vein size is balanced by Notch and ephrin B2/EphB4 during angiogenesis. Development 2008;135(22): 3755–64.
77. Bridge G, Monteiro R, Henderson S, et al. The microRNA-30 family targets DLL4 to modulate endothelial cell behavior during angiogenesis. Blood 2012;120(25): 5063–72.
78. Cascone T, Heymach JV. Targeting the angiopoietin/Tie2 pathway: cutting tumor vessels with a double-edged sword? J Clin Oncol 2012;30(4):441–4.
79. Baselga J, Cortes J, Kim SB, et al. Pertuzumab plus trastuzumab plus docetaxel for metastatic breast cancer. N Engl J Med 2012;366(2):109–19.
80. Flaherty KT, Robert C, Hersey P, et al. Improved survival with MEK inhibition in BRAF-mutated melanoma. N Engl J Med 2012;367(2):107–14.
81. Shimizu T, Tolcher AW, Papadopoulos KP, et al. The clinical effect of the dual-targeting strategy involving PI3K/AKT/mTOR and RAS/MEK/ERK pathways in patients with advanced cancer. Clin Cancer Res 2012;18(8):2316–25.
82. Marshall V, Martro E, Labo N, et al. Kaposi sarcoma (KS)-associated herpesvirus microRNA sequence analysis and KS risk in a European AIDS-KS case control study. J Infect Dis 2010;202(7):1126–35.
83. Pfeffer S, Sewer A, Lagos-Quintana M, et al. Identification of microRNAs of the herpesvirus family. Nat Methods 2005;2(4):269–76.
84. Italiano A, Chen CL, Thomas R, et al. Alterations of the p53 and PIK3CA/AKT/ mTOR pathways in angiosarcomas: a pattern distinct from other sarcomas with complex genomics. Cancer 2012;118(23):5878–87.

Desmoid Tumors

A Comprehensive Review of the Evolving Biology, Unpredictable Behavior, and Myriad of Management Options

Sumana Devata, MD, Rashmi Chugh, MD*

KEYWORDS

- Desmoid • Aggressive fibromatosis • Review • Familial adenomatous polyposis
- Tyrosine kinase inhibitors

KEY POINTS

- Desmoid tumors are rare tumors of mesenchymal origin that vary widely in presentation and behavior.
- Desmoid tumors can occur in association with familial adenomatous polyposis, trauma, prior surgery, or pregnancy.
- Sporadic desmoid tumors can be associated with somatic mutations in the β-catenin gene.
- Many treatment modalities have shown benefit ranging from conservative, nonsurgical approaches to aggressive cytotoxic chemotherapy.
- Ongoing studies on the biology of desmoid tumors are leading to more potential rational therapeutic strategies.

INTRODUCTION

Desmoid tumors, also known as aggressive fibromatosis, were first coined in the 1830s after the Greek word *desmos* meaning "tendon-like." These rare tumors arise from mesenchymal cells, similar to their malignant counterpart, sarcomas. Unlike sarcomas, there is no metastatic potential for desmoid tumors. However, despite their

Funding Sources: Biomarin, Infinity Pharmaceuticals, Mabvax Therapeutics, Morphotek, Novartis Pharmaceuticals (R. Chugh); None (S. Devata).
Conflict of Interest: None.
Division of Hematology/Oncology, Department of Internal Medicine, University of Michigan, C407 Med Inn Building, 1500 East Medical Center Drive, SPC 5848, Ann Arbor, MI 48109-5848, USA
* Corresponding author. Department of Internal Medicine, C407 Med Inn Building, 1500 East Medical Center Drive, SPC 5848, Ann Arbor, MI 48109-5848.
E-mail address: rashmim@med.umich.edu

benign classification, desmoid tumors can be multifocal, and locally infiltrate surrounding structures such that they can be a cause of both significant morbidity and, rarely, mortality.

Desmoid tumors vary widely in presentation and behavior. These collections of fibrous tissue range from being relatively indolent and asymptomatic to creating severe local symptoms with significant morbidity. Accordingly, treatments range in aggressiveness and include observation, surgery, radiation therapy, nonsteroidal anti-inflammatory drugs (NSAIDs), hormonal agents, tyrosine kinase inhibitors (TKIs), and cytotoxic chemotherapy. New molecular insights into desmoid tumors suggest potential therapeutic targets in an attempt to expand the arsenal of therapeutic options.

EPIDEMIOLOGY

Desmoid tumors are uncommon, with an estimated incidence of 2.4 to 4.3 per million per year,[1] accounting for less than 3% of soft-tissue lesions.[2] Although there is some variability, there is a 2- to 3.5-fold increased incidence in women.[3,4] A wide range of ages is affected, with most cases occurring between the ages of 15 and 60 years with an average age of 36.7 years.[4] The majority of cases are sporadic with no known predisposing factors. However, a sizeable minority of desmoid tumors occur as a consequence of the genetic syndrome familial adenomatous polyposis (FAP) or in association with pregnancy or trauma (see the section on predisposing factors).

PATHOGENESIS

The Wnt/β-catenin pathway drives the pathogenesis of both sporadic and FAP-associated desmoid tumors. FAP-associated tumors frequently have adenomatous polyposis coli gene (APC) mutations at or beyond 3′ of codon 1444.[5–9] One function of APC is to regulate the protein level of β-catenin. When β-catenin is present in high concentration it binds to APC, followed by binding of the serine-threonine kinase GSK3β. This binding eventually leads to phosphorylation of sites on APC and β-catenin degradation.[10,11] In cases of mutated APC a truncated APC protein is created, which is unable to degrade β-catenin appropriately.[11] This process results in accumulation of β-catenin and its target genes, which are implicated in loss of proliferation regulation.[10]

Approximately 85% to 90% of sporadic desmoid tumors are associated with somatic mutations in the β-catenin gene, CTNNB1.[12–14] In a study of 254 cases of sporadic desmoids, 88% had CTNNB1 mutations identified by direct sequencing, compared with no mutations detected in the control of 175 other spindle-cell lesions.[13] These gene mutations have been found in codons 41 and 45 of exon 3 of CTNNB1, which produce a stabilized β-catenin protein product leading to an accumulation of β-catenin in the cell.[15]

In endothelial cells β-catenin is not only a cell-adhesion molecule, but also plays a role in nuclear transcription.[16] Accumulation of β-catenin, by constitutive activation of the Wnt ligand pathway, loss of APC protein function, and inability to phosphorylate β-catenin or mutations in the CTNNB1 gene, allows translocation of cytoplasmic β-catenin into the nucleus and, in conjunction with other proteins, promotes abnormal proliferation.[15,17]

Recognizing the central role of β-catenin in desmoid tumors, the current value of CTNNB1 evaluation in an individual patient is unclear. Some advocate that pediatric desmoid patients with β-catenin accumulation in the nucleus be evaluated for the presence of CTNNB1 mutation. If negative, APC mutation analysis should be considered, as this could potentially be the initial manifestation of FAP.[18,19] Evaluation of

CTNNB1 could also be used as a potential diagnostic test in tumors that are challenging to identify.[20] In addition, targeting the Wnt/β-catenin pathway may be a future therapeutic option of value.

CLINICAL PRESENTATION AND BEHAVIOR

Desmoid tumors arise from a variety of connective tissues, including muscle, fascia, and aponeurosis, and can present at any site in the body, with extremities/trunk, abdominal wall, and intra-abdominal locations most commonly described. There is no metastatic potential for these tumors; however, they can be multifocal and locally infiltrate surrounding structures,[21] which may be due to their lack of a pseudocapsule and tendency to spread along fascial planes and muscle.[22]

Intra-abdominal tumors, occurring in the bowel, mesentery, or abdominal wall, are often associated with Gardner syndrome or FAP. The presentation can range from mass effect to more serious complications of mucosal ischemia, ulceration, and bleeding.[23] In any patient presenting with an abdominal desmoid tumor, a thorough family history and workup for FAP with colonoscopy should be considered.

Extra-abdominal tumors are typically sporadic non–FAP-associated lesions. Local invasion from these tumors can cause pain, weakness, paresthesias, and neuropathies, which can lead to debilitating symptoms.

DIAGNOSIS
Radiology

Because of the invasive nature of desmoid tumors, identifying the extent of tumor invasion onto vital structures is paramount for consideration of local therapies. Standard radiographs can provide limited information such as tumor size and location with findings that are generally nonspecific, poorly defined, and (rarely) with calcifications.[24,25] Underlying bone involvement may manifest as bone erosion or cortical scalloping.[25,26]

Computed tomography (CT) scans provide additional anatomic information; however, owing to variable muscle infiltration, margins or borders may be poorly identified (**Fig. 1**).[26] Lesions appear as either hyperdense and/or hypodense to skeletal muscle, and enhancement with contrast is not consistent.[27] In a study comparing CT appearance with histologic appearance of tumors, no relationship was found that could account for the variability seen on imaging.[27]

Magnetic resonance imaging (MRI) has been proved to be superior to other imaging modalities when characterizing desmoid tumors. MRI is able to show tumor infiltration

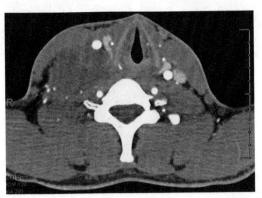

Fig. 1. Computed tomography image with contrast showing poorly defined borders.

into muscle and to distinguish boundaries between vital structures and fascial planes.[24] Central necrosis is not seen, and because of the variable cellular and collagen content of these tumors they are heterogeneous, with bands of low signal seen on standard sequencing.[24–26] T1-weighted images reveal hypointense or isointense lesions, whereas T2-weighted images show mixed hyperintense lesions.[24–26] Administration of intravenous gadolinium may lead to moderate or avid enhancement of the lesions; however, this is variable owing to the varying amount of collagen deposition in a tumor.[24–26,28] MRI provides information on tumor invasion, depth, and neurovascular encasement, which is necessary when determining the feasibility of surgery (**Fig. 2**).

Pathology

Histologically, desmoid tumors are composed of monoclonal fibroblasts[29,30] appearing as spindle-shaped cells separated by an abundant collagenous matrix (**Fig. 3**).[21,31] Few atypical, pleomorphic, or hyperchromic cells are seen, and the interlaced bundles of collagen and cells form dense tumors that are without pseudoencapsulation.[21,31] The infiltrating nature of these tumors is seen at muscle borders, where the tumors extend into muscle fascicles.[31]

Immunohistochemically these tumors show positivity for β-catenin and are negative for desmin, CD34, c-kit, and S-100.[32] In addition, desmoids can express cyclooxygenase-2 (COX-2)[32–35] and estrogen-β receptors.[33,36–38] The proliferation index, Ki-67, is typically low.[39] Cytogenetic analyses in sporadic tumors can reveal trisomy 8 and trisomy 20, which can occur individually or be present together.[40,41]

PREDISPOSING FACTORS
Familial Adenomatous Polyposis/Gardner Syndrome

FAP is associated with an autosomal dominant germline mutation in the *APC* gene. This mutation is associated with the development of hundreds of colon polyps, typically resulting in malignant transformation, osteomas, epidermoid cysts, and other soft-tissue and benign tumors. Of patients with FAP, approximately 10% develop desmoid tumors.[9,42] As prophylactic treatment, a majority of FAP patients undergo

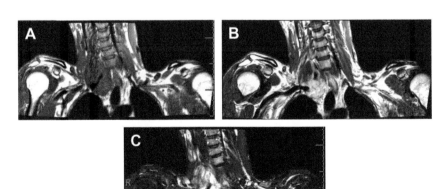

Fig. 2. Magnetic resonance images of desmoid tumor showing a heterogeneous mass surrounding vasculature. (*A*) T1-weighted image. (*B*) T2-weighted image showing heterogeneous mass. (*C*) Short-tau inversion recovery image.

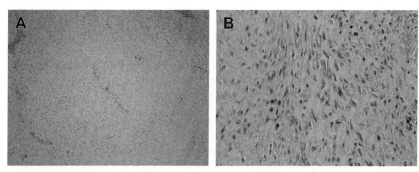

Fig. 3. (A) Low-power view (original magnification ×100) shows a proliferation of interlacing bundles of fibroblasts separated by dense, keloid-like collagen. At this magnification, small regularly distributed blood vessels are also conspicuous. (B) High-power view (original magnification ×400) demonstrates bland spindled nuclei with vesicular chromatin and small inconspicuous nucleoli. These cells are arranged between dense bundles of collagen.

colectomy for prevention of the future development of colon carcinoma. In these patients, desmoid tumors are a significant cause of morbidity and mortality because of their predilection for prior surgical sites,[7,23,43,44] and on average 77% of desmoid tumors occur 5 years after colectomy.[3] In one series, 50% of patients with FAP and prior abdominal surgery subsequently developed a desmoid tumor at surgical sites.[45] The median age at diagnosis is 31 years, with a 1:1 male/female ratio.[9]

In a retrospective review of registry data, 387 patients with FAP-associated desmoid tumors were identified, and within this population 53% were found to have intra-abdominal tumors, 24% abdominal wall tumors, and 9% extremity tumors.[9] Similar to prior publications, this study reported that family history, previous abdominal surgery, and specific APC mutations (3′ of codon 1444) were risk factors associated with the development of desmoid tumors in patients with FAP.[9]

Pregnancy

Desmoid tumors have been associated with elevated estrogen states, and have been well described as occurring in the abdominal wall during pregnancy or in the postpartum period.[46,47] The connection between estrogen levels and desmoids is based on case reports and anecdotal information, and estrogen receptors are not universally found in desmoids tumors, suggesting alternative mechanisms of growth.[48] Surgical trauma is also known to be associated with desmoid tumors, including prior cesarean sections, and this may add to the development of desmoid tumors during pregnancy.[48] Women who develop pregnancy-related desmoids are not at increased risk for recurrent or new tumors with subsequent pregnancies.[47,49]

Trauma and Prior Surgery

Surgical trauma, particularly abdominal surgeries, has been linked to the development of desmoid tumors in prior surgical areas.[50] This phenomenon is noted in patients with FAP, pregnancy, and sporadic tumors,[51–53] with one series reporting up to 28% of patients with prior surgical or penetrating trauma sites developing a desmoid tumor.[51] The etiology of these findings has been connected to mesenchymal stromal cells and dysregulation of β-catenin either through the APC gene or CTNNB1 gene mutations,[17] as well as to an abnormal increase in cytokines that are seen in wound healing leading to tumor growth.[37]

PROGNOSTIC FACTORS

The rarity of this disease, small cohorts of patients studied, and lack of randomized clinical trials leads to difficulties and variability in the identification of prognostic factors. In several series, age has been described as a prognostic factor, but results are inconsistent. Whereas some series report older age as a poor prognostic factor,[54] others indicate younger age,[55–57] and yet others did not identify age as having any prognostic significance.[22,58–60]

Recurrences are seen in 20% to 68% of patients, typically occurring within the first 1.5 to 5 years after treatment.[22,54,57–59,61,62] It is unclear as to what extent margin status after surgical excision contributes to local recurrence. Many studies cite positive margins as a negative prognostic factor,[22,55,56,63–67] whereas other series report no significant difference in relapse with positive or negative margins.[57,58,62,68,69] Unlike age and margin status, tumor location is more widely identified as affecting prognosis, with extra-abdominal tumors or limb and girdle tumors leading to increased risk of desmoid tumor recurrence after excision.[22,54,56,57,60,68,70–72]

In a study by Salas and colleagues,[69] 426 patients with sporadic aggressive fibromatosis were studied to determine desmoid tumor–related prognostic factors. Multivariate analysis identified age younger than 37 years, tumor size greater than 7 cm, and tumor location as factors for poor prognosis, and patients with all 3 factors had a significantly lower probability of progression-free survival.

MANAGEMENT

Desmoid tumors can be locally aggressive, leading to significant morbidity. Therapeutic management options are variable and include observation, surgery, radiation therapy, hormonal therapy, targeted therapy, and cytotoxic therapy. The overall survival rate is extremely good for these patients, with one study reporting a 96% 15-year survival.[73] However, the overall survival does not reflect the morbidity of this disease on afflicted patients, who are often young and otherwise healthy. Treatment approaches for patients require individualization and a multidisciplinary team approach.

Observation

Given the highly variable disease course, the wait-and-see approach has been advocated in select populations.[57,59,60,69,74] Prolonged stable disease and, less commonly, primary tumor regression has been reported,[49,59,69] often in patients with recurrent disease after surgery.[74] In a study of 142 patients with desmoid tumors treated without surgery or radiation, there was no significant difference in 5-year event-free survival (EFS) in patients treated with the wait-and-see approach in comparison with medical therapy (49.9% vs 58.6%, respectively; $P = .3196$), thus supporting observation as a more viable approach than systemic therapy.[59] Using a slightly different approach, a retrospective study by Bonvalot and colleagues[60] reported a 3-year EFS of 65% and 68% in patients with extra-abdominal desmoid tumors who were treated with R0 surgical resection in comparison with patients who were treated without surgery (observation or medical therapy). Based on these and other experiences, observation has become a very reasonable option for well-selected patients with desmoid tumors. Likewise, the latest consensus guidelines from the National Comprehensive Cancer Network (NCCN) recommends observation as a primary treatment option for surgically unresectable tumors or resectable tumors that are not symptomatic, life threatening, or causing significant impairment.[75]

Local Treatments

Local therapies such as surgery and radiation therapy are effective modalities for the treatment of desmoid tumors. Other emerging treatments, such as cryoablation, have shown potential improvement in small to medium-sized extra-abdominal desmoid tumors.[76]

Surgery

Surgical wide-margin resection is historically the frontline management for desmoid tumors.[22] However, recurrence rates after surgery for cases of either positive or negative margins are variable, ranging up to 40% in some series. The infiltrative nature and tendency to invade neurovascular structures can lead to difficulties in obtaining wide-margin resections when the goal of treatment is to preserve function, and the significance of margin status is unclear, as discussed earlier. It is reasonable to consider surgical resection as dependent on the expectant surgical functional outcome when these tumors cause impairment and excess morbidity. Specifically, NCCN consensus recommendations advocate that surgical resection with either positive or negative margins is acceptable in these situations.[75]

Radiation therapy

Radiation therapy (RT) in patients with desmoid tumors has been used in conjunction with surgery and as primary treatment in patients with unresectable tumors or in those patients for whom resection would significantly limit function. The role of adjuvant RT is unclear because there is no consensus on whether positive surgical margins are of prognostic significance, making it difficult to determine the benefit of RT after surgery.

In a review of 22 articles from 1983 to 1998, Nuyttens and colleagues[77] found that local tumor control was significantly improved with the addition of RT after surgery or with RT alone. In patients who underwent surgery, the addition of RT to those with positive margins improved local control rates from 41% to 75%.[77] Later reports also confirmed the benefit of adjuvant RT for local disease control and in those with positive surgical margins.[67,73,78–80]

By contrast, a retrospective analysis of 104 patients who underwent surgery, radiation, or surgery plus radiation demonstrated that all 3 modalities had similar local control rates 3 years after treatment.[81] Although there is no consensus regarding the benefit of RT used alone or in the adjuvant setting for local control, current studies report delivering a total of 50 to 60 Gy when administering radiation treatments, noting that increased doses cause significantly more complications.

As patients with desmoid tumors are often younger and have a very good long-term survival rate, the complications of RT require consideration. The most frequently reported radiation-related effects include pathologic fractures, range-of-motion limitations, limb contractures, pain, and in-field skin cancer.[73,77,81]

Systemic Therapies

Anti-inflammatory medications

NSAIDs were first noted to be active in desmoid tumors in 1977.[82] Desmoid tumors have been shown to overexpress cyclooxygenase, specifically COX-2, and inhibition with NSAIDs results in decreased proliferation of desmoid tumor cells.[34,35] Many small case series have demonstrated the utility of NSAIDs, including sulindac and indomethacin, both alone and in combination with other agents. In a series by Tsukada and colleagues,[83] 12 of 14 patients had a complete response, partial response, or stable disease while being treated with a median dose of sulindac, 300 mg daily. In another report by Klein and colleagues,[84] 3 patients with FAP were treated with indomethacin,

100 mg daily; 1 patient demonstrated a complete response whereas the 2 remaining patients had progressive disease (**Table 1**).

Although NSAIDs have been shown to have activity in desmoid tumors, reports incorporate both sporadic and FAP-associated tumors, assess small sample sizes, and do not provide comparisons between agents, all of which create limitations in the interpretation of these data.

Hormonal therapy

Antiestrogen treatments for desmoid tumors have been described as effective in many case reports, although it is unclear as to why this strategy is useful. In 1986, Lim and colleagues[85] analyzed 15 desmoid tumors, and found that 33% expressed estrogen receptors (ER) and 79% expressed antiestrogen binding sites (AEBS). In another study evaluating 40 desmoid tumors, all tumors specifically expressed ER-β, albeit to varying degrees.[36] Eighty-three percent of tumors had a greater than 50% ER-β expression, and all samples were ER-α negative.[36] In a subsequent study evaluating 59 desmoid cases, 89% were found to express ER-β and, similarly, all samples were ER-α negative.[38] However, correlation of ER status and response to antiestrogen therapy has yet to be reported.

Although the exact mechanism of action is not known, activity of a variety of antiestrogen therapies has been reported, including tamoxifen, toremifine, progesterone, goserelin, medroxyprogesterone acetate, testolactone, and prednisolone.[86] The largest published case series with antiestrogens was conducted by Brooks and colleagues,[87] who reported an overall 65% rate of stabilization of disease, partial response, or complete response to toremifene or tamoxifen (see **Table 1**). More recently toremifene was studied, and the data presented in abstract form indicated that 92.5% of patients had a partial response or stable disease, with an overall 81.5% of patients showing symptomatic improvement or radiographic response.[88] Many case reports have been published on the benefit of tamoxifen for these tumors.[86]

Given their relatively low toxicity profile independently, combination therapy of NSAIDs plus hormonal agents has been used with possible increased efficacy. In a

---

Table 1
Select case series of systemic NSAID and hormonal therapies used in the treatment of desmoid tumors

Therapy	No. of Patients	Outcome	Authors,[Ref.] Year
Sulindac	14	CR/PR: 57%; SD: 29%; PD: 14%	Tsukada et al,[83] 1992
Tamoxifen or toremifene	20	Overall 65% response rate	Brooks et al,[87] 1992
Toremifene	27	PR: 22.2%; SD: 70.3%; PD: 7.4%	Fiore et al,[88] 2011
Tamoxifen or raloxifen + sulindac	25 (17 FAP associated, 8 sporadic)	*FAP:* PR/CR: 29.4%; SD: 35.2%; PD: 23.5%; lost to follow-up: 11.7% *Sporadic:* CR: 12.5%; SD: 62.5%; PD: 12.5%; Remained in CR: 12.5%	Hansmann et al,[3] 2004

Abbreviations: CR, complete response; FAP, familial adenomatous polyposis; PD, progressive disease; PR, partial response; SD, stable disease.

series of 25 patients who received sulindac and tamoxifen, approximately 75% of sporadic tumors and 65% of FAP-associated tumors had benefit that ranged from stable disease to a complete response (see **Table 1**).[3] Major side effects included an increased incidence of ovarian cysts, chronic fatigue, and weight gain.[3] Although response rates are relatively high, it can take many months of treatment before benefit is seen, and available data are largely retrospective. Treatment with NSAIDs and/or hormonal agents should be considered in patients with tumors that are not life threatening or causing major functional limitations.

Tyrosine kinase inhibitors

For more than 10 years, the use of TKIs has been reported in the treatment of desmoid tumors, with success.[57,89–93] Imatinib, a selective TKI, inhibits several class-3 tyrosine kinase receptors, including abl, PDGFR, and c-KIT. The exact target of TKIs in desmoid tumors is not known, and response does not seem to correlate with c-KIT, PDGFR-α, PDGFR-β, CTNNB1, or APC mutations.[89–91,93] Other studies also demonstrated that the efficacy is unrelated to AKT, phosphatase and tension homologue,[89] and C-Src activity.[94]

Earlier studies indicated an approximate 15% response rate to imatinib,[91] but subsequent phase II trials favored stability of disease without robust tumor regression. The Sarcoma Alliance for Research through Collaboration conducted a phase II trial of imatinib in 51 patients with desmoid tumors, and demonstrated an overall response rate of 6% and 2-, 4-, and 12-month progression-free survival rates of 94%, 88%, and 66%, respectively.[89] Similar findings were reported in a phase II French Sarcoma Group trial, where 40 patients with progressive disease were treated with imatinib at 400 mg daily for 1 year and then increased to 800 mg for 8 additional months. The 3-, 6-, and 12-month progression-free survival was 91%, 80%, and 67%, respectively (**Table 2**).[93]

Sorafenib, a multitargeted kinase inhibitor of vascular endothelial growth factor receptor, among others, has also been evaluated in desmoid tumors. In a case series

Table 2			
Select trials and case series of tyrosine kinase inhibitor therapy in the treatment of desmoid tumors			
Therapy and Dosage	**No. of Patients**	**Outcomes**	**Authors,[Ref.] Year**
Imatinib BSA-based dosing (300 mg/200 mg/100 mg BID)	51	4-mo PFS: 88% 1-y PFS: 66% 3-y PFS: 58% PR 3, CR 0 Response rate: 6%	Chugh et al,[89] 2010
Imatinib 400 mg daily 800 mg if progression occurred	40	6-mo PFS: 80% 1-y PFS: 67% 2-y PFS: 55% PR 3, CR 1 Response rate: 11%	Penel et al,[93] 2011
Sorafenib 400 mg daily, adjusted for toxicities	26	PR 7, CR 0 Response rate: 25%	Gounder et al,[95] 2011

Abbreviations: BID, twice daily; BSA, body surface area; CR, complete response; PFS, progression-free survival; PR, partial response.

of 26 patients, 70% reported improvement of symptoms, and at 6 months 25% of patients had a partial response (see **Table 2**).[95]

Cytotoxic chemotherapy

Cytotoxic chemotherapy is reserved for patients with symptomatic tumors or tumors that are rapidly growing despite treatment with less toxic agents. Given the expectation of prolonged overall survival in desmoid patients, late-term side effects of cytotoxic therapy, including secondary malignancy and organ toxicity, are especially concerning in the management of this "benign" disease. However, in many clinical situations this becomes an important treatment option.

Although desmoid tumors have a low proliferation rate and low-grade features, cytotoxics are active agents in this setting. Single-agent regimens with doxorubicin or liposomal doxorubicin are reported to be effective, with one series reporting disease stability in 75% of patients with a median length of disease control of 14 months.[96] Multidrug combinations, including doxorubicin-based regimens with dacarbazine or cyclophosphamide and vincristine, or combinations of methotrexate with vinca alkaloids, have shown a median response rate of 50%.[86]

No randomized trials have compared chemotherapy options; however, the French Sarcoma Group reviewed cytotoxic chemotherapy treatment over 19 years and concluded that cytotoxic chemotherapy is a beneficial treatment option for desmoid tumors. Most patients were treated with combination regimens, including doxorubicin/dacarbazine, doxorubicin/ifosfamide/dacarbazine, methotrexate/vinblastine, and etoposide/cyclophosphamide. Independent of the agents used, the overall benefit, defined as an objective response or stable disease, was 80%.[97] Furthermore, a greater objective response rate was reported in patients who received anthracyclines, although overall progression-free survival was not different.[97] A durable benefit was seen in 45% of patients, as they did not require further treatment at a mean follow-up time of 36 months (**Table 3**).[97]

Given the dearth of clinical studies in this disease, there is no single most efficacious cytotoxic chemotherapeutic option. The most used agents are single-agent doxorubicin or liposomal doxorubicin, combination therapy with an anthracycline-based regimen, or methotrexate and vinblastine. Cytotoxic chemotherapy should be reserved for situations in which there are undesirable options for local therapies whereby the patient is symptomatic, requiring benefit in the short term. As opposed to hormonal and NSAID strategies, relief from desmoid-related symptoms can occur relatively quickly with cytotoxic therapies. The choice of therapy should be individualized, based on potential toxicities of therapy and the patient's comorbidities and preference.

Interferon

Interferon has been used as another possible systemic agent to control desmoid tumors. Similar to its effect in other diseases, the exact mechanism of action of interferon in desmoid tumors is unclear. There have been reports of regression with many different forms of interferon, including α2b, γ, and pegylated. A retrospective analysis of 13 patients treated with interferon-α with or without tretinoin showed local disease control in 85% of patients.[98] However, the limited case reports or series available, combined with the toxicities and availability of other options, severely limits the practical use of interferon.

FUTURE DIRECTIONS

With further understanding of the biology of desmoids and with new agents in development, there is much hope for the potential advent of nontoxic, targeted therapy for

Table 3
Select case series and studies of cytotoxic therapies in the treatment of desmoid tumors

Therapy	No. of Patients	Study Type	Median Age (Range)	Outcome	Authors,[Ref.] Year
Anthracycline-Based Regimens					
Doxorubicin, doxorubicin/ dacarbazine, or doxorubicin/ ifosfamide/ dacarbazine	13	Case series	NR	PR 7, CR 0 Response rate: 54%	Garbay et al,[97] 2012
Nonanthracycline-Based Regimens					
Etoposide, cyclophosphamide, methotrexate, vinorelbine, or methotrexate/ vinblastine	49	Case series	NR	PR 5, CR 1 Response rate: 12%	Garbay et al,[97] 2012
Pegylated liposomal doxorubicin (50 mg/m^2/4 wk)	11	Case series	29 y (3–53)	PR 4, CR 0 Response rate: 36%	Constantinidou et al,[96] 2009
Vinblastine (5 mg/m^2) and methotrexate (30 mg/m^2) weekly × 26 then every other week × 26	26	Phase II trial	11 y (7 mo–20 y)	PR 4, CR 1 Response rate: 19%	Skapek et al,[99] 2007
Vinblastine (6 mg/m^2) and methotrexate (30 mg/m^2) weekly × 1 y	30	Phase II trial	27 y	PR 12, CR: 0 Response rate: 40%	Azzarelli et al,[100] 2001
Cyclophosphamide/ ifosfamide, vincristine/ actinomycin-D/ cyclophosphamide, or vincristine/ doxorubicin/ ifosfamide/ actinomycin-D	19	Case series	NR	PR 5, CR: 4 Response rate: 47%	Pilz et al,[101] 1999
Doxorubicin/ dacarbazine × 7, then carboplatin/ dacarbazine	5	Case series, FAP only	36 y (29–45)	PR 3, CR 1 Response rate: 80%	Schnitzler et al,[102] 1997
Doxorubicin (60–90 mg/m^2) and dacarbazine (750–1000 mg/m^2)	12	Case series	29 y (16–66)	PR 4, CR 2 Response rate: 67%	Patel et al,[103] 1993

Abbreviations: CR, complete response; FAP, familial adenomatous polyposis; NR, not related; PR, partial response.

this disease. In desmoid-derived mesenchymal stem cells, expression of both the transcriptional regulator BMI-1 and the Hedgehog signaling effector Gli-1 has been noted.[17] Thus, the upstream Notch and Hedgehog pathways, both with agents under active investigation, have been implicated as possible therapeutic targets.

High-throughput screening and evaluation of signal-transduction pathways are evaluating other potential avenues of desmoid targeting. Ongoing investigation of desmoids on a molecular level will likely continue to offer greater understanding and options for afflicted patients. In the meantime, a multidisciplinary approach is key to the management of this complex disease given the breadth of manifestations, natural history of the disease, and multiple treatment modalities available.

REFERENCES

1. Reitamo JJ, Hayry P, Nykyri E, et al. The desmoid tumor. I. Incidence, sex-, age- and anatomical distribution in the Finnish population. Am J Clin Pathol 1982; 77(6):665–73.
2. Papagelopoulos PJ, Mavrogenis AF, Mitsiokapa EA, et al. Current trends in the management of extra-abdominal desmoid tumours. World J Surg Oncol 2006; 4:21.
3. Hansmann A, Adolph C, Vogel T, et al. High-dose tamoxifen and sulindac as first-line treatment for desmoid tumors. Cancer 2004;100(3):612–20.
4. Mankin HJ, Hornicek FJ, Springfield DS. Extra-abdominal desmoid tumors: a report of 234 cases. J Surg Oncol 2010;102(5):380–4.
5. Bertario L, Russo A, Sala P, et al. Genotype and phenotype factors as determinants of desmoid tumors in patients with familial adenomatous polyposis. Int J Cancer 2001;95(2):102–7.
6. Caspari R, Olschwang S, Friedl W, et al. Familial adenomatous polyposis: desmoid tumours and lack of ophthalmic lesions (CHRPE) associated with APC mutations beyond codon 1444. Hum Mol Genet 1995;4(3):337–40.
7. Durno C, Monga N, Bapat B, et al. Does early colectomy increase desmoid risk in familial adenomatous polyposis? Clin Gastroenterol Hepatol 2007;5(10): 1190–4.
8. Lefevre JH, Parc Y, Kerneis S, et al. Risk factors for development of desmoid tumours in familial adenomatous polyposis. Br J Surg 2008;95(9): 1136–9.
9. Nieuwenhuis MH, Lefevre JH, Bulow S, et al. Family history, surgery, and APC mutation are risk factors for desmoid tumors in familial adenomatous polyposis: an international cohort study. Dis Colon Rectum 2011;54(10):1229–34.
10. Li C, Bapat B, Alman BA. Adenomatous polyposis coli gene mutation alters proliferation through its beta-catenin-regulatory function in aggressive fibromatosis (desmoid tumor). Am J Pathol 1998;153(3):709–14.
11. Rubinfeld B, Albert I, Porfiri E, et al. Binding of GSK3beta to the APC-beta-catenin complex and regulation of complex assembly. Science 1996; 272(5264):1023–6.
12. Huss S, Nehles J, Binot E, et al. Beta-catenin (CTNNB1) mutations and clinicopathological features of mesenteric desmoid-type fibromatosis. Histopathology 2013;62(2):294–304.
13. Le Guellec S, Soubeyran I, Rochaix P, et al. CTNNB1 mutation analysis is a useful tool for the diagnosis of desmoid tumors: a study of 260 desmoid tumors and 191 potential morphologic mimics. Mod Pathol 2012;25(12):1551–8.
14. Tejpar S, Nollet F, Li C, et al. Predominance of beta-catenin mutations and beta-catenin dysregulation in sporadic aggressive fibromatosis (desmoid tumor). Oncogene 1999;18(47):6615–20.
15. Lazar AJ, Hajibashi S, Lev D. Desmoid tumor: from surgical extirpation to molecular dissection. Curr Opin Oncol 2009;21(4):352–9.

16. Barker N. The canonical Wnt/beta-catenin signalling pathway. Methods Mol Biol 2008;468:5–15.
17. Carothers AM, Rizvi H, Hasson RM, et al. Mesenchymal stromal cell mutations and wound healing contribute to the etiology of desmoid tumors. Cancer Res 2012;72(1):346–55.
18. Kattentidt Mouravieva AA, Geurts-Giele IR, de Krijger RR, et al. Identification of familial adenomatous polyposis carriers among children with desmoid tumours. Eur J Cancer 2012;48(12):1867–74.
19. Wang WL, Nero C, Pappo A, et al. CTNNB1 genotyping and APC screening in pediatric desmoid tumors: a proposed algorithm. Pediatr Dev Pathol 2012; 15(5):361–7.
20. Colombo C, Bolshakov S, Hajibashi S, et al. 'Difficult to diagnose' desmoid tumours: a potential role for CTNNB1 mutational analysis. Histopathology 2011;59(2):336–40.
21. Schlemmer M. Desmoid tumors and deep fibromatoses. Hematol Oncol Clin North Am 2005;19(3):565–71, vii–viii.
22. Ballo MT, Zagars GK, Pollack A, et al. Desmoid tumor: prognostic factors and outcome after surgery, radiation therapy, or combined surgery and radiation therapy. J Clin Oncol 1999;17(1):158–67.
23. Church JM. Mucosal ischemia caused by desmoid tumors in patients with familial adenomatous polyposis: report of four cases. Dis Colon Rectum 1998;41(5): 661–3.
24. Lee JC, Thomas JM, Phillips S, et al. Aggressive fibromatosis: MRI features with pathologic correlation. AJR Am J Roentgenol 2006;186(1):247–54.
25. Robbin MR, Murphey MD, Temple HT, et al. Imaging of musculoskeletal fibromatosis. Radiographics 2001;21(3):585–600.
26. Kingston CA, Owens CM, Jeanes A, et al. Imaging of desmoid fibromatosis in pediatric patients. AJR Am J Roentgenol 2002;178(1):191–9.
27. Francis IR, Dorovini-Zis K, Glazer GM, et al. The fibromatoses: CT-pathologic correlation. AJR Am J Roentgenol 1986;147(5):1063–6.
28. Romero JA, Kim EE, Kim CG, et al. Different biologic features of desmoid tumors in adult and juvenile patients: MR demonstration. J Comput Assist Tomogr 1995; 19(5):782–7.
29. Alman BA, Pajerski ME, Diaz-Cano S, et al. Aggressive fibromatosis (desmoid tumor) is a monoclonal disorder. Diagn Mol Pathol 1997;6(2):98–101.
30. Li M, Cordon-Cardo C, Gerald WL, et al. Desmoid fibromatosis is a clonal process. Hum Pathol 1996;27(9):939–43.
31. Enzinger FM, Shiraki M. Musculo-aponeurotic fibromatosis of the shoulder girdle (extra-abdominal desmoid). Analysis of thirty cases followed up for ten or more years. Cancer 1967;20(7):1131–40.
32. Owens CL, Sharma R, Ali SZ. Deep fibromatosis (desmoid tumor): cytopathologic characteristics, clinicoradiologic features, and immunohistochemical findings on fine-needle aspiration. Cancer 2007;111(3):166–72.
33. Mignemi NA, Itani DM, Fasig JH, et al. Signal transduction pathway analysis in desmoid-type fibromatosis: transforming growth factor-beta, COX2 and sex steroid receptors. Cancer Sci 2012;103(12):2173–80.
34. Poon R, Smits R, Li C, et al. Cyclooxygenase-two (COX-2) modulates proliferation in aggressive fibromatosis (desmoid tumor). Oncogene 2001;20(4):451–60.
35. Signoroni S, Frattini M, Negri T, et al. Cyclooxygenase-2 and platelet-derived growth factor receptors as potential targets in treating aggressive fibromatosis. Clin Cancer Res 2007;13(17):5034–40.

36. Deyrup AT, Tretiakova M, Montag AG. Estrogen receptor-beta expression in extraabdominal fibromatoses: an analysis of 40 cases. Cancer 2006;106(1): 208–13.

37. Mills BG, Frausto A, Brien E. Cytokines associated with the pathophysiology of aggressive fibromatosis. J Orthop Res 2000;18(4):655–62.

38. Santos GA, Cunha IW, Rocha RM, et al. Evaluation of estrogen receptor alpha, estrogen receptor beta, progesterone receptor, and cKIT expression in desmoids tumors and their role in determining treatment options. Biosci Trends 2010;4(1):25–30.

39. Dubova EA, Sidorenko TV, Shchyogolev AI, et al. Immunohistochemical characteristics of desmoid tumors. Bull Exp Biol Med 2012;152(6):743–7.

40. Dei Tos AP, Dal Cin P. The role of cytogenetics in the classification of soft tissue tumours. Virchows Arch 1997;431(2):83–94.

41. Qi H, Dal Cin P, Hernandez JM, et al. Trisomies 8 and 20 in desmoid tumors. Cancer Genet Cytogenet 1996;92(2):147–9.

42. Clark SK, Phillips RK. Desmoids in familial adenomatous polyposis. Br J Surg 1996;83(11):1494–504.

43. Penna C, Tiret E, Parc R, et al. Operation and abdominal desmoid tumors in familial adenomatous polyposis. Surg Gynecol Obstet 1993;177(3):263–8.

44. Quintini C, Ward G, Shatnawei A, et al. Mortality of intra-abdominal desmoid tumors in patients with familial adenomatous polyposis: a single center review of 154 patients. Ann Surg 2012;255(3):511–6.

45. Kadmon M, Moslein G, Buhr HJ, et al. Desmoid tumors in patients with familial adenomatous polyposis (FAP). Clinical and therapeutic observations from the Heidelberg polyposis register. Chirurg 1995;66(10):997–1005 [in German].

46. Johner A, Tiwari P, Zetler P, et al. Abdominal wall desmoid tumors associated with pregnancy: current concepts. Expert Rev Anticancer Ther 2009;9(11): 1675–82.

47. Way JC, Culham BA. Desmoid tumour. The risk of recurrent or new disease with subsequent pregnancy: a case report. Can J Surg 1999;42(1):51–4.

48. De Cian F, Delay E, Rudigoz RC, et al. Desmoid tumor arising in a cesarean section scar during pregnancy: monitoring and management. Gynecol Oncol 1999; 75(1):145–8.

49. Caldwell EH. Desmoid tumor: musculoaponeurotic fibrosis of the abdominal wall. Surgery 1976;79(1):104–6.

50. Reitamo JJ, Scheinin TM, Hayry P. The desmoid syndrome. New aspects in the cause, pathogenesis and treatment of the desmoid tumor. Am J Surg 1986; 151(2):230–7.

51. Lopez R, Kemalyan N, Moseley HS, et al. Problems in diagnosis and management of desmoid tumors. Am J Surg 1990;159(5):450–3.

52. Urist MR. Trauma and neoplasm; report of a case of desmoid tumor following simple fracture of the radius and ulna. Am J Surg 1957;93(4):682–8.

53. Wanjeri JK, Opeya CJ. A massive abdominal wall desmoid tumor occurring in a laparotomy scar: a case report. World J Surg Oncol 2011;9:35.

54. Rock MG, Pritchard DJ, Reiman HM, et al. Extra-abdominal desmoid tumors. J Bone Joint Surg Am 1984;66(9):1369–74.

55. Spear MA, Jennings LC, Mankin HJ, et al. Individualizing management of aggressive fibromatoses. Int J Radiat Oncol Biol Phys 1998;40(3):637–45.

56. Sorensen A, Keller J, Nielsen OS, et al. Treatment of aggressive fibromatosis: a retrospective study of 72 patients followed for 1-27 years. Acta Orthop Scand 2002;73(2):213–9.

57. Lev D, Kotilingam D, Wei C, et al. Optimizing treatment of desmoid tumors. J Clin Oncol 2007;25(13):1785–91.
58. Merchant NB, Lewis JJ, Woodruff JM, et al. Extremity and trunk desmoid tumors: a multifactorial analysis of outcome. Cancer 1999;86(10):2045–52.
59. Fiore M, Rimareix F, Mariani L, et al. Desmoid-type fibromatosis: a front-line conservative approach to select patients for surgical treatment. Ann Surg Oncol 2009;16(9):2587–93.
60. Bonvalot S, Eldweny H, Haddad V, et al. Extra-abdominal primary fibromatosis: aggressive management could be avoided in a subgroup of patients. Eur J Surg Oncol 2008;34(4):462–8.
61. Phillips SR, A'Hern R, Thomas JM. Aggressive fibromatosis of the abdominal wall, limbs and limb girdles. Br J Surg 2004;91(12):1624–9.
62. Pignatti G, Barbanti-Brodano G, Ferrari D, et al. Extraabdominal desmoid tumor. A study of 83 cases. Clin Orthop Relat Res 2000;(375):207–13.
63. Posner MC, Shiu MH, Newsome JL, et al. The desmoid tumor. Not a benign disease. Arch Surg 1989;124(2):191–6.
64. Meazza C, Bisogno G, Gronchi A, et al. Aggressive fibromatosis in children and adolescents: the Italian experience. Cancer 2010;116(1):233–40.
65. Leithner A, Gapp M, Leithner K, et al. Margins in extra-abdominal desmoid tumors: a comparative analysis. J Surg Oncol 2004;86(3):152–6.
66. Huang K, Fu H, Shi YQ, et al. Prognostic factors for extra-abdominal and abdominal wall desmoids: a 20-year experience at a single institution. J Surg Oncol 2009;100(7):563–9.
67. Goy BW, Lee SP, Eilber F, et al. The role of adjuvant radiotherapy in the treatment of resectable desmoid tumors. Int J Radiat Oncol Biol Phys 1997;39(3):659–65.
68. Gronchi A, Casali PG, Mariani L, et al. Quality of surgery and outcome in extraabdominal aggressive fibromatosis: a series of patients surgically treated at a single institution. J Clin Oncol 2003;21(7):1390–7.
69. Salas S, Dufresne A, Bui B, et al. Prognostic factors influencing progression-free survival determined from a series of sporadic desmoid tumors: a wait-and-see policy according to tumor presentation. J Clin Oncol 2011;29(26):3553–8.
70. Stoeckle E, Coindre JM, Longy M, et al. A critical analysis of treatment strategies in desmoid tumours: a review of a series of 106 cases. Eur J Surg Oncol 2009;35(2):129–34.
71. de Bree E, Keus R, Melissas J, et al. Desmoid tumors: need for an individualized approach. Expert Rev Anticancer Ther 2009;9(4):525–35.
72. Baumert BG, Spahr MO, Von Hochstetter A, et al. The impact of radiotherapy in the treatment of desmoid tumours. An international survey of 110 patients. A study of the Rare Cancer Network. Radiat Oncol 2007;2:12.
73. Rutenberg MS, Indelicato DJ, Knapik JA, et al. External-beam radiotherapy for pediatric and young adult desmoid tumors. Pediatr Blood Canc 2011;57(3):435–42.
74. Bonvalot S, Desai A, Coppola S, et al. The treatment of desmoid tumors: a stepwise clinical approach. Ann Oncol 2012;23(Suppl 10):x158–66.
75. von Mehren M, Benjamin R, Bui MM, et al. Soft tissue sarcoma. 2013; Version 3.2012. Available at: http://www.nccn.org/professionals/physician_gls/pdf/sarcoma.pdf. Accessed January 18, 2013.
76. Kujak JL, Liu PT, Johnson GB, et al. Early experience with percutaneous cryoablation of extra-abdominal desmoid tumors. Skeletal Radiol 2010;39(2):175–82.

77. Nuyttens JJ, Rust PF, Thomas CR Jr, et al. Surgery versus radiation therapy for patients with aggressive fibromatosis or desmoid tumors: a comparative review of 22 articles. Cancer 2000;88(7):1517–23.

78. Fontanesi J, Mott MP, Kraut MJ, et al. The role of postoperative irradiation in the treatment of locally recurrent incompletely resected extra-abdominal desmoid tumors. Sarcoma 2004;8(2–3):83–6.

79. Jelinek JA, Stelzer KJ, Conrad E, et al. The efficacy of radiotherapy as postoperative treatment for desmoid tumors. Int J Radiat Oncol Biol Phys 2001; 50(1):121–5.

80. Zlotecki RA, Scarborough MT, Morris CG, et al. External beam radiotherapy for primary and adjuvant management of aggressive fibromatosis. Int J Radiat Oncol Biol Phys 2002;54(1):177–81.

81. Gluck I, Griffith KA, Biermann JS, et al. Role of radiotherapy in the management of desmoid tumors. Int J Radiat Oncol Biol Phys 2011;80(3):787–92.

82. Waddell WR, Gerner RE. Indomethacin and ascorbate inhibit desmoid tumors. J Surg Oncol 1980;15(1):85–90.

83. Tsukada K, Church JM, Jagelman DG, et al. Noncytotoxic drug therapy for intra-abdominal desmoid tumor in patients with familial adenomatous polyposis. Dis Colon Rectum 1992;35(1):29–33.

84. Klein WA, Miller HH, Anderson M, et al. The use of indomethacin, sulindac, and tamoxifen for the treatment of desmoid tumors associated with familial polyposis. Cancer 1987;60(12):2863–8.

85. Lim CL, Walker MJ, Mehta RR, et al. Estrogen and antiestrogen binding sites in desmoid tumors. Eur J Cancer Clin Oncol 1986;22(5):583–7.

86. Janinis J, Patriki M, Vini L, et al. The pharmacological treatment of aggressive fibromatosis: a systematic review. Ann Oncol 2003;14(2):181–90.

87. Brooks MD, Ebbs SR, Colletta AA, et al. Desmoid tumours treated with triphenyl-ethylenes. Eur J Cancer 1992;28A(6–7):1014–8.

88. Fiore M, Colombo C, Radaelli S, et al. Activity of toremifene in sporadic desmoid-type fibromatosis. J Clin Oncol 2011;29 [abstract 10033].

89. Chugh R, Wathen JK, Patel SR, et al. Efficacy of imatinib in aggressive fibromatosis: results of a phase II multicenter Sarcoma Alliance for Research through Collaboration (SARC) trial. Clin Cancer Res 2010;16(19):4884–91.

90. Heinrich MC, Joensuu H, Demetri GD, et al. Phase II, open-label study evaluating the activity of imatinib in treating life-threatening malignancies known to be associated with imatinib-sensitive tyrosine kinases. Clin Cancer Res 2008; 14(9):2717–25.

91. Heinrich MC, McArthur GA, Demetri GD, et al. Clinical and molecular studies of the effect of imatinib on advanced aggressive fibromatosis (desmoid tumor). J Clin Oncol 2006;24(7):1195–203.

92. Mace J, Sybil Biermann J, Sondak V, et al. Response of extraabdominal desmoid tumors to therapy with imatinib mesylate. Cancer 2002;95(11):2373–9.

93. Penel N, Le Cesne A, Bui BN, et al. Imatinib for progressive and recurrent aggressive fibromatosis (desmoid tumors): an FNCLCC/French Sarcoma Group phase II trial with a long-term follow-up. Ann Oncol 2011;22(2):452–7.

94. Cho NL, Carothers AM, Rizvi H, et al. Immunohistochemical and molecular analysis of tyrosine kinase activity in desmoid tumors. J Surg Res 2012;173(2): 320–6.

95. Gounder MM, Lefkowitz RA, Keohan ML, et al. Activity of Sorafenib against desmoid tumor/deep fibromatosis. Clin Cancer Res 2011;17(12):4082–90.

96. Constantinidou A, Jones RL, Scurr M, et al. Pegylated liposomal doxorubicin, an effective, well-tolerated treatment for refractory aggressive fibromatosis. Eur J Cancer 2009;45(17):2930–4.

97. Garbay D, Le Cesne A, Penel N, et al. Chemotherapy in patients with desmoid tumors: a study from the French Sarcoma Group (FSG). Ann Oncol 2012;23(1): 182–6.

98. Leithner A, Schnack B, Katterschafka T, et al. Treatment of extra-abdominal desmoid tumors with interferon-alpha with or without tretinoin. J Surg Oncol 2000; 73(1):21–5.

99. Skapek S, Ferguson W, Granowetter L, et al. Vinblastine and methotrexate for desmoid fibromatosis in children: results of a Pediatric Oncology Group Phase II trial. J Clin Oncol 2007;25(5):501–6.

100. Azzarelli A, Gronchi A, Bertulli R, et al. Low-dose chemotherapy with methotrexate and vinblastine for patients with advanced aggressive fibromatosis. Cancer 2001;92(5):1259–64.

101. Pilz T, Pilgrim T, Bisogno G, et al. Chemotherapy in fibromatosis of childhood and adolescence: results from the Cooperative soft tissue sarcoma study (CWS) and the Italian Cooperative study group (ICG-AIEOP). Klin Padiatr 1999;211(4):291–5.

102. Shnitzler M, Cohen Z, Blackstein M, et al. Chemotherapy for desmoid tumors in association with familial adenomatous polyposis. Dis Colon Rectum 1997;40(7): 798–801.

103. Patel S, Evans H, Benjamin R. Combination chemotherapy in adult desmoid tumors. Cancer 1993;72(11):3244–7.

Update in Treatment and Targets in Ewing Sarcoma

Gregory M. Cote, MD, PhD, Edwin Choy, MD, PhD*

KEYWORDS

- Ewing sarcoma • Chemotherapy • Oncology • Treatment • Tumor

KEY POINTS

- The improvement in outcome for patients with localized and metastatic Ewing sarcoma since the development of cytotoxic chemotherapy remains one of the most profound advances in oncology.
- Vincristine, doxorubicin, and cyclophosphamide alternating with ifosfamide and etoposide (VDC/IE) remains the chemotherapeutic backbone of Ewing sarcoma therapy, and the addition of other cytotoxic agents to this regimen is unlikely to produce significant benefits.
- Identification of molecular targets for new treatments has become an intense area within Ewing sarcoma research.
- The development of improved preclinical Ewing sarcoma models and advanced molecular techniques, including high-throughput sequencing, will build on knowledge of EWS/FLI1 function, EWS/FLI1 transcription targets, and the other critical driver events in these tumors.

INTRODUCTION

The Ewing sarcomas are highly aggressive small round blue cell malignancies of the bone and soft tissue that primarily occur in the second decade of life. The so-called Ewing sarcoma family of tumors includes classical osseous Ewing sarcoma, extraosseous Ewing sarcoma, primitive neuroectodermal tumor, Askin tumor (now thought to be extraosseous Ewing sarcoma of the soft tissues of the chest wall or peripheral lung),[1] and atypical Ewing sarcoma. With variable degrees of neural differentiation, these were initially classified as distinct pathologic entities; however, with advances in molecular profiling, it became clear that these likely derive from the same neuroectodermal cell origin. For example, nearly all Ewing sarcoma family tumors have nonrandom chromosomal translocations involving the Ewing sarcoma breakpoint

Disclosures: The authors have nothing to disclose.
Division of Hematology Oncology, Yawkey Center for Outpatient Care, Massachusetts General Hospital, Harvard Medical School, 32 Fruit Street, Boston, MA 02114, USA
* Corresponding author.
E-mail address: echoy@partners.org

Hematol Oncol Clin N Am 27 (2013) 1007–1019
http://dx.doi.org/10.1016/j.hoc.2013.07.001   hemonc.theclinics.com
0889-8588/13/$ – see front matter © 2013 Elsevier Inc. All rights reserved.

region 1 gene (EWSR1) on chromosome 22 (described in more detail later). Multi-modality therapy, including aggressive neoadjuvant and adjuvant chemotherapy combined with surgery and/or radiation therapy (RT), has greatly improved the long-term survival of patients with localized disease up to greater than 70% at 5 years.[2–4] Unfortunately, almost 20% of have refractory or recurrent disease and approximatley one-quarter to one-third present with metastatic disease. Despite many attempts at intensifying treatment, survival remains poor in these patients.

Ewing sarcoma remains the second most common primary bone malignancy in the pediatric population, with an annual incidence of almost 3 cases per 1 million people.[3] Reported median age ranges from 12 to 19[3,5,6]; however, importantly, there is a wide distribution with patients seen at an age of only months up to the 5th and 6th decades of life. Ewing sarcoma is slightly more common in men than women. The incidence is much increased in whites compared with other ethnic backgrounds, which suggests a genetic contribution.[3,7] Because of its rarity, however, even a modest heritable factor contributing to the risk of developing Ewing sarcoma has not yet been able to be identified.[8]

Clinically, Ewing sarcoma most typically presents with localized symptoms of pain and swelling. In some cases, this is after a prior trauma or muscle strain.[9] Rarely, patients may develop constitutional symptoms, presumably due to cytokine release and inflammation. The most common sites of initial disease include axial and appendicular skeleton with, for example, approximately 20% to 25% originating in the pelvis and approximately 16% to 17% in the femur in some series.[5,10] Frequent sites of metastatic disease either at diagnosis or recurrence include the lungs and bone.

Adverse prognostic features include location (eg, pelvis[4,5,10–15]), size of the tumor (>8 cm),[4,5] high lactate dehydrogenase,[14] time to diagnosis,[12] age (<10–18 years old),[3–5,15] and, not surprisingly, evidence of metastatic disease at diagnosis.[3–5,14] An important caveat is that many of the negative prognostic factors were identified from somewhat dated patient series and thus are of unknown value with modern chemotherapy. In the authors' opinion, the most clinically useful negative prognostic factors are those identified in 2 randomized studies using modern chemotherapy regimens (discussed later), which include large tumors, pelvic site, and older age.[4,15]

In advanced disease, the location of metastases and time to relapse seems to factor into clinical outcome, with improved survival of those with lung versus bone (or bone plus lung) and those with late relapse.[5,16–18]

MOLECULAR BIOLOGY

Within the sarcomas, there are subsets with defined genetic alterations, including those with translocations involving members of the ten-eleven translocation (TET) family of RNA-binding proteins (including translocated in liposarcoma/fused in sarcoma [TLS/FUS], EWS, and TATA-binding protein–associated factor 15 [TAF15], reviewed by Tan and Manley[19] and by Jain and colleagues[20]). Examples include the Ewing family of tumors, desmoplastic small round cell tumor, clear cell sarcoma, angiomatoid fibrous histiocytoma, extraskeletal myxoid chondrosarcoma, and myxoid/round cell liposarcoma.

The TET gene products have multiple putative cellular functions, including roles in regulating transcription, RNA splicing, and intracellular signaling. In all TET family proteins, there is an RNA-binding domain localized to the C-terminus and an activation/regulatory domain is within the N-terminus.[19] These sarcomas are characterized by aberrant gene chimerisms, which bring together the TET amino terminal activation domain with the DNA-binding domain of a partner transcription factor. Thus, it is thought that this fusion protein may drive altered gene expression, cell differentiation, and ultimately tumor growth. The TET member and transcription factor member can be substituted within their subgroups while still resulting in similar histologic phenotypes. For example, in most (approximately 85%–90%) Ewing sarcoma tumors, the EWS gene 22 is aberrantly juxtaposed to the ETS transcription factor FLI1 on chromosome 11: t(11;22)(q24;q12).[21–24] Other ETS translocation partners with EWS, however, include ERG1 (10%),[25,26] ETV1,[27] ETV4 (also known as E1AF), and FEV. Additionally, the TET family member TLS/FUS is rarely seen to translocate to ERG1 and FEV in a phenotype indistinguishable from those with EWS.

INITIAL EVALUATION AND TREATMENT

Given the infrequency of this disease and the intricacies of clinical management, it is highly recommended that Ewing sarcoma patients undergo initial evaluation and treatment planning at a high-volume sarcoma treatment center. Histologic and molecular diagnosis should be confirmed by an expert pathologist. Ewing sarcomas are small blue round cell tumors (**Fig. 1**) typically positive for CD99 staining with variable degrees of neuronal differentiation. EWS rearrangement is either confirmed with fluorescence in situ hybridization (FISH) or by polymerase chain reaction. The FISH probe does not identify the translocation partner and (as discussed previously) EWS translocations can occur in other sarcomas. Moreover, in unpublished personal observation of a single patient under the authors' care, the EWS FISH probe was negative but molecular testing with DNA sequencing did identify EWS/FLI1 (Choy E, unpublished, 2012). Thus, if clinical suspicion is high, sequencing or polymerase chain reaction–based studies could be obtained.

The pretreatment evaluation should include full staging studies. Traditional plain films show a moth-eaten area of bone, revealing a confluence of finely destructive lesions that coalesce over time. Standard radiographs (**Fig. 2**) are now often supplanted by diagnostic CT scans in upfront imaging, which can assess the degree of bone cortex that is compromised by the tumor and predict the risk of developing pathologic fractures. MRI remains the gold standard for radiographic characterization of Ewing sarcoma because it can determine the relationship of tumor with critical anatomic structures, vessels, nerves, and surgical/fascial planes. All patients should also receive chest CT and technetium Tc 99m bone scanning or positron emission tomography scanning to identify metastases to the lungs and bones, respectively. Some practitioners perform bone marrow aspirates or MRI of the spine and pelvis to rule out occult marrow involvement. It is now the standard of care, however, to treat all chemotherapy-eligible patients with up to 1 year of systemic therapies regardless of proof of metastasis (discussed later), and as such, the bone marrow aspirate has recently played a lesser role in determining the clinical management of patients.

Localized Ewing Sarcoma

Despite up to 75% of patients having clinically and radiographic evidence of only localized tumors, it is known that without systemic chemotherapy most of these patients go on to develop overt metastatic disease. This has led to the hypothesis and clinical assumption in practice that patients with radiographically confirmed localized disease (with or without bone marrow biopsy) actually have micrometastatic Ewing sarcoma that is below the detection limits of staging techniques.

The current standard of care in the United States involves 17 cycles of chemotherapy using VDC/IE (vincrisine, doxorubicin, cyclophosphamide/ifosfamide, etoposide). Typically, patients receive 4 to 6 cycles of neoadjuvant therapy followed by

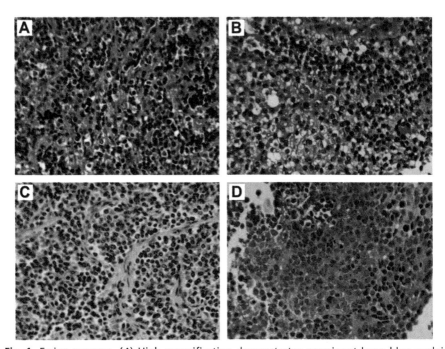

Fig. 1. Ewing sarcoma. (*A*) High magnification demonstrates prominent large blue nuclei with amphophilic cytoplasm. Note that a few nuclei at the periphery appear darker and more condensed; this may be because of early apoptosis. (*B*) A different high-power field demonstrates tumor cells with clear to amphophilic cytoplasm. A population of cells with round nuclei and finely divided chromatin and a subpopulation of cells with condensed chromatin that may be undergoing apoptosis are present. (*C*) Another high-power field demonstrates monotonous and uniformly appearing nuclei with solid groupings of viable tumor cells in an alveolar arrangement created by delicate vasculature. (*D*) A very-high-power photograph demonstrates that in the nonapoptotic tumor cells, nucleoli, when present, are single and not prominent. Note the lack of mitotic activity and poor cellular demarcations. (*From* Klein MJ. Ewing sarcoma. In: Folpe AL, Inwards CY, editors. Bone and soft tissue pathology: a volume in the series foundations in diagnostic pathology. Philadelphia: Saunders; 2010. p. 367–78; with permission.)

definitive local control (eg, surgery, RT, or surgery and RT) with continued chemotherapy for up to nearly a year, as long as there is evidence of sustained tumor response. This neoadjuvant/adjuvant strategy allows for rapid systemic and local control, the improvement of surgical options or radiation fields, and the assessment of tumor response on the surgical specimen. This intense, lengthy, and somewhat unusual regimen has been developed over several decades through several cooperative studies. A brief history is as follows.

The Intergroup Ewing's Sarcoma Study (IESS)-I recruited 342 children with localized tumors from 1973 to 1978.[13] Patients were randomized to radiation to the primary lesion plus (1) vincristine/doxorubicin/cyclophosphamide/dactinomycin (VDCA), (2) vincristine/cyclophosphamide/dactinomycin, or (3) vincristine/cyclophosphamide/dactinomycin plus bilateral prophylactic pulmonary RT. The 5-year relapse-free survival was superior for VDCA at 60% compared with 24% and 44% for treatments 2 and 3, respectively. Overall survival was similarly improved at 5 years: 65% alive in treatment group 1 and only 28% and 53% in treatments groups 2 and 3, respectively. Thus, doxorubicin was established as a key addition to the regimen.

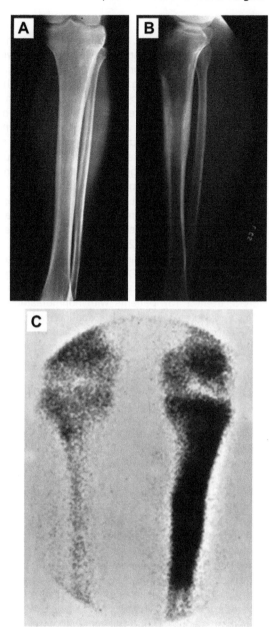

Fig. 2. Ewing sarcoma. (*A*) Anteroposterior and (*B*) lateral views of the left lower leg in an 18-year-old high-school football player who complained of lower leg pain persisting on exercise 3 months after football season but now present at rest. A slight increase in tibial metadiaphyseal radiodensity visible only in the lateral view is present. This is not due to the tumor permeating the medullary cavity but is because the tumor has caused the periosteum to form reactive new cortical bone. No visible soft tissue mass is present. The tumor is otherwise invisible on these conventional roentgenographs. (*C*) The technetium bone scan shows markedly increased uptake from the proximal tibia to the mid-diaphysis, corresponding to the areas in which the bone reacts to the tumor. These cannot be seen in the conventional views. (*From* Klein MJ. Ewing sarcoma. In: Folpe AL, Inwards CY, editors. Bone and soft tissue pathology: a volume in the series foundations in diagnostic pathology. Philadelphia: Saunders; 2010. p. 367–78; with permission.)

IESS-II, the subsequent intergroup study, was designed to determine if increasing the dose intensity could improve outcome in osteosarcoma and Ewing sarcoma patients.[28,29] This study randomized 214 nonmetastatic Ewing sarcoma patients to VDCA with a high-dose, intermittent dosing strategy compared with a lower weekly dosing schedule. Specifically, high-dose cyclophosphamide given every 3 weeks was compared with lower-dose weekly treatments. Additionally, doxorubicin was given every 6 weeks for 9 months compared with alternating doses with dactinomycin. The higher dose–intensity patients showed a 5-year disease-free survival of 68% compared with 48% in the less-intense treatment arm. Overall survival was 77% versus 63%. At this point, evidence suggested that upfront anthracycline and higher-dose alkylators were necessary to improve outcome.

There are several subsequent studies that demonstrated the benefit of adding ifosfamide and etoposide (IE) to the core regimen of VDC (the rationale of which was based on activity observed in the relapsed setting).[30–34] Two studies from the Rizzoli Orthopedic Institute in Bologna, Italy, REN-2 and REN-3, combined IE with VDCA. In REN-2, IE was combined with VDCA in a maintenance strategy.[35] In a single treatment arm, 82 patients received neoadjuvant VDC followed by alternating cycles incorporating IE. At 5 years, disease-free survival was 54% and overall survival 59%. The follow-up study, REN-3, treated 157 patients with nonmetastatic Ewing sarcoma with neoadjuvant VDC and vincristine/ifosfamide/dactinomycin followed by cycles of VDC, vincristine/ifosfamide/dactinomycin, IE, and vincristine/cytoxan/dactinomycin.[36] This complicated regimen first brought ifosfamide into the neoadjuvant stage of treatment and had an improved event-free survival of 71% and overall survival of 76.5% compared with historical controls.

The Children's Oncology Group (including the Pediatric Oncology Group [POG] and Children's Cancer Group [CCG]) designed a randomized trial of 518 patients with localized or metastatic Ewing sarcoma, ages 30 years and younger, where patients received 49 weeks (17 cycles) of VDC alone or alternating cycles of VDC with IE.[4] Dactinomycin replaced doxorubicin after patients received the 375 mg/m^2 of doxorubicin. Local control was planned at week 12 via RT or surgery or both. In the 398 patients without metastatic disease, the 5-year event-free survival was 69% for the VDC/IE arm versus 54% in the VDC arm (P = .005). Overall survival was similarly improved, at 72% and 61% (P = .01), respectively.

The POG/CCG attempted to build on to this VDC/IE regimen by compressing the same total doses of ifosfamide and cyclophosphamide into 11 high-dose cycles every 3 weeks compared with 17 standard doses every 3 weeks[2]; 487 participants were randomized to either arm. Unfortunately, there was no difference in event-free survival and, not surprisingly, toxicity was higher in the dose-intense regimen.

Given the disappointing results of dose intensification, the Children's Oncology Group designed another large randomized study to evaluate the efficacy of increasing dose frequency rather than intensity[15]; 568 patients without evidence of metastatic Ewing sarcoma were randomized to either the standard or dose-dense arm. In the standard arm, patients received VDC/IE every 3 weeks for 2 cycles (4 treatments) followed by local control and then VDC/IE every 3 weeks for 5 doses (10 more treatments). Doxorubicin was limited to a cumulative dose of 375 mg/m^2 and was dropped from subsequent cycles (ie, no dactinomycin was given in this trial). In the experimental arm, patients received VDC/IE every 2 weeks with growth factor support for 3 cycles (6 treatments) followed by local control and then VDC/IE every 2 weeks with growth factor for 4 more cycles (8 more treatments). Again doxorubicin was limited to 375 mg/m^2. The event-free survival at 5 years was 73% for the 14-day regimen and 65% for the 21-day regimen (P = .048). Overall survival was not significantly improved at 83% and 77% (P = .056), respectively, however. The toxicity of the regimens was similar between the arms. Subgroup analysis identified worse outcome in with patients with pelvic primaries and/or age over 18 years old. There were, however, only 67 patients over 18 years old in the study so it is impossible to extrapolate whether the intensified regimen improved outcomes in these high-risk subgroups.

Regarding the primary lesion, there is no current level 1 data on a head-to-head comparison of RT versus surgery versus both RT and surgery in the local management of Ewing sarcoma. Retrospective studies are inherently difficult to interpret due to selection bias. Practice patterns are clinician and center dependent. Many factors are weighed, including the location of disease, the ability to achieve an acceptable surgical outcome (eg, margins, function, and morbidity), and the risks of RT, such as a secondary malignancy and the effects on bone function and growth.

Thus, taken together, standard of care at the authors' institution is VDC/IE given either as dose dense (every 2 weeks) for 14 cycles or every 3 weeks for 17 cycles. There is variable practice between physicians of substituting dactinomycin for doxorubicin after 375 mg/m^2 versus dropping it all together. Although tempting, statistically, the first VDC/IE randomized study (which included dactinomycin) should not be compared with the dose-dense strategy (which omitted dactinomycin) despite the similar event-free and overall survival rates. Because the authors' practice treats primarily adult patients, the decision to attempt a dose-dense strategy is made on a patient-to-patient basis, depending on comorbidities, age, and tolerance of the regimen. Finally, regarding imaging during treatment, there is much variability between studies (discussed previously) and there are no formal United States guidelines. The authors believe, at minimum, that the generally accepted time points for staging include at diagnosis, before definitive tumor therapy (ie, surgery or RT or both), and at completion of treatment. Imaging should include targeting the primary site plus a chest CT; some practitioners include positron emission tomography or bone scans in these later time points. The authors typically repeat primary lesion imaging and a chest CT every 3 months after the completion of chemotherapy. During surveillance after therapy, the US National Comprehensive Cancer Network guidelines suggest physical examination, laboratory tests, and primary site plus chest imaging every 2 to 3 months for 2 years. Thereafter, intervals can be increased up to annually after 5 years. Special attention should be made to long-term complications at these late visits, including secondary RT or chemotherapy-associated malignancies and cardiovascular disease.

Metastatic and Recurrent Ewing Sarcoma

For the approximately 20% of patients with grossly metastatic Ewing sarcoma at presentation, survival remains poor.[3] For example, in the studies discussed previously, 5-year disease-free survival was disappointing and ranged from 9% to 30%. Surveillance, Epidemiology and End Results data suggest that even in the metastatic setting there are some patients that can achieve long-term survival.[3]

Published studies, albeit with small numbers, have explored similar systemic chemotherapy regimens (described previously) for localized disease, including doxorubicin/cylophosphamide, VDCA, and VDCA plus fluorouracil and VDC/IE. Probably the most important of these is the POG/CCG study, where 120 patients with metastatic disease were randomized to either VDC or VDC/IE.[4,16] The 5-year event-free survival was 22% in either treatment arm and overall survival was 34% to 35%. Thus, there was no statistically significant impact on mean overall survival by adding IE to the VDCA backbone. Similar data were seen in single-arm feasibility studies.[37]

Attempts at dose intensification with and without autologous or allogeneic stem cell rescue have been somewhat disappointing. The most recent, and largest, of these was the Euro-EWING 99 trial, which recruited 281 patients with metastatic Ewing sarcoma from 1999 to 2005.[38] Treatment included 6 cycles of vincristine/ifosfamide/doxorubicin/etoposide followed by 1 cycle of vincristine/dactinomycin/ifosfamide before local therapy. The patients were then conditioned with high-dose chemotherapy with busulfan and melphalan with autologous stem cell rescue. Safety was comparable to other regimens during induction and autologous stem cell rescue, with 1 patient dying during induction and 2 within the first 100 days of transplant. The event-free and overall survival rates were 27% and 34%, respectively. These results are comparable to other small reported studies. Thus, although there are some patients who can achieve a durable response, the authors believe that these studies should be reserved for the setting of a clinical trial.

At first diagnosis at the authors' institution, metastatic patients are typically treated with standard VDC/IE or VDC alone with the hope that some of these patients can be salvaged if they achieve responses.[39] The selection of the regimen is based on individual patient characteristics, including symptoms, age, and limited pulmonary metastases. Other regimens that could be considered include vincristine/doxorubicin/ifosfamide and vincristine/ifosfamide/doxorubicin/etoposide.[40] RT is used to treat the primary and other sites based on symptoms alone. Surgical resection may be considered depending on response and the ability to remove all sites of disease (eg, oligometastatic disease in the lung).

Outcomes in the progressive and recurrent setting also remain poor where there is no standard of care and complete responses are rare. In a single-center case series of 114 patients, only 12.3% remained alive at a median follow-up of 61 months.[6] Common regimens include ifosfamide/etoposide (if not given at first treatment),[33] ifosfamide/carboplatin/etoposide,[41] docetaxal/gemcitabine,[42] topotecan/cyclophosphamide,[43,44] and temozolomide/irinotecan.[45,46] The authors typically favor the latter 2 regimens, which combine topoisomerase I inhibitors (topotecan and irinotecan) with alkylators (cyclophosphamide and temozolomide), with reported objective response rates ranging from approximately 30% to 60%. With initial metastatic treatment or at relapse, however, the authors' bias is that early access to clinical trials should be offered to patients where available because, ultimately, it is clear that the limit of chemotherapy in the metastatic setting has been reached.

FUTURE DIRECTIONS

The absence of enzymatic kinase activity of the EWS/FLI1 transcription makes it inherently difficult to drug any protein-protein/protein-DNA interactions. Thus, developing targeted therapies has been a challenge for this disease and new treatment strategies are needed to improve survival for these patients.

Such strategies can be developed by identifying molecular targets that, when inhibited, can decrease the proliferative or metastatic ability of Ewing sarcoma tumor cells. One potential target is the EWS/FLI1 fusion gene product itself. Stegmaier and colleagues[47] screened a small-molecule library for drugs that would induce a gene expression signature for EWS/FLI1 repression. This screen identified cytosine arabinoside as an EWS/FLI1 modulator. Unfortunately, a phase II study of cytosine arabinoside (NCT00470275) did not observe drug activity in patients with relapsed/refractory Ewing sarcoma.[48] Similarly, Grohar and colleagues[49] identified mithramycin as an EWS/FLI1 modulator. A phase II study of mithramycin in refractory Ewing sarcoma is currently underway (NCT01610570). Other modulators of EWS/FLI1 are currently being studied.[50,51]

PARP-1 expression emerged as a potential target for treating Ewing's sarcoma when a high-throughput screen of cancer cell lines identified olaparib as a potent inhibitor of cell lines with EWS/FLI1 translocations.[52] Brenner and colleagues[53] postulated that the DNA damage response protein and transcriptional coregulator, PARP-1, was required for EWS/FLI1-mediated gene transcription. They showed that Ewing sarcoma cells and xenografts were sensitive to PARP-1 inhibition, and the addition of temozolomide to olaparib resulted in complete responses in mouse xenograft models. Phase II studies of olaparib (NCT01583543), a phase I study of olaparib and temozolomide (National Clinical Trial number is pending), and other PARP inhibition studies in recurrent/refractory Ewing sarcoma are under way.

Insulinlike growth factor type 1 receptor (IGF-1R) was identified as a potential target serendipitously when patients with Ewing sarcoma were included in several phase I clinical trials using various IGF-1R inhibitors: R1507[54] and CP-751,871.[55,56] There are currently 5 completed or ongoing phase II trials targeting IGF-1R in Ewing sarcoma: AMG 479 (NCT00563680), SCH 717454 (NCT00617890), CP-751,871 (NCT00560235, NCT00474760), IMC-A12 or cixutumumab (NCT00668148), and R1507 (NCT00642941). These studies show that a 10% to 15% subpopulation of patients with chemotherapy refractory Ewing sarcoma can experience a partial response to IGR-1R inhibition therapy.[57,58] Further studies are needed to determine how to identify this 10% to 15% of patients.

CONCLUDING REMARKS

The improvement in outcome for patients with localized and metastatic Ewing sarcoma since the development of cytotoxic chemotherapy remains one of the most profound advances in oncology and one of the proudest achievements of sarcoma researchers. Over the past decade, however, further progress in patients with recurrent, metastatic, or chemotherapy refractory disease has remained stagnant. VDC/IE remains the chemotherapeutic backbone of Ewing sarcoma therapy, and the addition of other cytotoxic agents to this regimen is unlikely to produce significant benefits. Therefore, identification of molecular targets for new treatments has become an intense area within Ewing sarcoma research. Such targets have been identified by studying (1) cell lines that were either introduced with EWS/FLI1 translocations or derived from tumor, (2) transgenic/xenograft animal models, or (3) human clinical trials. EWS/FLI1, IGF-1R, and PARP are all promising targets but currently do not have well-defined roles in standard clinical management. The development of improved preclinical Ewing sarcoma models and advanced molecular techniques, including high-throughput sequencing, will build on knowledge of EWS/FLI1 function, EWS/FLI1 transcription targets, and the other critical driver events in these tumors. The authors' hope is that these tools ultimately will help identify novel therapeutic strategies in the treatment of this disease.

REFERENCES

1. Askin FB, Rosai J, Sibley RK, et al. Malignant small cell tumor of the thoracopulmonary region in childhood: a distinctive clinicopathologic entity of uncertain histogenesis. Cancer 1979;43:2438–51.
2. Granowetter L, Womer R, Devidas M, et al. Dose-intensified compared with standard chemotherapy for nonmetastatic Ewing sarcoma family of tumors: a Children's Oncology Group Study. J Clin Oncol 2009;27:2536–41.

3. Esiashvili N, Goodman M, Marcus RB Jr. Changes in incidence and survival of Ewing sarcoma patients over the past 3 decades: Surveillance Epidemiology and End Results data. J Pediatr Hematol Oncol 2008;30:425–30.

4. Grier HE, Krailo MD, Tarbell NJ, et al. Addition of ifosfamide and etoposide to standard chemotherapy for Ewing's sarcoma and primitive neuroectodermal tumor of bone. N Engl J Med 2003;348:694–701.

5. Cotterill SJ, Ahrens S, Paulussen M, et al. Prognostic factors in Ewing's tumor of bone: analysis of 975 patients from the European Intergroup Cooperative Ewing's Sarcoma Study Group. J Clin Oncol 2000;18:3108–14.

6. Whelan J, McTiernan A, Cooper N, et al. Incidence and survival of malignant bone sarcomas in England 1979-2007. Int J Cancer 2012;131:E508–17.

7. Stiller CA, Parkin DM. Geographic and ethnic variations in the incidence of childhood cancer. Br Med Bull 1996;52:682–703.

8. Randall RL, Lessnick SL, Jones KB, et al. Is there a predisposition gene for Ewing's sarcoma? J Oncol 2010;2010:397632.

9. Widhe B, Widhe T. Initial symptoms and clinical features in osteosarcoma and Ewing sarcoma. J Bone Joint Surg Am 2000;82:667–74.

10. Craft A, Cotterill S, Malcolm A, et al. Ifosfamide-containing chemotherapy in Ewing's sarcoma: The Second United Kingdom Children's Cancer Study Group and the Medical Research Council Ewing's Tumor Study. J Clin Oncol 1998;16:3628–33.

11. Kissane JM, Askin FB, Foulkes M, et al. Ewing's sarcoma of bone: clinicopathologic aspects of 303 cases from the Intergroup Ewing's Sarcoma Study. Hum Pathol 1983;14:773–9.

12. Gupta AA, Pappo A, Saunders N, et al. Clinical outcome of children and adults with localized Ewing sarcoma: impact of chemotherapy dose and timing of local therapy. Cancer 2010;116:3189–94.

13. Nesbit ME Jr, Gehan EA, Burgert EO Jr, et al. Multimodal therapy for the management of primary, nonmetastatic Ewing's sarcoma of bone: a long-term follow-up of the First Intergroup study. J Clin Oncol 1990;8:1664–74.

14. Glaubiger DL, Makuch R, Schwarz J, et al. Determination of prognostic factors and their influence on therapeutic results in patients with Ewing's sarcoma. Cancer 1980;45:2213–9.

15. Womer RB, West DC, Krailo MD, et al. Randomized controlled trial of interval-compressed chemotherapy for the treatment of localized Ewing sarcoma: a report from the Children's Oncology Group. J Clin Oncol 2012;30:4148–54.

16. Miser JS, Krailo MD, Tarbell NJ, et al. Treatment of metastatic Ewing's sarcoma or primitive neuroectodermal tumor of bone: evaluation of combination ifosfamide and etoposide–a Children's Cancer Group and Pediatric Oncology Group study. J Clin Oncol 2004;22:2873–6.

17. Paulussen M, Ahrens S, Burdach S, et al. Primary metastatic (stage IV) Ewing tumor: survival analysis of 171 patients from the EICESS studies. European Intergroup Cooperative Ewing Sarcoma Studies. Ann Oncol 1998;9:275–81.

18. Paulussen M, Ahrens S, Craft AW, et al. Ewing's tumors with primary lung metastases: survival analysis of 114 (European Intergroup) Cooperative Ewing's Sarcoma Studies patients. J Clin Oncol 1998;16:3044–52.

19. Tan AY, Manley JL. The TET family of proteins: functions and roles in disease. J Mol Cell Biol 2009;1:82–92.

20. Jain S, Xu R, Prieto VG, et al. Molecular classification of soft tissue sarcomas and its clinical applications. Int J Clin Exp Pathol 2010;3:416–28.

21. Peter M, Couturier J, Pacquement H, et al. A new member of the ETS family fused to EWS in Ewing tumors. Oncogene 1997;14:1159–64.
22. Turc-Carel C, Aurias A, Mugneret F, et al. Chromosomes in Ewing's sarcoma. I. An evaluation of 85 cases of remarkable consistency of t(11;22)(q24;q12). Cancer Genet Cytogenet 1988;32:229–38.
23. Downing JR, Head DR, Parham DM, et al. Detection of the (11;22)(q24;q12) translocation of Ewing's sarcoma and peripheral neuroectodermal tumor by reverse transcription polymerase chain reaction. Am J Pathol 1993;143:1294–300.
24. Zucman J, Melot T, Desmaze C, et al. Combinatorial generation of variable fusion proteins in the Ewing family of tumours. EMBO J 1993;12:4481–7.
25. Sorensen PH, Lessnick SL, Lopez-Terrada D, et al. A second Ewing's sarcoma translocation, t(21;22), fuses the EWS gene to another ETS-family transcription factor, ERG. Nat Genet 1994;6:146–51.
26. Bielack SS, Paulussen M, Kohler G. A patient with two Ewing's sarcomas with distinct EWS fusion transcripts. N Engl J Med 2004;350:1364–5.
27. Jeon IS, Davis JN, Braun BS, et al. A variant Ewing's sarcoma translocation (7;22) fuses the EWS gene to the ETS gene ETV1. Oncogene 1995;10:1229–34.
28. Smith MA, Ungerleider RS, Horowitz ME, et al. Influence of doxorubicin dose intensity on response and outcome for patients with osteogenic sarcoma and Ewing's sarcoma. J Natl Cancer Inst 1991;83:1460–70.
29. Burgert EO Jr, Nesbit ME, Garnsey LA, et al. Multimodal therapy for the management of nonpelvic, localized Ewing's sarcoma of bone: intergroup study IESS-II. J Clin Oncol 1990;8:1514–24.
30. Antman KH, Ryan L, Elias A, et al. Response to ifosfamide and mesna: 124 previously treated patients with metastatic or unresectable sarcoma. J Clin Oncol 1989;7:126–31.
31. Jurgens H, Exner U, Kuhl J, et al. High-dose ifosfamide with mesna uroprotection in Ewing's sarcoma. Cancer Chemother Pharmacol 1989;24(Suppl 1):S40–4.
32. Magrath I, Sandlund J, Raynor A, et al. A phase II study of ifosfamide in the treatment of recurrent sarcomas in young people. Cancer Chemother Pharmacol 1986;18(Suppl 2):S25–8.
33. Miser JS, Kinsella TJ, Triche TJ, et al. Ifosfamide with mesna uroprotection and etoposide: an effective regimen in the treatment of recurrent sarcomas and other tumors of children and young adults. J Clin Oncol 1987;5:1191–8.
34. Kung FH, Pratt CB, Vega RA, et al. Ifosfamide/etoposide combination in the treatment of recurrent malignant solid tumors of childhood. A Pediatric Oncology Group Phase II study. Cancer 1993;71:1898–903.
35. Bacci G, Picci P, Ferrari S, et al. Neoadjuvant chemotherapy for Ewing's sarcoma of bone: no benefit observed after adding ifosfamide and etoposide to vincristine, actinomycin, cyclophosphamide, and doxorubicin in the maintenance phase–results of two sequential studies. Cancer 1998;82:1174–83.
36. Bacci G, Mercuri M, Longhi A, et al. Neoadjuvant chemotherapy for Ewing's tumour of bone: recent experience at the Rizzoli Orthopaedic Institute. Eur J Cancer 2002;38:2243–51.
37. Wexler LH, DeLaney TF, Tsokos M, et al. Ifosfamide and etoposide plus vincristine, doxorubicin, and cyclophosphamide for newly diagnosed Ewing's sarcoma family of tumors. Cancer 1996;78:901–11.
38. Ladenstein R, Potschger U, Le Deley MC, et al. Primary disseminated multifocal Ewing sarcoma: results of the Euro-EWING 99 trial. J Clin Oncol 2010;28:3284–91.

39. Choy E, Digumarthy SR, Koplin SA. Case records of the Massachusetts General Hospital. Case 36-2009. A 23-year-old man with cough, hoarseness, and abnormalities on chest imaging. N Engl J Med 2009;361:2080–7.

40. Juergens C, Weston C, Lewis I, et al. Safety assessment of intensive induction with vincristine, ifosfamide, doxorubicin, and etoposide (VIDE) in the treatment of Ewing tumors in the EURO-E.W.I.N.G. 99 clinical trial. Pediatr Blood Cancer 2006;47:22–9.

41. Van Winkle P, Angiolillo A, Krailo M, et al. Ifosfamide, carboplatin, and etoposide (ICE) reinduction chemotherapy in a large cohort of children and adolescents with recurrent/refractory sarcoma: the Children's Cancer Group (CCG) experience. Pediatr Blood Cancer 2005;44:338–47.

42. Navid F, Willert JR, McCarville MB, et al. Combination of gemcitabine and docetaxel in the treatment of children and young adults with refractory bone sarcoma. Cancer 2008;113:419–25.

43. Bernstein ML, Devidas M, Lafreniere D, et al. Intensive therapy with growth factor support for patients with Ewing tumor metastatic at diagnosis: Pediatric Oncology Group/Children's Cancer Group Phase II Study 9457–a report from the Children's Oncology Group. J Clin Oncol 2006;24:152–9.

44. Hunold A, Weddeling N, Paulussen M, et al. Topotecan and cyclophosphamide in patients with refractory or relapsed Ewing tumors. Pediatr Blood Cancer 2006;47:795–800.

45. Wagner LM, McAllister N, Goldsby RE, et al. Temozolomide and intravenous irinotecan for treatment of advanced Ewing sarcoma. Pediatr Blood Cancer 2007;48:132–9.

46. Casey DA, Wexler LH, Merchant MS, et al. Irinotecan and temozolomide for Ewing sarcoma: the Memorial Sloan-Kettering experience. Pediatr Blood Cancer 2009;53:1029–34.

47. Stegmaier K, Wong JS, Ross KN, et al. Signature-based small molecule screening identifies cytosine arabinoside as an EWS/FLI modulator in Ewing sarcoma. PLoS Med 2007;4:e122.

48. DuBois SG, Krailo MD, Lessnick SL, et al. Phase II study of intermediate-dose cytarabine in patients with relapsed or refractory Ewing sarcoma: a report from the Children's Oncology Group. Pediatr Blood Cancer 2009;52:324–7.

49. Grohar PJ, Woldemichael GM, Griffin LB, et al. Identification of an inhibitor of the EWS-FLI1 oncogenic transcription factor by high-throughput screening. J Natl Cancer Inst 2011;103:962–78.

50. Boro A, Pretre K, Rechfeld F, et al. Small-molecule screen identifies modulators of EWS/FLI1 target gene expression and cell survival in Ewing's sarcoma. Int J Cancer 2012;131:2153–64.

51. Erkizan HV, Kong Y, Merchant M, et al. A small molecule blocking oncogenic protein EWS-FLI1 interaction with RNA helicase A inhibits growth of Ewing's sarcoma. Nat Med 2009;15:750–6.

52. Garnett MJ, Edelman EJ, Heidorn SJ, et al. Systematic identification of genomic markers of drug sensitivity in cancer cells. Nature 2012;483:570–5.

53. Brenner JC, Feng FY, Han S, et al. PARP-1 inhibition as a targeted strategy to treat Ewing's sarcoma. Cancer Res 2012;72:1608–13.

54. Kurzrock R, Patnaik A, Aisner J, et al. A phase I study of weekly R1507, a human monoclonal antibody insulin-like growth factor-I receptor antagonist, in patients with advanced solid tumors. Clin Cancer Res 2010;16:2458–65.

55. Haluska P, Worden F, Olmos D, et al. Safety, tolerability, and pharmacokinetics of the anti-IGF-1R monoclonal antibody figitumumab in patients with refractory adrenocortical carcinoma. Cancer Chemother Pharmacol 2010;65:765–73.
56. Olmos D, Postel-Vinay S, Molife LR, et al. Safety, pharmacokinetics, and preliminary activity of the anti-IGF-1R antibody figitumumab (CP-751,871) in patients with sarcoma and Ewing's sarcoma: a phase 1 expansion cohort study. Lancet Oncol 2010;11:129–35.
57. Juergens H, Daw NC, Geoerger B, et al. Preliminary efficacy of the anti-insulin-like growth factor type 1 receptor antibody figitumumab in patients with refractory Ewing sarcoma. J Clin Oncol 2011;29:4534–40.
58. Pappo AS, Patel SR, Crowley J, et al. R1507, a monoclonal antibody to the insulin-like growth factor 1 receptor, in patients with recurrent or refractory Ewing sarcoma family of tumors: results of a phase II Sarcoma Alliance for Research through Collaboration study. J Clin Oncol 2011;29:4541–7.

Update on Targets and Novel Treatment Options for High-Grade Osteosarcoma and Chondrosarcoma

Jolieke G. van Oosterwijk, MSc[a], Jakob K. Anninga, MD, PhD[b],
Hans Gelderblom, MD, PhD[b], Anne-Marie Cleton-Jansen, PhD[a],
Judith V.M.G. Bovée, MD, PhD[a],*

KEYWORDS

- Osteosarcoma • Chondrosarcoma • Hypoxia • Sarcoma • Bone tumor
- Chemotherapy • Targeted therapy

KEY POINTS

- Since the introduction of conventional adjuvant chemotherapy 3 decades ago, survival of patients with osteosarcoma has reached a plateau of efficacy at 60% to 65%; patients with metastases at diagnosis have a poor fate.
- Immune stimulation is one of the few treatment options that may improve survival of patients with osteosarcoma.
- Chondrosarcoma is resistant to conventional chemotherapy and radiotherapy, and currently there are no curative options for patients with inoperable or metastatic disease.
- Targeting of apoptosis and survival pathways are promising approaches that may improve survival of patients with chondrosarcoma.

INTRODUCTION

Primary bone tumors are rare and have a specific age distribution (**Fig. 1**). Conventional osteosarcoma is the most frequent primary high-grade bone tumor in humans; there are 4 new cases per 10^6 population per year with the highest incidence in

Financial Support: Our research on bone tumors is financially supported by the Dutch Cancer Society (UL2010-4873: J.G. van Oosterwijk, J.V.M.G. Bovée), the Netherlands Organization for Scientific Research (917-67-315: J.V.M.G. Bovée) and EuroSARC, a collaborative project within the EC's 7th Framework programme under grant agreement 278742 (J.G. van Oosterwijk, A.M. Cleton-Jansen, H. Gelderblom, J.V.M.G. Bovée).
Disclosure: The authors have no conflicts of interest to disclose.
[a] Department of Pathology, Leiden University Medical Center, PO Box 9600, L1-Q, Leiden RC 2300, The Netherlands; [b] Department of Clinical Oncology, Leiden University Medical Center, PO Box 9600, K1, Leiden RC 2300, The Netherlands
* Corresponding author.
E-mail address: j.v.m.g.bovee@lumc.nl

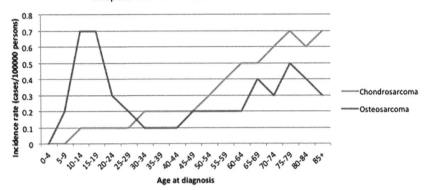

Age specific incidence rates
adapted from WHO classification of bone tumours

Fig. 1. Incidence of osteosarcoma and chondrosarcoma stratified by age group. Osteosarcoma is most common in adolescents, and a second incidence peak is observed after the sixth decade of life, in part caused by secondary osteosarcoma. Chondrosarcoma is the second most common primary bone malignancy in humans and occurs predominantly between the third and sixth decade of life. The increase in incidence observed after the sixth decade is attributed to recurrences. (*Adapted from* Fletcher CD, Bridge JA, Hogendoorn PC, et al. WHO classification of tumours of soft tissue and bone. 4th edition. 2013; with permission.)

adolescence.[1] The second most frequent primary bone malignancy, chondrosarcoma, accounts for approximately 3 new cases per 10^6 population per year predominantly affecting adults.[2] The clinical management of unresectable and metastatic disease as well as therapy resistance remain a clinical challenge.[3] This review discusses the molecular pathways that have been identified as a result of intensive genome-wide and basic biology analysis and the rationale for current clinical and preclinical targets for therapy for these 2 most frequent bone sarcomas.

OSTEOSARCOMA
Clinicopathologic Features

Conventional osteosarcoma is defined as a high-grade intraosseous malignant neoplasm in which the neoplastic cells produce bone.[1] Osteosarcoma represents about 55% of all malignant bone tumors and occurs predominantly in children and adolescents (see **Fig. 1**).[4] Most osteosarcomas are located around the knee (60%, **Fig. 2**) and other long tubular bones of the skeleton. Histologically, a broad spectrum of morphology can be seen, including varying amounts of osteoid, cartilage, and/or fibrous material.[1] In addition to conventional osteosarcoma, the World Health Organization 2013 classification recognizes low-grade central, parosteal, periosteal, and high-grade surface osteosarcoma as well as telangiectatic and small cell osteosarcoma as distinct, less frequent subtypes[1]; the latter 2 are also of high histologic grade. All high-grade osteosarcomas have a similar clinical behavior with a high risk of metastasis.

Osteosarcoma is primary when the underlying bone is normal and secondary when the bone is altered by conditions such as previous radiation or Paget disease. There is an increased incidence of primary osteosarcoma associated with several genetic syndromes, eg, Li-Fraumeni syndrome (TP53), hereditary retinoblastoma (Rb), or Rothmund-Thomson (RECQ-helicase); in older adults it is often secondary.[1] Although

Osteosarcoma   Chondrosarcoma

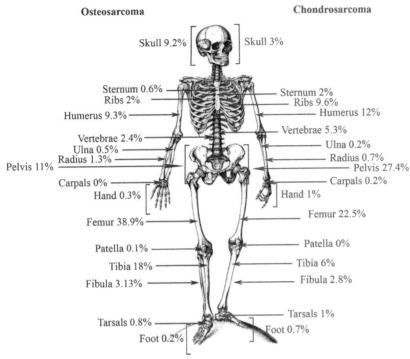

Skull 9.2%   Skull 3%

Sternum 0.6%   Sternum 2%
Ribs 2%   Ribs 9.6%
Humerus 9.3%   Humerus 12%

                                      Vertebrae 5.3%
Vertebrae 2.4%
Ulna 0.5%   Ulna 0.2%
Radius 1.3%   Radius 0.7%
Pelvis 11%   Pelvis 27.4%

Carpals 0%   Carpals 0.2%
Hand 0.3%   Hand 1%

                                      Femur 22.5%
Femur 38.9%

Patella 0.1%   Patella 0%

Tibia 18%   Tibia 6%

Fibula 3.13%   Fibula 2.8%

                                      Tarsals 1%
Tarsals 0.8%   Foot 0.7%
Foot 0.2%

Fig. 2. Distribution of osteosarcoma and chondrosarcoma across the skeleton. (*Adapted from* Unni KK, Inwards CY. Dahlin's bone tumors: general aspects and data on 10,165 cases. 6th edition. Philadelphia: Lippincott Williams & Wilkins; 2010. p. 7; with permission.)

rare, the incidence of osteosarcoma in these syndromes is manifold higher than in the general population, suggesting that the genes involved in these syndromes play an important role in the biology of osteosarcomas. Dismal prognostic factors for osteosarcoma are metastatic disease at diagnosis, proximal or axial tumor site, large size, and poor histologic response to preoperative chemotherapy.[5]

Current Management of Osteosarcoma and Resistance to Therapy

Osteosarcoma should be treated by an experienced multidisciplinary team and treatment consists of preoperative and postoperative chemotherapy and (complete) surgical resection of the tumor and, if present, metastatic tumor deposits.[6] Despite intensive treatment strategies, the chance of cure in patients with resectable osteosarcoma has remained around 60% to 65% in the past 3 decades,[7] indicating that a plateau of efficacy regarding conventional chemotherapy has been reached. In nearly all failures of treatment, the patients die from systemic spread of the disease, mainly to the lungs and bones.[8] Resistance to cytotoxic drugs has been recognized in osteosarcoma,[9] and is a marker for poor prognosis. However, patients with a good histologic response to chemotherapy may also develop metastases or recurrent disease, suggesting the presence of heterogeneous tumor cell populations. There is cumulating evidence that osteosarcomas contain cells with a tumor-initiating or so-called stem cell phenotype displaying a high tumorigenic capacity, and harboring multidrug resistance proteins contributing to resistance and recurrence of disease.[10–12]

Osteosarcoma is characterized by a highly instable and complex karyotype,[13] suggesting that genetic instability is the initial cause of osteosarcoma genesis. The recently described phenomenon chromothripsis, indicating scattering of chromosomes, is typical in osteosarcoma.[14] However, repair of genetic instability does not restore the damaged done. Several molecular pathways involved in osteosarcoma genesis are discussed as far as these are relevant and druggable (**Table 1**).

P53-related signaling

Mutational inactivation of the tumor suppressor gene *TP53* disrupts checkpoint responses to DNA damage, resulting in the potential for destabilization of the genome.[15] *TP53* mutations cause Li-Fraumeni syndrome; somatic *TP53* mutations also occur in 15% to 30% of osteosarcomas.[16] Presumed associations with prognosis are not reproducible.[17] MDM-family proteins that are involved in p53 protein degradation have been shown to be upregulated in many tumor types, although amplification of *MDM2* in osteosarcoma was especially found in the parosteal subtype.[18] Recently, an association with good prognosis and high expression of an MDM4 splice variation has been shown in osteosarcoma.[19] Both MDM2 and MDM4 are druggable targets through Nutlin-3[20]; RO5045337, and other drugs are in development (NCT01164033).

Retinoblastoma signaling

The tumor suppressor retinoblastoma gene *RB1* has a central role as a checkpoint in the cell cycle (**Fig. 4**). Loss of function as occurring in patients with an *RB1* germline mutation increases the risk of osteosarcoma up to 500-fold.[21,22] In osteosarcomas, *RB1* gene abnormalities have been found in 26% to 53% of patients.[23–26] Inactivation of the *RB1* gene also contributes to genomic instability in osteosarcomas.[27,28]

The product of the *CDKN2A/p16* gene is part of the Rb pathway inhibiting cell cycle progression by preventing the formation of the cyclin D-Cdk4 complex. Genomic loss, rather than inactivation by hypermethylation of *CDKN2A/p16* was strongly associated with a poor prognosis in osteosarcoma.[29,30] Homozygous deletion of the entire *CDKN2* locus, including *p16*, *p19*, and *p15* is always a recurrent event in oncogenic transformation of mouse mesenchymal stem cells, which form osteosarcomalike lesions on transplantation into mice.[29] However, only 10% of human osteosarcomas harbor a *CDKN2A* homozygous deletion.

Pharmacologic intervention to restore the defective RB signaling does not seem feasible. Identification of homozygous deletion of *CDKN2A* may serve as a useful prognostic marker to identify tumors with a very poor prognosis.

Developmental pathways: Wnt, TGF, bone morphogenetic protein, and hedgehog

Canonical Wnt signaling, through nuclear β-catenin, is important in many developmental processes, including osteogenic differentiation and many different cancer types.[31,32] Both upregulation and downregulation of the Wnt/β-catenin pathway has been reported in osteosarcoma.[33–35] Restoration of Wnt/β-catenin activation resulted in decreased proliferation and differentiation of the tumor cells, thereby suggesting a tumor suppressive role for this pathway in osteosarcoma.[35]

The noncanonical or β-catenin independent Wnt pathway has also been implicated in osteosarcoma, predominantly via the receptor tyrosine kinase ROR2. The Wnt5a ligand and ROR-2 receptor contribute to invasiveness of osteosarcoma cells, mediated via the matrix-metalloproteinase, MMP13.[36] Because the receptor tyrosine kinase ROR2 was found to be overexpressed in osteosarcomas, inhibition of this receptor could be a potential target.[37] Clinical phase 1 studies targeting the Wnt

Table 1

Overview of selected targets and trials in osteosarcoma

Target	Drug	Mechanism	Type of Trial and Clinical Results (n = Number of OS Cases)	Reference or Clinical Trial Identifier
IGF-1R	SCH717454/RG1507	MoAb anti-IGF-1R	Phase 1 (n = 3), NOR	182
EGF/EGF-R	Gefitinib	Small anti-EGF-R TK	Phase 1 (n = 9), NOR	183
PDGF/PDGF-R; KIT	Erlotinib	Small anti-EGF-R TK	Phase 1 (n = 6), NOR	
	Imatinib/STI571	Small anti-PDGF-R TK	Phase 2 (n = 38), NOR	
	Sorafenib	Small anti-VEGFR, anti-PDGFR and anti-KIT TK	Phase 2 (n = 35), 3 PR	140
	Pazopanib	Small anti-VEGFR1, -2, -3 PDGFRα/β and anti-Kit TK		NCT01759303
HER2	Trastuzumab	MoAb anti-HER2	Phase 2 (n = 41 HER2+), no difference in OAS/EFS between HER2+ and −	56
VEGF/VEGFR	Bevacizumab (+sorafenib/cyclo)	MoAb against 4 VEGF isoforms	Phase 1 (n = 5), NOR	184
	Endostatin	MoAb against VEGFR2		NCT01002092
	Cediranib/AZD2171	Small anti-VEGFR1, -2, -3 and anti-Kit TK	Phase 1 (n = 2), 1 PR	185

(continued on next page)

Table 1
(continued)

Target	Drug	Mechanism	Type of Trial and Clinical Results (n = Number of OS Cases)	Reference or Clinical Trial Identifier
DNA synthesis	Gemcitabine	Nucleoside analogue	Phase 2 (n = 10), NOR	186
	Gemcitabine + docetaxel	Nucleoside analogue	Phase 2 (n = 30), 6 PR	
	Pemetrexed (PMX)	Folate antagonist	Phase 2 (n = 32), 1 PR; phase 2 (n = 10), NOR	187
DNA minor groove	Ecteinascidin-743	Alkylating agent, inhibits cell cycle progression, enhances apoptosis	Phase 1 (n = 7), 2 PR; phase 2 (n = 23) NOR	188–190
Microtubules	Paclitaxel	Enhances microtubule polymerization, disrupts microtubule network, induces apoptosis	Phase 2 (n = 11), NOR	191
	Docetaxel		Phase 2 (n = 34), 1 CR, 2 PR	192,193
	Ixabepilone		Phase 2 (n = 11), NOR	194
RANK/RANKL	Zoledronic acid	Blocks mevalonate pathway, preventing isoprenylation of GTP-binding proteins, small, membrane-bound G-proteins cannot function		NTC00691236
	Pamidronate	See zoledronic acid	Phase 2 (n = 29), no efficacy reported, no serious side effects	82
SRC	Saracatinib	Inhibits tumor-induced SRC overexpression osteoclasts		NTC00752206
AKT/PI3K/mTOR	Deforolimus	mTOR inhibitor	Phase 1 (n = 1), NOR	195
	Ridaforolimus	mTOR inhibitor	Phase 2 (n = 212) 2 OS patients showed PR	196
	Sirolimus + cyclophosphamide	Antiproliferative, cell cycle arrest, antiapoptotic	Phase 2 (n = 6), NOR	197
	Everolimus	Binds to mTORC1 complex, inhibits downstream signaling; inhibits VEGF and HIF		NCT01216826

Multiple	Curcumin	Cell cycle arrest in G2/M, increased apoptosis (decrease Bcl-2, increase Bax IC), inhibition migration/adhesion. Antagonizing growth factors, protein kinases, cytokine signaling, cyclin D, and upregulates p53		NCT00689195
INF-α/β	INF-α/β	Activation of Ifn type 1-specific response elements via the TK/JAK-STAT1/2 pathway, activating T cells, macrophages, and NK cells	Phase 2 (n = 20), 4 PR; phase 3 (n = 89), 10y-EFS 39%	72
Immune-competent cells	MTP-PE	MTP binds NOD2 receptor in monocytes, dendritic cells, and macrophages leading to NF-κB activation	Phase 2 (n = 28), TTR 9.0 vs 4.5 mo (P<.03); phase 3 (OS IIb, n = 338), OAS 78% vs 70% (P<.03); phase 3 (OSIII, n = 46), OAS 53% vs 40% (P = .27)	64,198,199
GM-CSF	Sargramostim	Increase number/cytotoxicity of macrophages, T cells, NK cells, and dendritic cells	Phase 2 (n = 43); NOR	74
	GM-CSF + gemcitabine	Increase immunologic response and FAS expression		
T cell	105AD7 vaccine	Immune response against CD55	Phase 2 (n = 14), n = 5 have response	
	Anti-GD2	Immune response against disialoganglioside (GD2)	Phase 1 (n = 1), NOR	NCT00743496

Abbreviations: AKT, protein kinase B; CR, complete response; EFS, event-free survival; EGF, epidermal growth factor; GM-CSF, granulocyte-macrophage colony-stimulating factor; HER, human epidermal growth factor receptor; HIF, hypoxia inducible factor; IGF-1, insulinlike growth factor 1; Ifn, interferon; JAK, Janus kinase; MoAB, Monoclonal Antibody; mTOR, mammalian target of rapamycin; MTP-PE, muramyl tripeptide phosphatidylethanolamine; NK, natural killer; NOR, no objective response; OAS, overall survival; OS, osteosarcoma; PDGF, platelet-derived growth factor-α; PI3K, phosphoinositide 3-kinase; PR, partial response; R, receptor; RANK, receptor activator of NF-kappa B; RANKL, receptor activator of NF-kappa B ligand; STAT, signal transducer and activator of transcription; TK, tyrosine kinase; TTR, time to relapse; VEGF, vascular endothelial growth factor.

pathway are under way, such as the Wnt-pathway antagonist OMP-54F28 (NCT01608867).

Other developmental pathways in osteogenesis include the SMAD-mediated TGFβ and bone morphogenetic protein pathways and the hedgehog pathways. Decreased expression of phosphorylated SMAD2, indicating decreased TGFβ signaling, was shown to be associated with poor survival in osteosarcoma.[38] Activity of the hedgehog pathway is variable in osteosarcoma and cyclopamine, an inhibitor of hedgehog signaling was shown to inhibit osteosarcoma cell line proliferation, but this was independent of hedgehog signal transduction and could most likely be attributed to a specific toxicity of this compound.[38] Other drugs targeting the hedgehog pathway are currently under development in (osteo)sarcoma; eg, IPI-906, LDE225, and GDC-0449.

Proliferative pathways: insulin growth factor

In vertebrates, insulinlike growth factor 1 (IGF-1) is a major growth-promoting signal for skeletal development.[39] Aberrant signaling of the IGF-1 pathway through its receptors IGF-1R and IR (insulin receptor) has been implicated in various cancer types, including sarcomas.[40,41] Treatment with different monoclonal antibodies against IGF-1R has been performed in xenograft models of osteosarcoma, in which a response was detected in at least 60% of all cases studied.[42–44]

Proliferative pathways: platelet-derived growth factor

Platelet-derived growth factor-α (PDGF-AA) and its receptor (PDGFRA) were found to be expressed on osteosarcoma cells, suggesting an autocrine/paracrine loop of growth stimulation,[45,46] although mutations were absent.[47] Inhibition of PDGFRA using imatinib in osteosarcoma cell lines blocked intracellular PDGFRA-induced cell signaling, but the downstream target, mitogen-activated protein kinase, was constitutively activated, indicating an escape route of induction.[46] Expression of KIT, another tyrosine kinase receptor blocked by imatinib, was found in 20% of osteosarcomas, although KIT mutations were absent.[48] The multi (including PDGFRA) tyrosine kinase inhibitor sorafenib was found to be active in preclinical osteosarcoma models[49,50] and in a phase 2 study.[51] These results warrant further studies of this (class of) drugs in osteosarcoma.

Proliferative pathways: human epidermal growth factor

The human epidermal growth factor receptor 2 (HER2) is a 185-kDa membrane-bound glycoprotein, encoded by the *ErbB2* protooncogene.[52,53] Overexpression of the HER2 gene by *ErbB2* amplification results in oncogenic transformation of cells. In osteosarcomas, HER2 overexpression is associated with metastasis[54] and with increased expression of P-glycoprotein.[55] Targeted treatment with the monoclonal antibody trastuzumab is an effective treatment in HER2-overexpressing breast cancers, and is supposed to have a beneficial effect in osteosarcomas. Therefore, a phase 2 trial in patients with osteosarcomas has been launched.[56] However, not all groups could confirm HER2 overexpression in osteosarcoma,[57–59] and the theoretic backbone for the use of trastuzumab is debatable. The phase 2 trial did not show a difference in outcome among presumed HER2+ and HER2− patients, suggesting that HER2 should not be regarded as a target for treatment of osteosarcoma.[56]

Immune modulation

The role of immunotherapy in osteosarcoma has not been elucidated yet, but has been regarded as a magic box since the use of Coley's toxin, which produced a regression in osteosarcomas that were not amenable to surgery.[60] The recent insights in the complex immunologic interplay of immune-competent cells in cancer, the plasticity of this immune response,[61] and diverse effects of infiltrating macrophages in carcinomas versus sarcomas[62] have increased the interest in immunomodulation of osteosarcomas. It has been shown that the presence of tumor-infiltrating macrophages in biopsy samples of osteosarcoma was associated with reduced metastatic propensity and better survival.[63] This observation could be a rationale for adjuvant treatment with muramyl tripeptide phosphatidylethanolamine (MTP-PE), an immune stimulatory drug.[64] However, the results of the landmark phase 3 study investigating the benefit of MTP-PE in frontline treatment of osteosarcoma has been a matter of debate, leaving the indication for this drug unsure or unregistered in many countries.[64–66]

In addition, the cytotoxic potential of natural killer cells against osteosarcoma cells was demonstrated to be activated by IL15[67] or cetuximab.[68] Other drugs that can activate macrophage activity in tumors that have not been investigated yet in osteosarcoma, such as paclitaxel, are reported to activate the macrophage response in vitro, through a mechanism similar to bacterial liopopolysaccharides.[69]

Immune stimulation by interferon (Ifn) was supported by in vitro studies, demonstrating a more intensive effect of Ifn-α compared with the type-2 Ifn, Ifn-γ.[70] Nonrandomized clinical experience with Ifn-α showed a long-term event-free survival of 40% in a patient group treated with Ifn-α as adjuvant to local treatment with surgery.[71] Limited clinical experience had shown a transient effect of Ifn-α in patients with lung metastases[72] and advanced disease.[73] The recently closed EURAMOS-1 study will provide a more definitive answer about the contribution of immune modulation later in 2013, as this study included an arm with Ifn-α in addition to conventional chemotherapy in good responders after primary osteosarcoma treatment (www.euramos. org).

Other immunologic approaches, for example, inhalation of granulocyte-macrophage colony-stimulating factor (GM-CSF), did not seem effective in patients,[74] and addition of interleukin-1α to etoposide has an unwarranted spectrum of side effects, too serious to use on a large scale in patients.[75] Vaccination with the antiidiotype vaccine 105AD7 showed measurable T-cell responses in patients,[76] but the advantage for patients with osteosarcoma in the clinic needs to be established.

Other therapies: bisphosphonates and tyrosine kinase inhibitors

Bisphosphonates such as zoledronic acid or pamidronate inhibit osteoclast activity and are found to be effective in avoiding complications caused by bone metastases. However, (pre)clinical experience with these compounds proved that bisphosphonates also exerted antineoplastic effects.[77] In osteosarcoma cells, a caspase-independent apoptosis was reported after exposure to zoledronic acid.[78] This P53-independent apoptosis occurred via mitochondrial pathways in these osteosarcoma cells. In another study, the presence of the drug-resistance protein P-glycoprotein did not impair the anticancer activity of the bisphosphonates.[79] In addition, osteosarcoma cells could be inhibited in their migration capacity[80] and lung metastases could be suppressed by bisphosphonates.[81] These antitumor effects have led to the initiation of a phase 2 clinical trial with pamidronate in addition to the routine chemotherapy schedule for patients with localized or metastatic osteosarcoma.[82] Event-free survival in this uncontrolled trial for patients with localized disease after 5 years was 72% and overall survival was 93%, whereas 45% of the patients with metastatic disease survived without recurrence. Currently, the French led OS2006 trial is investigating the addition of pamidronate to frontline chemotherapy in patients with resectable osteosarcoma in a randomized fashion.

CHONDROSARCOMA
Clinicopathologic Features

Chondrosarcomas are hyaline cartilaginous tumors most often arising in bones that develop during endochondral ossification. Incidence and location are shown in **Figs. 1** and **2**. Conventional chondrosarcoma accounts for approximately 85% of all primary chondrosarcomas[3] and prognosis is strongly correlated with histologic grading. Grade I chondrosarcoma, now reclassified as an atypical cartilaginous tumor, shows low cellularity and is locally aggressive, but typically does not metastasize.[2] Grade II and grade III conventional chondrosarcomas show increased cellularity with mitoses and reduced cartilaginous matrix, and a corresponding increase in metastasizing capacity alongside poor patient survival.[2,83] Amongst the rare chondrosarcoma subtypes, dedifferentiated chondrosarcoma accounts for up to 10% of all chondrosarcomas and has a dismal prognosis. Dedifferentiated chondrosarcoma is composed of 2 histologically distinct components: a high-grade dedifferentiated component and a seemingly low-grade cartilaginous component.[84] Mesenchymal chondrosarcoma is considered high grade and accounts for approximately 3% of primary chondrosarcomas, histologically showing undifferentiated small round cells admixed with well-differentiated cartilage.[85] Clear cell chondrosarcoma is considered low grade and accounts for 2% of all primary chondrosarcomas, demonstrating tumor cells with a clear empty cytoplasm.[86] Extraskeletal myxoid chondrosarcoma is primarily located in soft tissue and is considered a misnomer because it lacks cartilaginous differentiation, and is therefore out of the scope of this review.

Current Management of Chondrosarcoma and Resistance to Therapy

The firstline treatment of chondrosarcoma is surgical resection with local adjuvant treatment such as phenol or cryosurgery, followed by filling the cavity with bone graft, showing long-term local control in atypical cartilaginous tumor/grade I chondrosarcoma.[87] Because of the necessity for wide resection margins to prevent recurrence in grade II and III chondrosarcomas, the patient often needs to undergo mutilating surgery. In the event of tumor location at a nonresectable site, such as in the skull or pelvis, or metastatic disease, there is still no curative treatment.[3,66] Chondrosarcoma is notorious for its resistance to conventional chemotherapy and radiotherapy.[3] Recently, a phase 2 study including 25 patients with chondrosarcoma using the nucleoside analogue gemcitabine (657 mg/m^2 on day 1 and day 8) followed by the antimitotic docetaxel (75 mg/m^2 on day 8) over a course of 21 days was aborted because only 2 patients showed partial response.[88] In a recent study including 9 patients with dedifferentiated chondrosarcoma treated with surgery and chemotherapy (adriamycin, ifosfamide, cisplatin, and methotrexate), all patients died of metastatic disease.[89] These results illustrate the need for new targeted treatments in chondrosarcoma, because the conventional chemotherapeutics targeting the DNA machinery are not effective.

Primary chemoresistance of chondrosarcoma has long been ascribed to the phenotypic properties, such as hyaline cartilaginous matrix surrounding the cells prohibiting access to the cells, poor vascularization, and a slow division rate.[90,91] As these properties are less prominent in high-grade chondrosarcomas, which typically show less matrix, increased vascularization, and increased mitotic rate, the resistance to therapy could also be due to activated antiapoptosis or prosurvival pathways.[90] Moreover, nuclear accumulation of doxorubicin was shown despite the presence of matrix and multidrug resistance pump activity. In addition, inhibition of the antiapoptotic Bcl-2 family members was found to overcome resistance to doxorubicin and cisplatin in chondrosarcoma cell lines.[92]

Targets and Novel Treatment Options in Chondrosarcoma

In recent years, advances have been made in identifying multiple active pathways in chondrosarcoma, and preclinical work has led to the identification of potential targets for clinical trials (**Table 2**). Here, the recent identification of *IDH* mutations is discussed in relation to active survival pathways and HIF1α expression found in high-grade chondrosarcomas, as well as growth plate signaling pathways including antiapoptotic signaling, and retinoblastoma pathway alterations.

Survival pathways: isocitrate dehydrogenase mutations

Mutations in the isocitrate dehydrogenases (IDH) are found in 87% of benign enchondromas, 38% to 70% of primary conventional central chondrosarcomas, and 54% of dedifferentiated chondrosarcomas, but not in clear cell or mesenchymal chondrosarcomas.[93–98] IDH is involved in the tricarboxylic acid cycle (Krebs cycle)[99] and mutations in IHD1/2 lead to a diminished capacity to convert isocitrate to α-ketoglutarate (α-KG) and an acquired ability to convert αKG to D-2-hydroxyglutarate (D2HG), which is considered an oncometabolite.[97,99–103]

The exact mechanism by which D2HG causes tumor formation is unknown although increasing evidence points toward epigenetic mechanisms.[104–109] D2HG impairs the function of the αKG-dependent dioxygenase TET2, leading to inhibition of DNA demethylation causing CpG island hypermethylation.[105,110,111] Enchondromas carrying *IDH* mutations were hypermethylated.[95] In addition, D2HG was shown to impair histone demethylation.[111] Moreover, mutations in IDH are postulated to inhibit the prolyl/lysyl/hydroxylation of collagen proteins and thereby their maturation as an *IDH1* R132H conditional knock-in mouse model showed a reduction in collagen IV maturation.[112] D2HG was postulated to induce pseudohypoxia (**Fig. 3**) by inhibition of the HIF proline hydroxylases although this is controversial.[100,112,113]

HIF-1α is upregulated by a multitude of malignancies to cope with reduced perfusion, and is associated with increased proliferation, vascular endothelial growth factor (VEGF) production, and resistance to chemotherapy and radiotherapy.[114–118] High-grade conventional chondrosarcomas show activation of the hypoxia pathway through HIF1α.[119] Most drugs targeting hypoxia, are designed either to target VEGF, the downstream target of HIF1α, or the phosphoinositide 3-kinase (PI3K)/protein kinase B (AKT)/mammalian target of rapamycin (mTOR) pathway, which can induce HIF1α independent of oxygen conditions (see **Fig. 3**).[114,120]

Survival pathways: PI3K, AKT, mTOR, VEGF

The PI3K/AKT pathway is often upregulated in cancer and can either inhibit apoptosis or promote cell proliferation (see **Fig. 3**).[121] Active AKT signaling was shown in chondrosarcoma[122] and the PI3K/AKT pathway has been shown to be involved in proliferation in mesenchymal chondroprogenitor cells.[123] In chondrocytes, the PI3K/AKT can be activated by the chondrogenic transcription factor SOX9,[124] which is also expressed in chondrosarcoma.[125,126] SOX9 siRNA in a chondrosarcoma cell line (SW1353) induced apoptosis that could be rescued by phosphatase and tensin homolog (PTEN) expression.[124] Mutations in the tumor suppressor *PTEN* are rare in chondrosarcoma.[127] Perifosine, an AKT inhibitor inhibiting AKT membrane recruitment, showed a 17% decrease in tumor size in 1 patient with chondrosarcoma after 2 cycles (Steinert, CTOS 2006). A larger phase 2 study was conducted including patients with chemoinsensitive sarcomas but the results have not yet been posted (NCT00401388).

mTOR is a point of convergence of many pathways involved in protein synthesis and cell proliferation, including the PI3K/AKT pathway (see **Fig. 3**). The first suggestion of activation of the mTOR pathway was in mesenchymal chondrosarcoma,

Table 2
Overview of targets and selected trials in chondrosarcoma

Target	Drug	Mechanism	Clinical Results	Clinical Trial Identifier or Reference
DNA synthesis	Gemcitabine	Nucleoside analogue	Phase 2 (n = 53) combination with docetaxel. Terminated due to lack of evidence of efficacy	[88]
	Permetrexed	Prevents formation of DNA and RNA	Study completed, no results posted	NCT00107419
AKT/PI3K	Perifosine	Inhibits AKT membrane recruitment	Phase 1 (n = 10) combination with gemcitabine Patient with CS showed 17% decrease in tumor size after 2 cycles	NCT00401388 (Steinert CTOS 2006)
mTOR	Sirolimus	mTOR inhibitor	Combination with cyclophosphamide in 10 patients Disease control rate of 70%	[131]
SRC	Dasatinib	Small molecule kinase inhibitor	Phase 2, ongoing, NOR in CS	NCT00464620 (Schuetze CTOS 2006)
PDGF	Sunitinib (SU11248)	Multitargeted receptor tyrosine kinase inhibitor	Phase 2, completed, no results posted Case study: Antitumor activity in 2 patients with extraskeletal myxoid CS Case study: Durable response after combination with proton beam radiation in 1 patient with metastatic clear cell CS	NCT00474994,[141,200]
	Imatinib	Competitive tyrosine kinase inhibitor	Phase 2 (n = 26), NOR	[140]
	Pazopanib	Blocks autophosphorylation of PDGF receptors, VEGF receptors, FGF receptors 1 and 3; inhibits Kit and Lck	Recruiting	NCT01330966

Pathway	Drug	Mechanism	Result	Reference
Hedgehog	Saridegib (IPI-926)	Smoothened inhibitor	Study terminated due to lack of evidence of efficacy	NCT01609179
	Vismodegib (GDC-0449)	Smoothened inhibitor	Ongoing Ongoing	NCT01310816 NCT01267955
Apoptosis	Dulanermin rhAPO2L/TRAIL (AMG 951)	Induces apoptosis through binding to DR4 and DR5	Phase 1 study (n = 71) 2 patients with CS durable PR Case study: near CR over 78 mo in 1 patient with metastatic disease	159,201
	PRO95780	Monoclonal IgG1 antiantibody that triggers extrinsic apoptotic pathway through DR5	Phase 1 study (n = 50), terminated due to lack of evidence of efficacy Patient with CS 20% reduction in measurable disease	160
Rb pathway	Alvespimycin	HSP90 inhibitor	Phase 1 study (n = 25) CS patient CR with reduction in CDK4 levels	169

Abbreviations: CR, complete response; CS, chondrosarcoma; FGF, fibroblast growth factor; NOR, no objective response; PR, partial response.

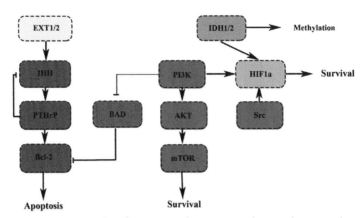

Fig. 3. Apoptosis and survival pathways. AKT (PKB, protein kinase B); BAD, Bcl-2 associated protein 2; Bcl-2, B-cell lymphoma 2; EXT1/2, exostosin 1/2; HIF1a, hypoxia inducible factor 1a; IDH1/2, isocitrate 1/2; IHH, Indian hedgehog; mTOR, mammalian target of rapamycin; PI3K, phosphoinositide 3-kinase; PTHrP, parathyroid protein; Src, sarcoma.

showing strong cytoplasmic p-AKT, p-mTOR, and PDGFR-alpha staining.[128] In an adjuvant rat orthotopic Swarm rat chondrosarcoma model, everolimus alone or in combination with doxorubicin after curettage showed inhibition of mTORC1 and decreased cell proliferation, however, the combination with doxorubicin showed an antagonistic effect with activation of the mTORC2 pathway.[129] Allosteric inhibitors of the mTOR pathway, rapalogs (rapamycin [sirolimus], everolimus, and temsirolimus), have limited efficacy in the clinic, but show high synergy with dual PI3K/mTOR inhibitors such as BEZ235.[130] A clinical trial with temsirolimus and liposomal doxorubicin included patients with chondrosarcoma (NCT00949325). While awaiting the results of this trial, a study including 10 patients with unresectable chondrosarcoma who were treated with sirolimus and cyclophosphamide showed a disease control rate of 70%.[131] However, the resistance to rapalogs observed in other malignancies suggests that, in chondrosarcoma, a strategy including dual PI3K/mTOR inhibitors such as BEZ235 should be considered for future clinical trials.

Activated Src signaling can also lead to HIF1α expression (see **Fig. 3**)[90,132,133] and promote cell survival. Src signaling was shown to be increased in chondrosarcoma,[122] and the tyrosine kinase inhibitor dasatinib showed a decrease in cell proliferation in 7 of 9 cell lines.[122] However, in a phase 2 study, no objective response was obtained with dasatinib single agent (70 mg twice a day as starting dose) in patients with chondrosarcoma (Schuetze CTOS 2010).

Activation of survival pathways can be through stimulation of the receptor tyrosine kinases by IGF-1 or PDGF. IGF-1 pathway activation was shown to be involved in chondrosarcoma proliferation, migration, apoptosis,[134–136] as well as progression to malignancy.[136] Activation of the PDGF pathway has been shown to be related to worse prognosis in chondrosarcoma.[137–139] Inhibition with imatinib, however, showed no effect in vitro in 4 chondrosarcoma cell lines,[122] and in a clinical study including 26 patients no objective response was measured.[140] HIF1α expression is suggested to result in increased VEGF expression in chondrosarcoma.[118] Sunitinib and pazopanib are tyrosine kinase inhibitors, targeting multiple kinases including PDGF and VEGF. In combination with proton beam radiation, sunitinib was reported to achieve complete symptomatic relief and durable response in a patient with metastatic clear cell chondrosarcoma.[141] A clinical study with pazopanib is currently recruiting patients with chondrosarcoma (NCT01330966).

Developmental pathways: hedgehog

In osteochondroma, a benign cartilaginous tumor at the surface of bone that can give rise to secondary peripheral chondrosarcoma, mutations in the genes encoding either exostosin-1 (EXT1) or exostosin-2 (EXT2) have been identified.[142] EXT1 and EXT2 are involved in the biosynthesis of heparan sulfate proteoglycans, which are necessary for the diffusion of the morphogen Indian hedgehog (IHH).[143] Recently, osteochondromas were shown to contain a mixture of both EXT mutant as well wildtype tumor cells (with functional EXT), and the latter were shown to be the precursor cells of peripheral chondrosarcoma[144] because peripheral chondrosarcomas have functional EXT, pointing toward a pathogenesis in chondrosarcoma independent of EXT.

IHH is part of a negative feedback loop with parathyroid hormone-related protein (PTHrP), creating a tight balance between proliferation and differentiation (see **Fig. 3**) (for review see Refs.[145,146]). Aberrant hedgehog signaling is also found in central chondrosarcoma,[147,148] despite the absence of EXT mutations. Blocking of the hedgehog pathway with triparanol was shown to be effective,[148] but reports on the effect of cylopamine are conflicting.[147–149]

A recent randomized phase 2 clinical trial with IPI-926 (saridegib), a potent cyclopamine analogue,[150] for patients with metastatic or locally advanced conventional chondrosarcoma was terminated as the primary end point, progression-free survival, was not met (NCT01609179). A second trial is currently ongoing with vismodegib, a cyclopamine-competitive smoothened inhibitor (NCT01267955). Preliminary results show stable disease in 4 out of 17 patients (Italiano, ASCO 2012). In osteochondroma, primary cilia were found to retain their normal length but lose their orientation contributing to loss of chondrocyte directionality[151]; 70% to 100% of human enchondromas and chondrosarcomas were found to lack primary cilia.[152] In Ift88−/− mice lacking primary cilia, increased hedgehog signaling and enchondroma and chondrosarcoma formation, was observed. As cyclopamine depends on the primary cilia for smoothened accumulation, chondrosarcoma cells lacking primary cilia were unresponsive to cyclopamine treatment.[152] These results support the role for IHH in initiation of chondrosarcoma, and suggest that when inhibiting the hedgehog pathway in chondrosarcoma, targets should be carefully selected.

Developmental pathways: antiapoptosis

The antiapoptotic protein Bcl-2 is under direct regulation of PTH1R and is upregulated in chondrosarcoma (see **Fig. 3**).[153] Moreover, Bcl-xl, another antiapoptotic protein belonging to the Bcl-2 family, was shown to be overexpressed in 18 chondrosarcoma tissues,[154] indicating a specific defense mechanism contributing to chemoresistance in chondrosarcoma. siRNA against Bcl-2, Bcl-xl, and x-linked inhibitor of apoptosis protein showed an enhanced sensitivity to doxorubicin and radiation,[155,156] and treatment with the BH-3 mimetic ABT-737, was shown to synergistically overcome resistance to doxorubicin and cisplatin.[92] Another antiapoptotic protein, not related to the Bcl-2 family, survivin, was also found to be highly expressed in chondrosarcoma[157,158] and inhibition experiments in 2 cell lines resulted in overcoming resistance to doxorubicin.[157] These data point toward an effective defense mechanism in which chondrosarcoma cells prevent programmed cell death in response to stress signals such as DNA damage.

Treatment with dulanermin (rhApo2L/TRAIL), a death receptor 4 (DR4) and 5 (DR5) agonist, showed complete remission in 1 patient,[159] and treatment with apomab, a

DR5 agonist, showed a 20% reduction in measureable disease in 1 patient with chondrosarcoma,[160] but showed no efficacy in a follow-up phase 2 trial designed to ultimately enroll 90 patients with chondrosarcoma (NCT00543712). These (pre)clinical results combined with this promising result with dulanermin show that restoring the defect in the apoptotic machinery could have strong therapeutic potential in chondrosarcoma. However, because multiple antiapoptotic proteins are upregulated in chondrosarcoma, a multitargeted approach may be more effective, considering that dulanermin, targeting both DR4 and DR5, was more effective than PRO95780, targeting only DR5.

Retinoblastoma signaling

The retinoblastoma protein pRb is a tumor suppressor controlling the cell cycle. In the absence of p16^{INK4A}, RB-1 is released from E2F transcription factors and cell cycle progression and gene transcription can occur (see **Fig. 4**).[161] Recently *Rb* was shown to be required for hypertrophic chondrocyte differentiation, and Rb$^{c/c}$/p107$^{-/-}$ mice were shown to develop enchondromas, indicating an important role for cell cycle regulation during tumor development.[162]

Ninety-six percent of conventional central high-grade chondrosarcomas show alterations in the retinoblastoma pathway[163]; not only through loss of the tumor suppressor *CDKN2A/p16*[164,165] along with increased *CDK4*[166] but also through amplifications of *CDK6* and *E2F3*.[167] In dedifferentiated chondrosarcoma, p16 aberrations were found to be common (85%) and associated with loss of chromosome 9p[94] or promoter methylation.[168] In mesenchymal and clear cell chondrosarcoma, p16 alterations were found in 70% and 95% of cases, respectively.[94] Inhibition of CDK4 using shRNA against CDK4 was found to inhibit cell proliferation in 3 central chondrosarcoma cell lines.[163] In a phase 1 dose-defining study of the HSP90 inhibitor alvespimycin, 1 patient with chondrosarcoma showed prolonged stable disease (>6 months) with reduction in CDK4 levels,[169] supporting further exploration of HSP90 or CDK4 inhibitors in chondrosarcoma.

In close proximity to the *CDKN2* locus on chromosome 9 is methylthioadenosine phosphorylase (*MTAP*), an enzyme vital for the recycling of adenine and methionine synthesis. Deletions involving the MTAP locus (9p21) have been reported in 50% of cases of chondrosarcoma.[167,170–172] In MTAP-deficient cells, adenine and methionine

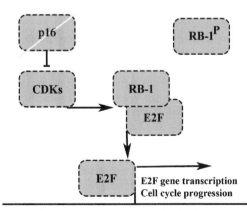

Fig. 4. RB-1 pathway: p16 is a tumor suppressor and inhibits the cyclin-dependent kinases (CDKs). On loss of p16, active CDKs phosphorylate RB-1 and release it from the E2F transcription factors, allowing for E2F target gene transcription and uncontrolled cell cycle progression.

are not metabolized rendering these cells more sensitive to selective inhibition of de novo purine synthesis. Permetrexed disodium is a multitargeted antifolate preventing the formation of precursor purine and pyrimidine nucleotides.[173] A phase 2 trial with permetrexed disodium, has been performed in patients with metastatic or locally advanced chondrosarcoma (NCT00107419). No results have been posted yet.

Other therapies: cyclooxygenase-2 and aromatase inhibitors
Estrogen signaling plays a role in skeletal maturation and was found to be active in all chondrosarcoma subtypes.[174–176] Even though the initial results were promising,[174,177] a recent retrospective series including 6 patients with locally advanced or metastatic chondrosarcoma treated with aromatase inhibitors did not show an increase in progression-free survival compared with historically untreated patients.[176] The prostaglandin synthase cyclooxygenase-2 (COX-2) is upregulated during inflammation and in, for example, colorectal, breast, and prostate cancer.[178] COX-2 upregulation was shown in chondrosarcoma[179,180] and found to be associated with poor survival.[181] COX-2 inhibition with celecoxib showed decreased cell viability in 4 chondrosarcoma cell lines, however, in chondrosarcoma xenografts, a relapse was observed after 6 weeks.[180] The negative results obtained with aromatase inhibitors in patients and COX-2 inhibitors in mice do not support clinical implementation of these therapeutic strategies.

REFERENCES

1. Fletcher CD, Bridge JA, Hogendoorn PC, et al. World Health Organization classification of tumours of soft tissue and bone. 4th edition. Lyon: IARC Press; 2013.
2. Hogendoorn PC, Bovée JV, Nielsen GP. Chondrosarcoma (grades I-III), including primary and secondary variants and periosteal chondrosarcoma. In: Fletcher CD, Bridge JA, Hogendoorn PC, et al, editors. World Health Organization classification of tumours. Pathology and genetics of tumours of soft tissue and bone. 4th edition. Lyon: IARC Press; 2013. p. 264–8.
3. Gelderblom H, Hogendoorn PC, Dijkstra SD, et al. The clinical approach towards chondrosarcoma. Oncologist 2008;13(3):320–9.
4. Savage SA, Mirabello L. Using epidemiology and genomics to understand osteosarcoma etiology. Sarcoma 2011;2011:548151.
5. Bielack S, Carrle D, Jost L. Osteosarcoma: ESMO clinical recommendations for diagnosis, treatment and follow-up. Ann Oncol 2008;19(Suppl 2):ii94–6.
6. Ferrari S, Palmerini E. Adjuvant and neoadjuvant combination chemotherapy for osteogenic sarcoma. Curr Opin Oncol 2007;19(4):341–6.
7. Anninga JK, Gelderblom H, Fiocco M, et al. Chemotherapeutic adjuvant treatment for osteosarcoma: where do we stand? Eur J Cancer 2011;47(16):2431–45.
8. Kempf-Bielack B, Bielack SS, Jurgens H, et al. Osteosarcoma relapse after combined modality therapy: an analysis of unselected patients in the Cooperative Osteosarcoma Study Group (COSS). J Clin Oncol 2005;23(3):559–68.
9. Serra M, Pasello M, Manara MC, et al. May P-glycoprotein status be used to stratify high-grade osteosarcoma patients? Results from the Italian/Scandinavian Sarcoma Group 1 treatment protocol. Int J Oncol 2006;29(6):1459–68.
10. Martins-Neves SR, Lopes AO, do Carmo A, et al. Therapeutic implications of an enriched cancer stem-like cell population in a human osteosarcoma cell line. BMC Cancer 2012;12:139.
11. Yang M, Yan M, Zhang R, et al. Side population cells isolated from human osteosarcoma are enriched with tumor-initiating cells. Cancer Sci 2011;102(10): 1774–81.

12. Li J, Zhong XY, Li ZY, et al. CD133 expression in osteosarcoma and derivation of CD133(+) cells. Mol Med Rep 2013;7(2):577–84.
13. Szuhai K, Cleton-Jansen AM, Hogendoorn PC, et al. Molecular pathology and its diagnostic use in bone tumors. Cancer Genet 2012;205(5):193–204.
14. Stephens PJ, Greenman CD, Fu B, et al. Massive genomic rearrangement acquired in a single catastrophic event during cancer development. Cell 2011; 144(1):27–40.
15. Overholtzer M, Rao PH, Favis R, et al. The presence of p53 mutations in human osteosarcomas correlates with high levels of genomic instability. Proc Natl Acad Sci U S A 2003;100(20):11547–52.
16. Calvert GT, Randall RL, Jones KB, et al. At-risk populations for osteosarcoma: the syndromes and beyond. Sarcoma 2012;2012:152382.
17. Wunder JS, Gokgoz N, Parkes R, et al. TP53 mutations and outcome in osteosarcoma: a prospective, multicenter study. J Clin Oncol 2005;23(7):1483–90.
18. Duhamel LA, Ye H, Halai D, et al. Frequency of Mouse Double Minute 2 (MDM2) and Mouse Double Minute 4 (MDM4) amplification in parosteal and conventional osteosarcoma subtypes. Histopathology 2012;60(2):357–9.
19. Lenos K, Grawenda AM, Lodder K, et al. Alternate splicing of the p53 inhibitor HDMX offers a superior prognostic biomarker than p53 mutation in human cancer. Cancer Res 2012;72(16):4074–84.
20. Vassilev LT, Vu BT, Graves B, et al. In vivo activation of the p53 pathway by small-molecule antagonists of MDM2. Science 2004;303(5659):844–8.
21. Burkhart DL, Sage J. Cellular mechanisms of tumour suppression by the retinoblastoma gene. Nat Rev Cancer 2008;8(9):671–82.
22. Marees T, Moll AC, Imhof SM, et al. Risk of second malignancies in survivors of retinoblastoma: more than 40 years of follow-up. J Natl Cancer Inst 2008; 100(24):1771–9.
23. Patino-Garcia A, Pineiro ES, Diez MZ, et al. Genetic and epigenetic alterations of the cell cycle regulators and tumor suppressor genes in pediatric osteosarcomas. J Pediatr Hematol Oncol 2003;25(5):362–7.
24. Pellin A, Boix-Ferrero J, Carpio D, et al. Molecular alterations of the RB1, TP53, and MDM2 genes in primary and xenografted human osteosarcomas. Diagn Mol Pathol 1997;6(6):333–41.
25. Benassi MS, Molendini L, Gamberi G, et al. Alteration of pRb/p16/cdk4 regulation in human osteosarcoma. Int J Cancer 1999;84(5):489–93.
26. Heinsohn S, Evermann U, Zur SU, et al. Determination of the prognostic value of loss of heterozygosity at the retinoblastoma gene in osteosarcoma. Int J Oncol 2007;30(5):1205–14.
27. Zheng L, Lee WH. Retinoblastoma tumor suppressor and genome stability. Adv Cancer Res 2002;85:13–50.
28. Knudsen ES, Sexton CR, Mayhew CN. Role of the retinoblastoma tumor suppressor in the maintenance of genome integrity. Curr Mol Med 2006;6(7):749–57.
29. Mohseny AB, Szuhai K, Romeo S, et al. Osteosarcoma originates from mesenchymal stem cells in consequence of aneuploidization and genomic loss of Cdkn2. J Pathol 2009;219(3):294–305.
30. Mohseny AB, Tieken C, Van der Velden PA, et al. Small deletions but not methylation underlie CDKN2A/p16 loss of expression in conventional osteosarcoma. Genes Chromosomes Cancer 2010;49(12):1095–103.
31. Holcombe RF, Marsh JL, Waterman ML, et al. Expression of Wnt ligands and Frizzled receptors in colonic mucosa and in colon carcinoma. Mol Pathol 2002;55(4):220–6.

32. Wan X, Liu J, Lu JF, et al. Activation of beta-catenin signaling in androgen receptor-negative prostate cancer cells. Clin Cancer Res 2012;18(3):726–36.
33. Haydon RC, Deyrup A, Ishikawa A, et al. Cytoplasmic and/or nuclear accumulation of the beta-catenin protein is a frequent event in human osteosarcoma. Int J Cancer 2002;102(4):338–42.
34. Cleton-Jansen AM, Anninga JK, Briaire-de Bruijn IH, et al. Profiling of high-grade central osteosarcoma and its putative progenitor cells identifies tumourigenic pathways. Br J Cancer 2009;101(11):1909–18.
35. Cai Y, Mohseny AB, Karperien M, et al. Inactive Wnt/beta-catenin pathway in conventional high-grade osteosarcoma. J Pathol 2010;220:24–33.
36. Enomoto M, Hayakawa S, Itsukushima S, et al. Autonomous regulation of osteosarcoma cell invasiveness by Wnt5a/Ror2 signaling. Oncogene 2009;28(36): 3197–208.
37. Morioka K, Tanikawa C, Ochi K, et al. Orphan receptor tyrosine kinase ROR2 as a potential therapeutic target for osteosarcoma. Cancer Sci 2009;100(7): 1227–33.
38. Mohseny AB, Cai Y, Kuijjer M, et al. The activities of Smad and Gli mediated signalling pathways in high-grade conventional osteosarcoma. Eur J Cancer 2012; 48(18):3429–38.
39. Baker J, Liu JP, Robertson EJ, et al. Role of insulin-like growth factors in embryonic and postnatal growth. Cell 1993;75(1):73–82.
40. Maki RG. Small is beautiful: insulin-like growth factors and their role in growth, development, and cancer. J Clin Oncol 2010;28(33):4985–95.
41. Kolb EA, Gorlick R. Development of IGF-IR inhibitors in pediatric sarcomas. Curr Oncol Rep 2009;11(4):307–13.
42. Kolb EA, Gorlick R, Houghton PJ, et al. Initial testing (stage 1) of a monoclonal antibody (SCH 717454) against the IGF-1 receptor by the pediatric preclinical testing program. Pediatr Blood Cancer 2008;50(6):1190–7.
43. Kolb EA, Kamara D, Zhang W, et al. R1507, a fully human monoclonal antibody targeting IGF-1R, is effective alone and in combination with rapamycin in inhibiting growth of osteosarcoma xenografts. Pediatr Blood Cancer 2010;55(1):67–75.
44. Kolb EA, Gorlick R, Maris JM, et al. Combination testing (Stage 2) of the Anti-IGF-1 receptor antibody IMC-A12 with rapamycin by the pediatric preclinical testing program. Pediatr Blood Cancer 2012;58(5):729–35.
45. Sulzbacher I, Traxler M, Mosberger I, et al. Platelet-derived growth factor-AA and -alpha receptor expression suggests an autocrine and/or paracrine loop in osteosarcoma. Mod Pathol 2000;13(6):632–7.
46. Kubo T, Piperdi S, Rosenblum J, et al. Platelet-derived growth factor receptor as a prognostic marker and a therapeutic target for imatinib mesylate therapy in osteosarcoma. Cancer 2008;112(10):2119–29.
47. Sulzbacher I, Birner P, Dominkus M, et al. Expression of platelet-derived growth factor-alpha receptor in human osteosarcoma is not a predictor of outcome. Pathology 2010;42(7):664–8.
48. Sulzbacher I, Birner P, Toma C, et al. Expression of c-kit in human osteosarcoma and its relevance as a prognostic marker. J Clin Pathol 2007;60(7):804–7.
49. Pignochino Y, Grignani G, Cavalloni G, et al. Sorafenib blocks tumour growth, angiogenesis and metastatic potential in preclinical models of osteosarcoma through a mechanism potentially involving the inhibition of ERK1/2, MCL-1 and ezrin pathways. Mol Cancer 2009;8:118.
50. Wang CT, Lin CS, Shiau CW, et al. SC-1, a sorafenib derivative, shows anti-tumor effects in osteogenic sarcoma cells. J Orthop Res 2013;31(2):335–42.

51. Grignani G, Palmerini E, Dileo P, et al. A phase II trial of sorafenib in relapsed and unresectable high-grade osteosarcoma after failure of standard multimodal therapy: an Italian Sarcoma Group study. Ann Oncol 2012;23(2):508–16.

52. Park JW, Neve RM, Szollosi J, et al. Unraveling the biologic and clinical complexities of HER2. Clin Breast Cancer 2008;8(5):392–401.

53. Tafe LJ, Tsongalis GJ. The human epidermal growth factor receptor 2 (HER2). Clin Chem Lab Med 2012;50(1):23–30.

54. Morris CD, Gorlick R, Huvos G, et al. Human epidermal growth factor receptor 2 as a prognostic indicator in osteogenic sarcoma. Clin Orthop Relat Res 2001; 382:59–65.

55. Scotlandi K, Manara MC, Hattinger CM, et al. Prognostic and therapeutic relevance of HER2 expression in osteosarcoma and Ewing's sarcoma. Eur J Cancer 2005;41(9):1349–61.

56. Ebb D, Meyers P, Grier H, et al. Phase II trial of trastuzumab in combination with cytotoxic chemotherapy for treatment of metastatic osteosarcoma with human epidermal growth factor receptor 2 overexpression: a report from the children's oncology group. J Clin Oncol 2012;30(20):2545–51.

57. Anninga JK, Van de Vijver MJ, Cleton-Jansen AM, et al. Overexpression of the Her-2 oncogene does not play a role in high-grade osteosarcomas. Eur J Cancer 2004;40:963–70.

58. Somers GR, Ho M, Zielenska M, et al. HER2 amplification and overexpression is not present in pediatric osteosarcoma: a tissue microarray study. Pediatr Dev Pathol 2005;8(5):525–32.

59. Willmore-Payne C, Holden JA, Zhou H, et al. Evaluation of Her-2/neu gene status in osteosarcoma by fluorescence in situ hybridization and multiplex and monoplex polymerase chain reactions. Arch Pathol Lab Med 2006;130(5):691–8.

60. Coley WB. The treatment of malignant tumors by repeated inoculations of erysipelas. With a report of ten original cases. 1893. Clin Orthop Relat Res 1991;(262):3–11.

61. Biswas SK, Sica A, Lewis CE. Plasticity of macrophage function during tumor progression: regulation by distinct molecular mechanisms. J Immunol 2008; 180(4):2011–7.

62. Cleton-Jansen AM, Buddingh EP, Lankester AC. Immunotherapy: is it different for sarcomas? Oncoimmunology 2012;1(2):255–7.

63. Buddingh' EP, Kuijjer ML, Duim RA, et al. Tumor-infiltrating macrophages are associated with metastasis suppression in high-grade osteosarcoma: a rationale for treatment with macrophage-activating agents. Clin Cancer Res 2011; 17:2010–9.

64. Meyers PA, Schwartz CL, Krailo MD, et al. Osteosarcoma: the addition of muramyl tripeptide to chemotherapy improves overall survival–a report from the Children's Oncology Group. J Clin Oncol 2008;26(4):633–8.

65. Bielack SS, Marina N, Ferrari S, et al. Osteosarcoma: the same old drugs or more? J Clin Oncol 2008;26(18):3102–3.

66. ESMO/European Sarcoma Network Working Group. Bone sarcomas: ESMO clinical practice guidelines for diagnosis, treatment and follow-up. Ann Oncol 2012;23(Suppl 7):vii100–9.

67. Buddingh EP, Schilham MW, Ruslan SE, et al. Chemotherapy-resistant osteosarcoma is highly susceptible to IL-15-activated allogeneic and autologous NK cells. Cancer Immunol Immunother 2011;60(4):575–86.

68. Pahl JH, Ruslan SE, Buddingh EP, et al. Anti-EGFR antibody cetuximab enhances the cytolytic activity of natural killer cells toward osteosarcoma. Clin Cancer Res 2012;18(2):432–41.

69. Manthey CL, Brandes ME, Perera PY, et al. Taxol increases steady-state levels of lipopolysaccharide-inducible genes and protein-tyrosine phosphorylation in murine macrophages. J Immunol 1992;149(7):2459–65.
70. Brosjo O, Bauer HC, Nilsson OS, et al. Effect of human interferon-alpha and interferon-gamma on growth, histology, and DNA content of human osteosarcomas in nude mice. J Interferon Res 1989;9(4):475–89.
71. Muller CR, Smeland S, Bauer HC, et al. Interferon-alpha as the only adjuvant treatment in high-grade osteosarcoma: long term results of the Karolinska Hospital series. Acta Oncol 2005;44(5):475–80.
72. Ito H, Murakami K, Yanagawa T, et al. Effect of human leukocyte interferon on the metastatic lung tumor of osteosarcoma: case reports. Cancer 1980;46(7):1562–5.
73. Edmonson JH, Long HJ, Frytak S, et al. Phase II study of recombinant alfa-2a interferon in patients with advanced bone sarcomas. Cancer Treat Rep 1987;71(7–8):747–8.
74. Arndt CA, Koshkina NV, Inwards CY, et al. Inhaled granulocyte-macrophage colony stimulating factor for first pulmonary recurrence of osteosarcoma: effects on disease-free survival and immunomodulation. A report from the Children's Oncology Group. Clin Cancer Res 2010;16(15):4024–30.
75. Worth LL, Jaffe N, Benjamin RS, et al. Phase II study of recombinant interleukin 1alpha and etoposide in patients with relapsed osteosarcoma. Clin Cancer Res 1997;3(10):1721–9.
76. Ullenhag GJ, Spendlove I, Watson NF, et al. T-cell responses in osteosarcoma patients vaccinated with an anti-idiotypic antibody, 105AD7, mimicking CD55. Clin Immunol 2008;128(2):148–54.
77. Clezardin P. Bisphosphonates' antitumor activity: an unravelled side of a multifaceted drug class. Bone 2011;48(1):71–9.
78. Nilsson S, Huelsenbeck J, Fritz G. Mevalonate pathway inhibitors affect anticancer drug-induced cell death and DNA damage response of human sarcoma cells. Cancer Lett 2011;304(1):60–9.
79. Kubista B, Trieb K, Sevelda F, et al. Anticancer effects of zoledronic acid against human osteosarcoma cells. J Orthop Res 2006;24(6):1145–52.
80. Molinuevo MS, Bruzzone L, Cortizo AM. Alendronate induces anti-migratory effects and inhibition of neutral phosphatases in UMR106 osteosarcoma cells. Eur J Pharmacol 2007;562(1–2):28–33.
81. Ory B, Heymann MF, Kamijo A, et al. Zoledronic acid suppresses lung metastases and prolongs overall survival of osteosarcoma-bearing mice. Cancer 2005;104(11):2522–9.
82. Meyers PA, Healey JH, Chou AJ, et al. Addition of pamidronate to chemotherapy for the treatment of osteosarcoma. Cancer 2011;117(8):1736–44.
83. Evans HL, Ayala AG, Romsdahl MM. Prognostic factors in chondrosarcoma of bone. A clinicopathologic analysis with emphasis on histologic grading. Cancer 1977;40:818–31.
84. Inwards CY, Hogendoorn PC. Dedifferentiated chondrosarcoma. In: Fletcher CD, Bridge JA, Hogendoorn PC, et al, editors. World Health Organization classification of tumours. Pathology and genetics of tumours of soft tissue and bone. 4th edition. Lyon: IARC Press; 2013. p. 269–70.
85. Nakashima Y, de Pinieux G, Ladanyi M. Mesenchymal chondrosarcoma. In: Fletcher CD, Bridge JA, Hogendoorn PC, et al, editors. World Health Organization classification of tumours. Pathology and genetics of tumours of soft tissue and bone. Lyon: IARC Press; 2013. p. 271–2.

86. McCarthy EF, Hogendoorn PC. Clear cell chondrosarcoma. In: Fletcher CD, Bridge JA, Hogendoorn PC, et al, editors. World Health Organization classification of tumours. Pathology and genetics of tumours of soft tissue and bone. 4th edition. Lyon: IARC Press; 2013. p. 273–4.

87. Verdegaal SH, Brouwers HF, van Zwet EW, et al. Low-grade chondrosarcoma of long bones treated with intralesional curettage followed by application of phenol, ethanol, and bone-grafting. J Bone Joint Surg Am 2012;94(13): 1201–7.

88. Fox E, Patel S, Wathen JK, et al. Phase II study of sequential gemcitabine followed by docetaxel for recurrent Ewing sarcoma, osteosarcoma, or unresectable or locally recurrent chondrosarcoma: results of Sarcoma Alliance for Research Through Collaboration Study 003. Oncologist 2012;17(3): 321–e329.

89. Yokota K, Sakamoto A, Matsumoto Y, et al. Clinical outcome for patients with dedifferentiated chondrosarcoma: a report of 9 cases at a single institute. J Orthop Surg Res 2012;7(1):38.

90. Bovée JV, Hogendoorn PC, Wunder JS, et al. Cartilage tumours and bone development: molecular pathology and possible therapeutic targets. Nat Rev Cancer 2010;10(7):481–8.

91. David E, Blanchard F, Heymann MF, et al. The bone niche of chondrosarcoma: a sanctuary for drug resistance, tumour growth and also a source of new therapeutic targets. Sarcoma 2011;2011:932451.

92. van Oosterwijk JG, Herpers B, Meijer D, et al. Restoration of chemosensitivity for doxorubicin and cisplatin in chondrosarcoma in vitro: BCL-2 family members cause chemoresistance. Ann Oncol 2012;23(6):1617–26.

93. Schaap FG, French PJ, Bovee JV. Mutations in the isocitrate dehydrogenase genes IDH1 and IDH2 in tumors. Adv Anat Pathol 2013;20(1):32–8.

94. Meijer D, de JD, Pansuriya TC, et al. Genetic characterization of mesenchymal, clear cell, and dedifferentiated chondrosarcoma. Genes Chromosomes Cancer 2012;51(10):899–909.

95. Pansuriya TC, van ER, d'Adamo P, et al. Somatic mosaic IDH1 and IDH2 mutations are associated with enchondroma and spindle cell hemangioma in Ollier disease and Maffucci syndrome. Nat Genet 2011;43(12):1256–61.

96. Amary MF, Bacsi K, Maggiani F, et al. IDH1 and IDH2 mutations are frequent events in central chondrosarcoma and central and periosteal chondromas but not in other mesenchymal tumours. J Pathol 2011;224(3):334–43.

97. Amary MF, Damato S, Halai D, et al. Ollier disease and Maffucci syndrome are caused by somatic mosaic mutations of IDH1 and IDH2. Nat Genet 2011;43(12): 1262–5.

98. Damato S, Alorjani M, Bonar F, et al. IDH1 mutations are not found in cartilaginous tumours other than central and periosteal chondrosarcomas and enchondromas. Histopathology 2012;60(2):363–5.

99. Leonardi R, Subramanian C, Jackowski S, et al. Cancer-associated isocitrate dehydrogenase mutations inactivate NADPH-dependent reductive carboxylation. J Biol Chem 2012;287(18):14615–20.

100. Zhao S, Lin Y, Xu W, et al. Glioma-derived mutations in IDH1 dominantly inhibit IDH1 catalytic activity and induce HIF-1alpha. Science 2009;324(5924):261–5.

101. Dang L, White DW, Gross S, et al. Cancer-associated IDH1 mutations produce 2-hydroxyglutarate. Nature 2009;462(7274):739–44.

102. Luchman HA, Stechishin OD, Dang NH, et al. An in vivo patient-derived model of endogenous IDH1-mutant glioma. Neuro Oncol 2012;14(2):184–91.

103. Ward PS, Patel J, Wise DR, et al. The common feature of leukemia-associated IDH1 and IDH2 mutations is a neomorphic enzyme activity converting alpha-ketoglutarate to 2-hydroxyglutarate. Cancer Cell 2010;17(3):225–34.
104. Dang L, Jin S, Su SM. IDH mutations in glioma and acute myeloid leukemia. Trends Mol Med 2010;16(9):387–97.
105. Figueroa ME, Abdel-Wahab O, Lu C, et al. Leukemic IDH1 and IDH2 mutations result in a hypermethylation phenotype, disrupt TET2 function, and impair hematopoietic differentiation. Cancer Cell 2010;18(6):553–67.
106. Hartmann C, Meyer J, Balss J, et al. Type and frequency of IDH1 and IDH2 mutations are related to astrocytic and oligodendroglial differentiation and age: a study of 1,010 diffuse gliomas. Acta Neuropathol 2009;118(4):469–74.
107. Kang MR, Kim MS, Oh JE, et al. Mutational analysis of IDH1 codon 132 in glioblastomas and other common cancers. Int J Cancer 2009;125(2):353–5.
108. Murugan AK, Bojdani E, Xing M. Identification and functional characterization of isocitrate dehydrogenase 1 (IDH1) mutations in thyroid cancer. Biochem Biophys Res Commun 2010;393(3):555–9.
109. Yan H, Parsons DW, Jin G, et al. IDH1 and IDH2 mutations in gliomas. N Engl J Med 2009;360(8):765–73.
110. Noushmehr H, Weisenberger DJ, Diefes K, et al. Identification of a CpG island methylator phenotype that defines a distinct subgroup of glioma. Cancer Cell 2010;17(5):510–22.
111. Lu C, Ward PS, Kapoor GS, et al. IDH mutation impairs histone demethylation and results in a block to cell differentiation. Nature 2012;483(7390):474–8.
112. Sasaki M, Knobbe CB, Itsumi M, et al. D-2-hydroxyglutarate produced by mutant IDH1 perturbs collagen maturation and basement membrane function. Genes Dev 2012;26(18):2038–49.
113. Koivunen P, Lee S, Duncan CG, et al. Transformation by the (R)-enantiomer of 2-hydroxyglutarate linked to EGLN activation. Nature 2012;483(7390):484–8.
114. Greer SN, Metcalf JL, Wang Y, et al. The updated biology of hypoxia-inducible factor. EMBO J 2012;31(11):2448–60.
115. Robey IF, Lien AD, Welsh SJ, et al. Hypoxia-inducible factor-1alpha and the glycolytic phenotype in tumors. Neoplasia 2005;7(4):324–30.
116. O'Donnell JL, Joyce MR, Shannon AM, et al. Oncological implications of hypoxia inducible factor-1alpha (HIF-1alpha) expression. Cancer Treat Rev 2006;32(6):407–16.
117. Fang J, Yan L, Shing Y, et al. HIF-1alpha-mediated up-regulation of vascular endothelial growth factor, independent of basic fibroblast growth factor, is important in the switch to the angiogenic phenotype during early tumorigenesis. Cancer Res 2001;61(15):5731–5.
118. Lin C, McGough R, Aswad B, et al. Hypoxia induces HIF-1alpha and VEGF expression in chondrosarcoma cells and chondrocytes. J Orthop Res 2004;22(6):1175–81.
119. Boeuf S, Bovee JV, Lehner B, et al. Correlation of hypoxic signalling to histological grade and outcome in cartilage tumours. Histopathology 2010;56(5):641–51.
120. Agani F, Jiang BH. Oxygen-independent regulation of HIF-1: novel involvement of PI3K/AKT/mTOR pathway in cancer. Curr Cancer Drug Targets 2013;13(3):245–51.
121. Maddika S, Ande SR, Panigrahi S, et al. Cell survival, cell death and cell cycle pathways are interconnected: implications for cancer therapy. Drug Resist Updat 2007;10(1–2):13–29.

122. Schrage YM, Briaire-de Bruijn IH, de Miranda NF, et al. Kinome profiling of chondrosarcoma reveals Src-pathway activity and dasatinib as option for treatment. Cancer Res 2009;69(15):6216–22.
123. Akiyama H, Furukawa S, Wakisaka S, et al. Cartducin stimulates mesenchymal chondroprogenitor cell proliferation through both extracellular signal-regulated kinase and phosphatidylinositol 3-kinase/Akt pathways. FEBS J 2006;273(10): 2257–63.
124. Ikegami D, Akiyama H, Suzuki A, et al. Sox9 sustains chondrocyte survival and hypertrophy in part through Pik3ca-Akt pathways. Development 2011;138(8): 1507–19.
125. Cajaiba MM, Jianhua L, Goodman MA, et al. Sox9 expression is not limited to chondroid neoplasms: variable occurrence in other soft tissue and bone tumors with frequent expression by synovial sarcomas. Int J Surg Pathol 2010;18(5): 319–23.
126. Wehrli BM, Huang W, De CB, et al. Sox9, a master regulator of chondrogenesis, distinguishes mesenchymal chondrosarcoma from other small blue round cell tumors. Hum Pathol 2003;34(3):263–9.
127. Lin C, Meitner PA, Terek RM. PTEN mutation is rare in chondrosarcoma. Diagn Mol Pathol 2002;11(1):22–6.
128. Brown RE, Boyle JL. Mesenchymal chondrosarcoma: molecular characterization by a proteomic approach, with morphogenic and therapeutic implications. Ann Clin Lab Sci 2003;33(2):131–41.
129. Perez J, Decouvelaere AV, Pointecouteau T, et al. Inhibition of chondrosarcoma growth by mTOR inhibitor in an in vivo syngeneic rat model. PLoS One 2012; 7(6):e32458.
130. Yang S, Xiao X, Meng X, et al. A mechanism for synergy with combined mTOR and PI3 kinase inhibitors. PLoS One 2011;6(10):e26343.
131. Bernstein-Molho R, Kollender Y, Issakov J, et al. Clinical activity of mTOR inhibition in combination with cyclophosphamide in the treatment of recurrent unresectable chondrosarcomas. Cancer Chemother Pharmacol 2012;70(6): 855–60.
132. Aligayer H, Boyd DD, Heiss MM, et al. Activation of Src kinase in primary colorectal carcinoma: an indicator of poor clinical prognosis. Cancer 2002;94(2): 344–51.
133. Fizazi K. The role of Src in prostate cancer. Ann Oncol 2007;18(11):1765–73.
134. Matsumura T, Whelan MC, Li XQ, et al. Regulation by IGF-I and TGF-beta1 of Swarm-rat chondrosarcoma chondrocytes. J Orthop Res 2000;18(3):351–5.
135. Wu CM, Li TM, Hsu SF, et al. IGF-I enhances alpha5beta1 integrin expression and cell motility in human chondrosarcoma cells. J Cell Physiol 2011;226(12): 3270–7.
136. Ho L, Stojanovski A, Whetstone H, et al. Gli2 and p53 cooperate to regulate IGFBP-3- mediated chondrocyte apoptosis in the progression from benign to malignant cartilage tumors. Cancer Cell 2009;16(2):126–36.
137. Masui F, Ushigome S, Fujii K. Clear cell chondrosarcoma: a pathological and immunohistochemical study. Histopathology 1999;34(5):447–52.
138. Sulzbacher I, Birner P, Trieb K, et al. Platelet-derived growth factor-alpha receptor expression supports the growth of conventional chondrosarcoma and is associated with adverse outcome. Am J Surg Pathol 2001;25(12):1520–7.
139. Franchi A, Baroni G, Sardi I, et al. Dedifferentiated peripheral chondrosarcoma: a clinicopathologic, immunohistochemical, and molecular analysis of four cases. Virchows Arch 2012;460(3):335–42.

140. Grignani G, Palmerini E, Stacchiotti S, et al. A phase 2 trial of imatinib mesylate in patients with recurrent nonresectable chondrosarcomas expressing platelet-derived growth factor receptor-alpha or -beta: an Italian Sarcoma Group study. Cancer 2011;117(4):826–31.

141. Dallas J, Imanirad I, Rajani R, et al. Response to sunitinib in combination with proton beam radiation in a patient with chondrosarcoma: a case report. J Med Case Rep 2012;6:41.

142. Jennes I, Pedrini E, Zuntini M, et al. Multiple osteochondromas: mutation update and description of the multiple osteochondromas mutation database (MOdb). Hum Mutat 2009;30(12):1620–7.

143. Stickens D, Brown D, Evans GA. EXT genes are differentially expressed in bone and cartilage during mouse embryogenesis. Dev Dyn 2000;218(3):452–64.

144. de Andrea CE, Reijnders CM, Kroon HM, et al. Secondary peripheral chondrosarcoma evolving from osteochondroma as a result of outgrowth of cells with functional EXT. Oncogene 2012;31(9):1095–104.

145. Chung UI, Lanske B, Lee K, et al. The parathyroid hormone/parathyroid hormone-related peptide receptor coordinates endochondral bone development by directly controlling chondrocyte differentiation. Proc Natl Acad Sci U S A 1998;95:13030–5.

146. Chung UI, Schipani E, McMahon AP, et al. Indian hedgehog couples chondrogenesis to osteogenesis in endochondral bone development. J Clin Invest 2001; 107(3):295–304.

147. Schrage YM, Hameetman L, Szuhai K, et al. Aberrant heparan sulfate proteoglycan localization, despite normal exostosin, in central chondrosarcoma. Am J Pathol 2009;174(3):979–88.

148. Tiet TD, Hopyan S, Nadesan P, et al. Constitutive hedgehog signaling in chondrosarcoma up-regulates tumor cell proliferation. Am J Pathol 2006;168(1): 321–30.

149. Oji GS, Gomez P, Kurriger G, et al. Indian hedgehog signaling pathway differences between swarm rat chondrosarcoma and native rat chondrocytes. Iowa Orthop J 2007;27:9–16.

150. Tremblay MR, Lescarbeau A, Grogan MJ, et al. Discovery of a potent and orally active hedgehog pathway antagonist (IPI-926). J Med Chem 2009;52(14): 4400–18.

151. de Andrea CE, Wiweger M, Prins F, et al. Primary cilia organization reflects polarity in the growth plate and implies loss of polarity and mosaicism in osteochondroma. Lab Invest 2010;90(7):1091–101.

152. Ho L, Ali SA, Al-Jazrawe M, et al. Primary cilia attenuate hedgehog signalling in neoplastic chondrocytes. Oncogene 2012. [Epub ahead of print].

153. Rozeman LB, Hameetman L, Cleton-Jansen AM, et al. Absence of IHH and retention of PTHrP signalling in enchondromas and central chondrosarcomas. J Pathol 2005;205(4):476–82.

154. Shen ZN, Nishida K, Doi H, et al. Suppression of chondrosarcoma cells by 15-deoxy-Delta 12,14-prostaglandin J2 is associated with altered expression of Bax/Bcl-xL and p21. Biochem Biophys Res Commun 2005;328(2):375–82.

155. Kim DW, Kim KO, Shin MJ, et al. siRNA-based targeting of antiapoptotic genes can reverse chemoresistance in P-glycoprotein expressing chondrosarcoma cells. Mol Cancer 2009;8:28.

156. Kim DW, Seo SW, Cho SK, et al. Targeting of cell survival genes using small interfering RNAs (siRNAs) enhances radiosensitivity of Grade II chondrosarcoma cells. J Orthop Res 2007;25(6):820–8.

157. Lechler P, Renkawitz T, Campean V, et al. The antiapoptotic gene survivin is highly expressed in human chondrosarcoma and promotes drug resistance in chondrosarcoma cells in vitro. BMC Cancer 2011;11:120.

158. Machado I, Giner F, Mayordomo E, et al. Tissue microarrays analysis in chondrosarcomas: light microscopy, immunohistochemistry and xenograft study. Diagn Pathol 2008;3(Suppl 1):S25.

159. Subbiah V, Brown RE, Buryanek J, et al. Targeting the apoptotic pathway in chondrosarcoma using recombinant human Apo2L/TRAIL (dulanermin), a dual proapoptotic receptor (DR4/DR5) Agonist. Mol Cancer Ther 2012;11(11): 2541–6.

160. Camidge DR. Apomab: an agonist monoclonal antibody directed against Death Receptor 5/TRAIL-Receptor 2 for use in the treatment of solid tumors. Expert Opin Biol Ther 2008;8(8):1167–76.

161. Witkiewicz AK, Knudsen KE, Dicker AP, et al. The meaning of p16(ink4a) expression in tumors: functional significance, clinical associations and future developments. Cell Cycle 2011;10(15):2497–503.

162. Landman AS, Danielian PS, Lees JA. Loss of pRB and p107 disrupts cartilage development and promotes enchondroma formation. Oncogene 2012. [Epub ahead of print].

163. Schrage YM, Lam S, Jochemsen AG, et al. Central chondrosarcoma progression is associated with pRb pathway alterations; CDK4 downregulation and p16 overexpression inhibit cell growth in vitro. J Cell Mol Med 2008;13(9A): 2843–52.

164. Hallor KH, Staaf J, Bovée JV, et al. Genomic profiling of chondrosarcoma: chromosomal patterns in central and peripheral tumors. Clin Cancer Res 2009;15(8): 2685–94.

165. van Beerendonk HM, Rozeman LB, Taminiau AH, et al. Molecular analysis of the INK4A/INK4A-ARF gene locus in conventional (central) chondrosarcomas and enchondromas: indication of an important gene for tumour progression. J Pathol 2004;202(3):359–66.

166. Asp J, Inerot S, Block JA, et al. Alterations in the regulatory pathway involving p16, pRb and cdk4 in human chondrosarcoma. J Orthop Res 2001;19(1): 149–54.

167. Niini T, Scheinin I, Lahti L, et al. Homozygous deletions of cadherin genes in chondrosarcoma-an array comparative genomic hybridization study. Cancer Genet 2012;205(11):588–93.

168. Ropke M, Boltze C, Neumann HW, et al. Genetic and epigenetic alterations in tumor progression in a dedifferentiated chondrosarcoma. Pathol Res Pract 2003;199(6):437–44.

169. Pacey S, Wilson RH, Walton M, et al. A phase I study of the heat shock protein 90 inhibitor alvespimycin (17-DMAG) given intravenously to patients with advanced solid tumors. Clin Cancer Res 2011;17(6):1561–70.

170. Jagasia AA, Block JA, Qureshi A, et al. Chromosome 9 related aberrations and deletions of the CDKN2 and MTS2 putative tumor suppressor genes in human chondrosarcomas. Cancer Lett 1996;105:91–103.

171. Jagasia AA, Block JA, Diaz MO, et al. Partial deletions of the CDKN2 and MTS2 putative tumor suppressor genes in a myxoid chondrosarcoma. Cancer Lett 1996;105:77–90.

172. Chow WA, Bedell V, Gaytan P, et al. Methylthioadenosine phosphorylase gene deletions are frequently detected by fluorescence in situ hybridization in conventional chondrosarcomas. Cancer Genet Cytogenet 2006;166(2):95–100.

173. Bertino JR, Waud WR, Parker WB, et al. Targeting tumors that lack methylthioadenosine phosphorylase (MTAP) activity: current strategies. Cancer Biol Ther 2011;11(7):627–32.

174. Cleton-Jansen AM, van Beerendonk HM, Baelde HJ, et al. Estrogen signaling is active in cartilaginous tumors: implications for antiestrogen therapy as treatment option of metastasized or irresectable chondrosarcoma. Clin Cancer Res 2005; 11(22):8028–35.

175. Grifone TJ, Haupt HM, Podolski V, et al. Immunohistochemical expression of estrogen receptors in chondrosarcomas and enchondromas. Int J Surg Pathol 2008;16(1):31–7.

176. Meijer D, Gelderblom H, Karperien M, et al. Expression of aromatase and estrogen receptor alpha in chondrosarcoma, but no beneficial effect of inhibiting estrogen signaling both in vitro and in vivo. Clin Sarcoma Res 2011;1(1):5.

177. Fong YC, Yang WH, Hsu SF, et al. 2-Methoxyestradiol induces apoptosis and cell cycle arrest in human chondrosarcoma cells. J Orthop Res 2007;25(8):1106–14.

178. Rizzo MT. Cyclooxygenase-2 in oncogenesis. Clin Chim Acta 2011;412(9–10): 671–87.

179. Sutton KM, Wright M, Fondren G, et al. Cyclooxygenase-2 expression in chondrosarcoma. Oncology 2004;66(4):275–80.

180. Schrage YM, Machado I, Meijer D, et al. COX-2 expression in chondrosarcoma: a role for celecoxib treatment? Eur J Cancer 2010;46:616–24.

181. Endo M, Matsumura T, Yamaguchi T, et al. Cyclooxygenase-2 overexpression associated with a poor prognosis in chondrosarcomas. Hum Pathol 2006; 37(4):471–6.

182. Bagatell R, Herzog CE, Trippett TM, et al. Pharmacokinetically guided phase 1 trial of the IGF-1 receptor antagonist RG1507 in children with recurrent or refractory solid tumors. Clin Cancer Res 2011;17(3):611–9.

183. Daw NC, Furman WL, Stewart CF, et al. Phase I and pharmacokinetic study of gefitinib in children with refractory solid tumors: a Children's Oncology Group Study. J Clin Oncol 2005;23(25):6172–80.

184. Glade Bender JL, Adamson PC, Reid JM, et al. Phase I trial and pharmacokinetic study of bevacizumab in pediatric patients with refractory solid tumors: a Children's Oncology Group Study. J Clin Oncol 2008;26(3):399–405.

185. van CH, Voest EE, Punt CJ, et al. Phase I evaluation of cediranib, a selective VEGFR signalling inhibitor, in combination with gefitinib in patients with advanced tumours. Eur J Cancer 2010;46(5):901–11.

186. Merimsky O, Meller I, Flusser G, et al. Gemcitabine in soft tissue or bone sarcoma resistant to standard chemotherapy: a phase II study. Cancer Chemother Pharmacol 2000;45(2):177–81.

187. Warwick AB, Malempati S, Krailo M, et al. Phase 2 trial of pemetrexed in children and adolescents with refractory solid tumors: a Children's Oncology Group study. Pediatr Blood Cancer 2013;60(2):237–41.

188. Delaloge S, Yovine A, Taamma A, et al. Ecteinascidin-743: a marine-derived compound in advanced, pretreated sarcoma patients–preliminary evidence of activity. J Clin Oncol 2001;19(5):1248–55.

189. Lau L, Supko JG, Blaney S, et al. A phase I and pharmacokinetic study of ecteinascidin-743 (Yondelis) in children with refractory solid tumors. A Children's Oncology Group study. Clin Cancer Res 2005;11(2 Pt 1):672–7.

190. Laverdiere C, Kolb EA, Supko JG, et al. Phase II study of ecteinascidin 743 in heavily pretreated patients with recurrent osteosarcoma. Cancer 2003;98(4): 832–40.

191. Patel SR, Papadopoulos NE, Plager C, et al. Phase II study of paclitaxel in patients with previously treated osteosarcoma and its variants. Cancer 1996;78(4): 741–4.
192. McTiernan A, Whelan JS. A phase II study of docetaxel for the treatment of recurrent osteosarcoma. Sarcoma 2004;8(2–3):71–6.
193. Zwerdling T, Krailo M, Monteleone P, et al. Phase II investigation of docetaxel in pediatric patients with recurrent solid tumors: a report from the Children's Oncology Group. Cancer 2006;106(8):1821–8.
194. Jacobs S, Fox E, Krailo M, et al. Phase II trial of ixabepilone administered daily for five days in children and young adults with refractory solid tumors: a report from the Children's Oncology Group. Clin Cancer Res 2010;16(2):750–4.
195. Mita MM, Mita AC, Chu QS, et al. Phase I trial of the novel mammalian target of rapamycin inhibitor deforolimus (AP23573; MK-8669) administered intravenously daily for 5 days every 2 weeks to patients with advanced malignancies. J Clin Oncol 2008;26(3):361–7.
196. Chawla SP, Staddon AP, Baker LH, et al. Phase II study of the mammalian target of rapamycin inhibitor ridaforolimus in patients with advanced bone and soft tissue sarcomas. J Clin Oncol 2012;30(1):78–84.
197. Schuetze SM, Zhao L, Chugh R, et al. Results of a phase II study of sirolimus and cyclophosphamide in patients with advanced sarcoma. Eur J Cancer 2012;48(9):1347–53.
198. Kleinerman ES, Gano JB, Johnston DA, et al. Efficacy of liposomal muramyl tripeptide (CGP 19835A) in the treatment of relapsed osteosarcoma. Am J Clin Oncol 1995;18(2):93–9.
199. Chou AJ, Kleinerman ES, Krailo MD, et al. Addition of muramyl tripeptide to chemotherapy for patients with newly diagnosed metastatic osteosarcoma: a report from the Children's Oncology Group. Cancer 2009;115(22):5339–48.
200. Stacchiotti S, Dagrada GP, Morosi C, et al. Extraskeletal myxoid chondrosarcoma: tumor response to sunitinib. Clin Sarcoma Res 2012;2(1):22.
201. Herbst RS, Eckhardt SG, Kurzrock R, et al. Phase I dose-escalation study of recombinant human Apo2L/TRAIL, a dual proapoptotic receptor agonist, in patients with advanced cancer. J Clin Oncol 2010;28(17):2839–46.

Targeted Therapies in Rare Sarcomas: IMT, ASPS, SFT, PEComa, and CCS

Silvia Stacchiotti, MD[a],[*], Andrea Marrari, MD[a],
Angelo P. Dei Tos, MD[b], Paolo G. Casali, MD[a]

KEYWORDS

- Sarcoma • Inflammatory myofibroblastic tumor • Alveolar soft part sarcoma
- Solitary fibrous tumor • Hemangiopericytoma • Perivascular epithelioid cell tumor
- Clear cell sarcoma • Chemotherapy

KEY POINTS

- A subgroup of rare entities within a family of rare cancers was selected for responsiveness to a set of molecularly targeted agents.
- Low-grade tumors may respond much less to standard chemotherapy, while their higher degree of differentiation may be associated with a higher relevance of cellular pathways, which may well serve as drug-susceptible targets.
- Inflammatory myofibroblastic tumor carries a translocation-related target, which is strongly related to the mechanism of action of the drugs employed, while in the case of alveolar soft part sarcoma and clear cell sarcoma, the activation of MET seems to be paralleled by a lower activity of the relevant drugs.
- In perivascular epithelioid cell tumors, a translocation resulting in MET activation was found in a small proportion of cases, while mammalian target of rapamycin (mTOR) inhibitors were shown to have some activity, in the absence of major genetic alterations of the mTOR pathway, though in the presence of a degree of its disruption.
- It is possible that some of the effects seen in the clinic are caused by an unspecific mechanism of action for these targeted agents, ranging from an antiangiogenic effect to an effect on pathways that may be more or less crucial for the tumor cell.

Disclosures: S. Stacchiotti–Advisory: Novartis; Lectures: Pfizer; Travel coverage for medical meetings: Novartis, Pfizer; Research funding for clinical studies in which I was involved: Bayer, Glaxo SK, Lilly, Novartis, Pfizer, Roche. A. Marrari–Research funding for clinical studies in which I was involved: Bayer, Glaxo SK, Lilly, Novartis, Pfizer, Roche. A.P. Dei Tos–None. P.G. Casali–Advisory: Bayer, Glaxo SK, Novartis, Pfizer; Travel coverage for medical meetings: Bayer, Glaxo SK, Novartis, Pfizer; Research funding for clinical studies in which I was involved: Bayer, Glaxo SK, Lilly, Novartis, Pfizer, Roche.
[a] Adult Sarcoma Medical Oncology Unit, Department of Cancer Medicine, Fondazione IRCCS Istituto Nazionale Tumori, via Venezian 1, Milan 20133, Italy; [b] Anatomic Pathology, Department of Oncology, General Hospital of Treviso, Piazza Ospedale 1, Treviso 31100, Italy
* Corresponding author.
E-mail address: silvia.stacchiotti@istitutotumori.mi.it

INTRODUCTION

Inflammatory myofibroblastic tumor (IMT), alveolar soft part sarcoma (ASPS), solitary fibrous tumor (SFT), perivascular epithelioid cell tumor (PEComa), and clear cell sarcoma (CCS) are among rarer soft tissue sarcomas (STS), each of them accounting for less than 1 case per 1,000,000 population per year.[1,2] They all represent translocated STS, characterized by the presence of relatively specific recurrent translocation, yet not always in the same proportion of cases. In the case of IMT and SFT, the cytogenetic aberration is responsible for the activation of 2 different proteins, anaplastic lymphoma kinase (ALK) and signal transducers and activators of transcription 6 (STAT6), respectively.[3–5] Curiously, in case of ASPS, PEComa, and CCS, the 3 different histotype-specific translocations have the common feature to induce the dysregulation of the microphthalmia transcription factor (MITF) family proteins.[6–12] In turn, these proteins up-regulate the transcription of MET, thus being responsible for the high metastatic rate of these sarcomas. Based on this shared molecular characteristic, ASPS, PEComa, and CCS belong to the MIT family tumors.[1]

IMT, SFT, ASPS, PEComas, and CCS are characterized by a low (if any) sensitivity to conventional cytotoxic chemotherapy. Given the rarity of these tumors, few prospective studies focusing on their medical treatment are available. However, the well-characterized mechanisms of oncogenesis make each histotype potentially sensitive to appropriate targeted treatments. In addition, other molecular and/or morphologic peculiar characteristics (eg, the particular vascular pattern in the case of ASPS and SFT, or the activation of mammalian target of rapamycin (mTOR) in PEComas) suggest a role for new targeted agents.

This article aims to review the data currently available in the literature on the activity of targeted medical treatment in each of these histologies.

INFLAMMATORY MYOFIBROBLASTIC TUMOR

IMT is a mesenchymal spindle cell neoplasm associated with plasma cells, lymphocytes, and granulocytes in variable amount, and featuring myofibroblastic differentiation.[3] Almost half of IMT carries a recurrent clonal aberration involving the *ALK* locus on chromosome 2p23.[4,13] ALK is a receptor tyrosine kinase implicated in the normal development and function of the nervous system, and whatever the partner genes, the resulting chimeric protein induces a hyperactivation of the kinase activity leading to uncontrolled cell growth. IMT is a low-grade sarcoma that arises predominantly in the lung, mesentery, retroperitoneum, and pelvis of children and young adults with a propensity for local recurrences, although infrequently, IMT may metastasize. Interestingly, the more aggressive variants of IMT usually are not associated with ALK rearrangement.[1] Surgery is the treatment of choice for localized disease; patients with unresectable IMT may benefit from steroids and chemotherapy.[14,15]

Among molecular target agents, the ALK/MET-inhibitor crizotinib (Xalkori) is currently the only agent found to be potentially active in this disease.

Crizotinib is an orally available inhibitor of MET and ALK tyrosine kinases; its antiproliferative activity is derived from the competitive inhibition of the adenosine triphosphate (ATP)-binding site of both kinases.[16] The activity of crizotinib in IMT was recently described by Butrynski and colleagues.[17] Two patients with unresectable recurrent IMT received crizotinib within a dose escalation phase 1 trial (NCT00585195). Interestingly, 1 patient, who suffered from an ALK-negative disease, progressed to the drug, while the other patient, whose disease carried the *ALK-RANBP2* fusion gene, achieved sustained partial response (PR). As for tyrosine kinase inhibitor (TKI), despite initial impressive clinical activity, resistance to crizotinib occurred; after 8 months of therapy, some of the responding abdominal masses restarted to grow. The patient had debulking surgery. Genetic analyses on the surgical specimens confirmed the presence of *ALK-RANBP2* fusion gene; however, sequencing analysis showed the presence of a mutation in the kinase domain of ALK, F1174L, in one of the nonresponding lesions, which was not present in the pretreatment specimen.[18] In vitro studies demonstrated that the presence of the F1174L conferred growth advantage over the *ALK-RANBP2* genotype; this was mirrored by a higher phosphorylation of ALK. Moreover, the ALK-RANBP2 F1174L conferred lower sensibility to crizotinib compared with ALK-RANBP2. Searching for a way to overcome resistance, other drugs were tested on the ALK-RANBP2 F1174L mutant; TAE684, a structurally unrelated second generation ALK inhibitor, and the HSP90 inhibitor 17AAG proved active, opening new possibilities for sequential or combination therapy. Given the clinical activity of crizotinib in patients with IMT, a European phase 2 clinical trial is actively enrolling patients with advanced disease (NCT01524926).

ALVEOLAR SOFT TISSUE SARCOMA

ASPS mainly affects young patients and is composed of a distinctive epithelioid cell population organized in an alveolar growth pattern.[1] It is characterized by an unbalanced recurrent t(X;17)(p11;q25) translocation[6,7] that leads to MET transcriptional up-regulation by means of the transcription factor ASPL-TFE3. ASPS is marked by a peculiar tumor-associated vasculature and by the expression of vascular endothelial growth factor (VEGFR) and platelet derived growth factor receptor (PDGFR) on both tumor vessels and tumor cells.[1] The natural history of ASPS is marked by an indolent behavior in spite of a greater than 60% risk of metastasis and fewer than 50% of patients disease-free at 10 years (1). ASPS is known for its resistance to conventional chemotherapy, and no standard active medical options are available for the advanced phase (**Figs. 1** and **2**).[19]

Given the molecular profile and preclinical data,[6,7,20] MET represents a potential therapeutic target. Furthermore, the activity of antiangiogenic agents such as interferon-alfa,[21,22] bevacizumab[23] (Avastin), sunitinib[24,25] (Sutent) and cediranib[26] (*AZD2171*) was reported, too.

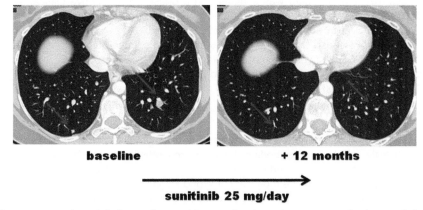

baseline   + 12 months

sunitinib 25 mg/day

Fig. 1. CT scan (arterial phase after contrast medium). Lung metastases (*red arrows*) from retroperitoneal ASPS at baseline and after 12 months of treatment with sunitinib, 25 mg/d, with evidence a complete response to therapy.

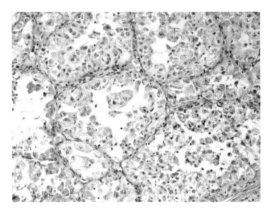

Fig. 2. Alveolar soft part sarcoma with nested groups of cells showing a central loss of cohesion producing a pseudoalveolar pattern. (*From* Horvai AE, Link T. High-yield pathology: bone and soft tissue pathology. Philadelphia: Saunders; 2012. p. 426–7; with permission.)

In detail, a phase 2 study on the selective MET inhibitor tivantinib (*ARQ197,*) in advanced patients recently showed a modest antitumor activity of this agent in ASPS. No PR by response evaluation criteria in solid tumor (RECIST) were observed out of 27 ASPS patients who entered the study, with a 5.5-month median progression-free survival (PFS) in a slow-growing disease.[20] Another phase 2 trial on the MET inhibitor crizotinib has just started in Europe (NCT01524926), open to patients with ALK and MET-related tumors, included cases of ASPS, CCS, and IMT. No preliminary data on crizotinib in ASPS are available. Among multitargeted TKIs, the authors reported on a series of 9 patients with progressive metastatic ASPS treated with sunitinib with RECIST PR in 5 cases, and a 17-month median PFS.[25] The sunitinib antitumor effect looked to be mediated by PDGFRB, VEGFR2, and RET and were found to be expressed on tumor vessels and also on tumor cells. A direct antitumor effect of sunitinib was also confirmed in a short-term cell culture. Following preliminary data in early phase clinical trials showing its activity in ASPS,[26] the VEGF/KIT TKI cediranib was evaluated in a phase 2 prospective clinical study (NCT00942877). The results were recently published, confirming that this agent is active in ASPS. The authors detected 35% PR plus 60% stable disease (SD) by RECIST, with a disease control rate of 84% at 24 weeks. Interestingly, most patients with a RECIST SD showed a tumor shrinkage, even if less than 30%.[27] A randomized phase 3 study comparing sunitinib and cediranib is ongoing in the United States (NCT01391962).

SOLITARY FIBROUS TUMOR

SFT has been initially reported as a primary mesenchymal tumor of the pleura and consequently labeled as a benign localized mesothelioma. It shows complete morphologic and genetic overlap with hemangiopericytoma (HPC), an entity that has formally abolished by the most recent World Health Organization (WHO) classification of mesenchymal neoplasm and is grouped within fibroblastic tumors.[1] SFT can arise at almost all anatomic sites; the name HPC is still (and erroneously) retained only for tumors arising from the central nervous system (CNS).[28] Very recently a recurrent *NAB2-STAT6* gene fusion has been detected in the vast majority of SFT, regardless of anatomic location.[5] Interestingly the same aberration has been observed in meningeal HPCs, further proving that they represent the same entity.[29] SFT is characterized by a broad spectrum of malignancy degree. Three clinical–pathologic variants can be schematically recognized: classical (or usual) SFT (CSFT), malignant (MSFT), and dedifferentiated (DSFT).[30,31] CSFT is characterized by bland morphologic appearance and usually a favorable outcome. Unexpected recurrences with aggressive behavior can be rarely observed.[31] MSFT is characterized by a mitotic index of at least per 10 high-power field, hypercellularity, necrosis and/or pleomorphism.[1] DSFT's hallmark is the presence of a sarcomatous overgrowth mimicking not otherwise specified or distinct high-grade sarcoma types.[30,31] DSFT shows an increasing Ki-67 labeling and mTOR pathway activation.[32] Other studies have emphasized the frequent expression of platelet-derived growth factor receptor (PDGFR) family members, MET, DDR1, ERBB2, and FGFR1, as well as insulin-like growth factor (IGF)2 and IGF1.[33] Among sarcomas, SFT has the most prominent expression of IGF2.[34] In addition, IGF2 production can be responsible for paraneoplastic hypoglycemia.[1] SFT natural history is characterized by a high cure rate after complete surgery, with a 10% to 15% risk of metastasis.[1] DSFT shows an aggressive behavior with a higher metastatic potential.[31] The standard treatment of localized SFT is complete surgical resection, while medical treatment is needed in the advanced phase. Unfortunately, the expected response rate (RR) to doxorubicin-based chemotherapy is low.[35]

Among molecular target agents, the activity of antiangiogenics such as bevacizumab in combination with temozolomide,[36] sorafenib[37] (Nexavar), sunitinib[37–40] and pazopanib[41] (Votrient) has been described in recent years. Responses were nondimensional in the majority of patients, and the molecular mechanisms by which the drugs inhibit tumor growth are still not well understood. The antitumor effect of IGF1R inhibitors was also reported.[32,42]

In detail, bevacizumab is an anti-VEGF-A recombinant humanized monoclonal antibody. The group from MD Anderson reported on its effect in combination with temozolomide in 14 patients suffering of advanced SFT, with 14% PR and 76% SD by RECIST, for a median PFS of 10.8 months. Of interest, when Choi criteria were applied, 79% PR were classified.[36] After the first case-reports,[32,37,38] sunitinib activity in SFT was confirmed in a retrospective study on 31 progressive advanced patients treated at the National Cancer Institute, Milan.[40] Best responses by RECIST were 6.5% PR and 50% SD, with 6-month median PFS. Again, a superior RR could be detected when nondimensional response evaluation criteria were applied, with 48% PR according to Choi criteria. Of interest, while PDGFRB and VEGFR2 as evaluated by immunohistochemistry were positive in all cases (PDGFRB in both tumor cells and vessels; VEGFR2 only in tumor vessels) and not predictive of response, a less aggressive morphology corresponded to an increased RR. Among antiangiogenics, pazopanib is another VEGFR1/2/3, PDGFR, and KIT inhibitor, recently approved for treatment of advanced STS. In the phase 2 study on pazopanib in STS, 3 patients suffering SFT were enrolled. Their responses were not all detailed, but at least 1 SFT patient was shown to have a computed tomography (CT) density reduction without tumor shrinkage after 3 months of therapy.[43] No details are currently available on SFT treated with pazopanib in the recently completed phase 3 trial.[40] Anti-IGF1R inhibitors also sound interesting in this tumor, given the molecular profile of the disease. Preliminary data on 2 patients support this hypothesis. The first report is on a dimensional response to figitumumab, a fully human immunoglobulin (Ig)G2 anti-IGF1R monoclonal antibody in an SFT patient with molecular evidence of IGF1R activation.[32] A second patient had an impressive response to figitumumab plus everolimus (Afinitor), an mTOR inhibitor she received within a phase 1 study.[42] A phase 2 study on the IGF1R inhibitor cituxumumab in combination with the mTOR inhibitor temsirulimus (Torisel) in STS including SFT (NCT01016015) was recently published, again showing the activity of the combination in the subgroup of SFT patients.[44]

PERIVASCULAR EPITHELIOID CELL

PEComas are rare mesenchymal neoplasms of myomelanocytic differentiation that share a distinctive cell type, descriptively named perivascular epithelioid cell (PEC).[45] This cell, which is of unknown lineage, expresses both smooth muscle and melanocytic markers. The PEComa family includes different entities such as angio-myolipoma (AML), lymphangioleiomyomatosis (LAM), clear cell sugar tumor of the lung, and PEComa. The term PEComa practically refers to all PEComas other than AML and LAM. The clinical behavior of these diseases is extremely heterogeneous. LAM, although pathologically benign, causes cystic degeneration of the lungs, leading to progressive respiratory failure; similarly, renal AML may lead to abdominal hemorrhage or kidney failure. Epithelioid AMLs frequently display aggressive clinical behavior with local and distant recurrences. The presence of mitotic activity and necrosis correlates with aggressive behavior (malignant PEComa); however, criteria of malignancy need further validation. The evidence that PEComas may be associated with tuberous sclerosis complex (TSC), an autosomal-dominant disease caused by inactivating mutation in the tumor suppressor genes *TSC1* or *TSC2*, not only helped in the molecular characterization of the disease but also opened up new therapeutic opportunities.[46] The TSC1/TSC2 complex inhibits the proliferative signals of the mTOR complex 1 (mTORC1) through inhibition of Rheb, a Guanosine-5′-triphosphate (GTP) hydrolase enzyme (ase) of the rat sarcoma family that activates mTORC1.[46] Mutation in *TSC1* or *TSC2* leads to hyperactivation of the mTOR pathway. Although the molecular mechanisms responsible for the development of sporadic PEComas are only partially understood, preliminary data suggest activation of mTORC1 due to loss of TSC1 or TSC2.[47] However, a subset of biologically distinct PEComas has been described.[48,49] These PEComas, showing strong TFE3 immunoreactivity, carry rearrangements in *TFE3* and have intact *TSC2*, thus potentially influencing clinical history and sensitivity to therapy.[48,49] Malignant PEComas arise ubiquitously. Standard treatment for patients with localized disease is wide surgery. Despite surgery, malignant PEComa may recur locally or metastasize. Anthracycline- or gemcitabine-based chemotherapy is administered in the advanced phase of disease, with unsatisfactory RR.[50]

In addition to the randomized evidence of mTOR inhibitors' efficacy in LAM patients,[51] preliminary data suggest that of mTOR inhibitors can be active also in malignant PEComa.[47,52–54]

So far, 4 different mTOR inhibitors are available for clinical purposes: rapamycin, (Rapamune) and its 3 derivatives, namely temsirolimus, everolimus, and ridaforolimus (Ariad). A randomized phase 3 placebo-controlled trial of sirolimus in patients with LAM confirmed early data; sirolimus was effective in stabilizing forced expiratory volume, improving force vital capacity and quality of life.[51,55] Moreover, everolimus proved to be active in reducing the volume of subependymal giant-cell astrocytomas in a group of 28 patients with TSC,[56] together with improvement in symptomatic patients. Afterward, Wagner and Wolff described the activity of mTOR inhibitors in single patients carrying malignant PEComa.[47,52] This was followed by many other reports confirming the activity of these compounds in the disease.[53,54] However, a recent retrospective analysis presented in abstract form showed responses to mTOR to be short lasting, with a 4-month median PFS.[50] Cases of primary resistant disease were also reported.[57,58] The mechanisms responsible for resistance to mTOR inhibitors in malignant PEComa are currently unknown. Based on these results, a phase 2 study on BEZ235 (Novartis, Basel, Switzerland), an orally available dual inhibitor of mTOR and PI3K inhibitors, in metastatic or unresectable malignant PEComa (NCT01690871), is ongoing in Europe.

CLEAR CELL SARCOMA

CCS is another very rare STS mainly affecting adolescents and young adults, with a female predominance, potentially arising from any site of the body, lower limbs being the most common primary location.[1] A rather distinctive subset arises in the gastrointestinal (GI) tract and has been recently renamed as malignant GI neuroectodermal tumor.[59] CCS is also known as malignant melanoma of the soft part, because it displays morphologic and immunohistochemical features very similar to malignant melanoma. In fact, these 2 malignancies have overlapping immunohistochemical characteristics like the expression of melanocytic markers.[1] CCS is marked in the majority of cases by 2 recurrent chromosomal translocations that do not occur in melanoma. The translocation *t(12;22)(q13;q12)* results in fusion of the *EWSR1* and the *ATF1* genes. Of note, 7 different types of EWSR1-ATF1 fusion transcript have been described to date.[9–12] Less frequently, the translocation t(2;22)(q34;q12) has been found resulting in the *EWSR1-CREB1* fusion-gene.[9,60] Curiously, *EWSR1-ATF1* and *EWSR1-CREB1* are gene fusions described in several histopathologically and behaviorally diverse neoplasms: CCS, angiomatoid fibrous histiocytoma, hyalinizing CCS of the salivary gland, and primary pulmonary myxoid sarcoma.[61] A proportion of CCS does not carry any chromosomic rearrangements. In these cases, the presence of structural and numerical aberrations of chromosomes 22 and 8 was reported.[62,63] Recently, cases with the V600E BRAF mutation in translocated CCS were reported, too, thus underlining the similarities with melanoma.[63,64] Clinically, CCS is characterized by an aggressive behavior and greater than 60% incidence of metastases, with a subsequent very poor prognosis. CCS is poorly sensitive to chemotherapy (**Figs. 3** and **4**).[65]

Molecular target agents with a marked activity in this disease are yet to be identified, even if MET inhibitors[20] and antiangiogenics have shown some degree of activity.[66–68]

MET inhibitors were found to be active both in CCS cell lines and xenograft model.[69] Unfortunately the phase 2 study on tivantinib in MIT family tumors detected only 1 PR

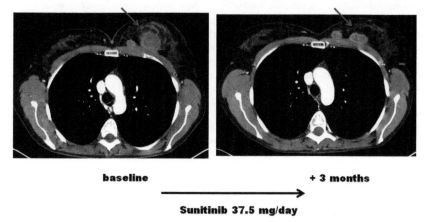

baseline   + 3 months

Sunitinib 37.5 mg/day

Fig. 3. CT scan (arterial phase after contrast medium). Soft tissue metastasis (*red arrow*) from leg CCS at baseline and after 3 months of treatment with sunitinib, 37.5 mg/d, with evidence a RECIST partial response.

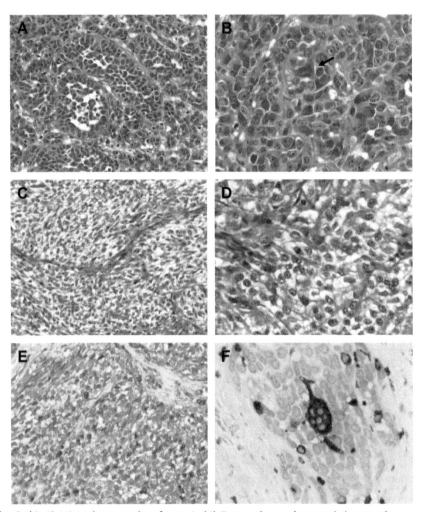

Fig. 4. (*A, B*) Microphotographs of case 1. (*A*) Tumor shows characteristic nested or pseu-doalveolar pattern. (*B*) Tumor cells are mostly epithelioid with prominent nucleoli and eosinophilic cytoplasm. Osteoclast-type multinucleated giant cell (*arrow*) is focally present. (*C, D*) Microphotographs of case 2. (*C*) The tumor is composed of sheets or nests of predominantly epithelioid cells. (*D*) Tumor cells have small but prominent nucleoli and clear cytoplasm with occasional mitotic figures. Some plasma cells are found within the tumor. (*E, F*) Microphotographs of immunostaining. (*E*) Immunostaining for S-100 protein is diffusely positive in the tumor cells of case 1 and 2. (*F*) CD68 immunostaining is positive in osteoclast-like giant cells. (*From* Joo M, Chang SH, Kim H, et al. Primary gastrointestinal clear cell sarcoma: report of 2 cases, 1 case associated with IgG4-related sclerosing disease, and review of literature. Ann Diagn Pathol 2009;13(1):30–5; with permission.)

of 11 CCS patients who entered the study, with a 1.9-month median PFS.[20] Of note, no correlation between MET protein expression levels in tumor samples and response was found. Among antiangiogenics, the authors reported initially on a patient with an advanced CCS responsive to sunitinib.[66] Recently, the authors updated their series with evidence of a PR RECIST in 4 cases among 8 advanced CCS patients treated with the same agent, and a median PFS of 4 months. Response was confirmed pathologically in 1 case.[67] A response to sorafenib in an advanced CCS patient was reported, too.[68]

DISCUSSION

This article refers to a subgroup of rare entities within a family of rare cancers, such as sarcomas. They have been selected for their responsiveness to a set of molecularly targeted agents. Interestingly, they are rather insensitive to cytoxics.

In part, this may be due to the fact that most of these entities, with the exception of CCS, fall within the category of relatively low-grade STS. Obviously, low-grade tumors may respond much less to standard chemotherapy, while their higher degree of differentiation may be associated with a higher relevance of cellular pathways, which may well serve as drug-susceptible targets. In addition, all entities mentioned herein have been translocation-related sarcomas (ie, they belong to the growing subset of sarcomas whose pathogenetic mechanism can be associated with a specific genetic defect). Sometimes, this results in obvious targets, such as another translocation-related sarcoma such as dermatofibrosarcoma protuberans (DFSP).[70] Within these entities, IMT carries a translocation-related target (ie, ALK), which is strongly related to the mechanism of action of the drugs employed. On the other hand, in the case of ASPS and CCS, the activation of MET seems to be paralleled by a lower activity of the relevant drugs (ie, anti-MET agents). In the case of SFT, agents targeting STAT6 have not been tested. In PEComas, a translocation resulting in MET activation was found in a small proportion of cases, while mTOR inhibitors were shown to have some activity, in the absence of major genetic alterations of the mTOR pathway (with the exception of LAM), although in the presence of a degree of its disruption. For these reasons, even across these entities, true biomarkers are not available (with an ongoing study testing ALK and MET as biomarkers in IMT, ASPS, and CCS). Thus, the models of GI stromal tumor (GIST) and DFSP remain far off, although in the context of highly interesting entities for targeted therapies.

Some of the agents used for these entities are antiangiogenics. They are also TKI, affecting specific targets, including PDGFRA and PDGFRB, which have been shown to be potentially involved in some sarcomas (eg, ASPS). However, this article discusses activation of pathways in the absence of mutations, and the like, so that it is possible that some of the effects that were seen in the clinic were caused by a rather unspecific mechanism of action for these targeted agents, from an antiangiogenic effect to an effect on pathways that may be more or less crucial for the tumor cell.

Intriguingly, patterns of tumor response are not the same across all these entities. For example, the authors saw tumor shrinkages to sunitinib in ASPS and mainly nondimensional responses to the same agent in SFT, and preclinical data would point to a more direct antitumor effect in the former compared with a less specific effect in the latter. Even response duration is different, from a medium-/long-term effect in ASPS to a shorter effect in CCS. Responses may be short also in malignant PEComas responding to mTOR inhibitors. This raises the issue of tumor response assessment, since this might not be an exclusively clinical difficulty but also something related to the mechanism of action of these agents (ie, to something more inherently linked to the nature of the antitumor effect). In other words, patterns of tumor response might tell more about the antitumor effect than is known today.

This has to do with the clinical methodology and the methodology of clinical research. The latter is challenged by the small numbers of these sarcomas. Indeed, the evidence that has been provided so far is rather suboptimal, from case reports to small case series analyses. In some instances, prospective clinical studies are ongoing, and this is worth mentioning, because it may point to an improvement in the way rare sarcoma subgroups are currently addressed by clinical research. However, with the lack of improvements in the methodology of clinical research itself, these rare entities will always entail an additional difficulty, compared with more frequent types.

This is also important for clinical practice today. In fact, in the face of the same quality of evidence, discrepancies do exist as to how much these drugs are accessible across different countries and health systems. This will only continue as the economic crisis continues. The quality of evidence must improve. This can be done by carrying out clinical studies more systematically also in these rare entities, and by improving the methodology of research in such a way as to better accommodate small population studies.

REFERENCES

1. Fletcher CD, Bridge JA, Pancras CW, editors. World Health Organization classification of tumours of soft tissue and bone. Lyon (France): IARC Press; 2013.
2. Stiller CA, Trama A, Serraino D, et al. Descriptive epidemiology of sarcomas in Europe: report from the RARECARE project. Eur J Cancer 2013;49(3):684–95.
3. Gleason BC, Hornick JL. Inflammatory myofibroblastic tumours: where are we now? J Clin Pathol 2008;61:428–37.
4. Coffin CM, Patel A, Perkins S, et al. ALK1 and p80 expression and chromosomal rearrangements involving 2p23 in inflammatory myofibroblastic tumor. Mod Pathol 2001;14:569–76.
5. Robinson DR, Wu YM, Kalyana-Sundaram S, et al. Identification of recurrent NAB2-STAT6 gene fusions in solitary fibrous tumor by integrative sequencing. Nat Genet 2013;45:180–5.
6. Landanyi M, Lui MY, Antonescu CR, et al. The der(17)t(X;17)(p11;q25) of human alveolar soft part sarcoma fuses the TFE3 transcription factor gene to ASPL, a novel gene at 17q25. Oncogene 2001;20:48–57.
7. Tsuda M, Davis IJ, Argani P, et al. TFE3 fusions activate MET signaling by transcriptional up-regulation, defining another class of tumors as candidates for therapeutic MET inhibition. Cancer Res 2007;67:919–29.
8. Chang IW, Huang HY, Sung MT. Melanotic Xp11 translocation renal cancer: a case with PSF-TFE3 gene fusion and up-regulation of melanogenetic transcripts. Am J Surg Pathol 2009;33:1894–901.
9. WangW-L ME, Zhang W, Hernandez VS, et al. Detection and characterization of EWSR1/ATF1 and EWSR1/CREB1 chimeric transcripts in clear cell sarcoma (melanoma of soft parts). Mod Pathol 2009;22:1201–9.
10. Jakubauskas A, Valceckiene V, Andrekute K, et al. Discovery of two novel EWSR1/ATF1 transcripts in four chimerical transcripts-expressing clear cell sarcoma and their quantitative evaluation. Exp Mol Pathol 2011;90:194–200.
11. Panagopoulos I, Mertens F, Dêbiec-Rychter M, et al. Molecular genetic characterization of the EWS/ATF1 fusion gene in clear cell sarcoma of tendons and aponeuroses. Int J Cancer 2002;99:560–7.
12. Gineikiene E, Seinin D, Brasiuniene B, et al. Clear cell sarcoma expressing a novel chimerical transcript EWSR1 exon 7/ATF1 exon 6. Virchows Arch 2012; 461:339–43.
13. Griffin CA, Hawkins AL, Dvorak C, et al. Recurrent involvement of 2p23 in inflammatory myofibroblastic tumors. Cancer Res 1999;59:2776–80.
14. Coffin CM, Hornick JL, Fletcher CD. Inflammatory myofibroblastic tumor: comparison of clinicopathologic, histologic, and immunohistochemical features

including ALK expression in atypical and aggressive cases. Am J Surg Pathol 2007;31:509–20.

15. Su W, Ko A, O'Connell T, et al. Treatment of pseudotumors with nonsteroidal anti-inflammatory drugs. J Pediatr Surg 2000;35:1635–7.

16. Rodig SJ, Shapiro GI. Crizotinib, a small-molecule dual inhibitor of the c-Met and ALK receptor tyrosine kinases. Curr Opin Investig Drugs 2010;11:1477–90.

17. Butrynski JE, D'Adamo DR, Hornick JL, et al. Crizotinib in ALK-rearranged inflammatory myofibroblastic tumor. N Engl J Med 2010;363:1727–33.

18. Sasaki T, Okuda K, Zheng W, et al. The neuroblastoma-associated F1174L ALK mutation causes resistance to an ALK kinase inhibitor in ALK-translocated cancers. Cancer Res 2010;70:10038–43.

19. Reichardt P, Lindner T, Pink D, et al. Chemotherapy in alveolar soft part sarcomas. What do we know? Eur J Cancer 2003;39:1511–6.

20. Wagner AJ, Goldberg JM, Dubois SG, et al. Tivantinib (ARQ 197), a selective inhibitor of MET, in patients with microphthalmia transcription factor-associated tumors: results of a multicenter phase 2 trial. Cancer 2012;118: 5894–902.

21. Bisogno G, Rosolen A, Carli M. Interferon alpha for alveolar soft part sarcoma. Pediatr Blood Cancer 2005;44:687–8.

22. Roozendaal KJ, de Valk B, ten Velden JJ, et al. Alveolar soft-part sarcoma responding to interferon alpha-2b. Br J Cancer 2003;89:243–5.

23. Azizi AA, Haberler C, Czech T, et al. Vascular-endothelial-growth-factor (VEGF) expression and possible response to angiogenesis inhibitor bevacizumab in metastatic alveolar soft part sarcoma. Lancet Oncol 2006;7:521–3.

24. Stacchiotti S, Tamborini E, Marrari A, et al. Response to sunitinib malate in advanced alveolar soft part sarcoma. Clin Cancer Res 2009;15:1096–104.

25. Stacchiotti S, Negri T, Zaffaroni N, et al. Sunitinib in advanced alveolar soft part sarcoma: evidence of a direct antitumor effect. Ann Oncol 2011;22:1682–90.

26. Gardner K, Judson I, Leahy M, et al. Activity of cediranib, a highly potent and selective VEGF signaling inhibitor, in alveolar soft part sarcoma [abstract 10523]. J Clin Oncol 2009;27:541.

27. Kummar S, Allen D, Monks A, et al. Cediranib for metastatic alveolar soft part sarcoma. J Clin Oncol 2013;31:2296–302.

28. Louis DN, Ohgaki H, Wiestler OD, et al. WHO classification of tumours of the central nervous system. World health organization classification of tumours. 4th edition. Lyon (France): International Agency for Research on Cancer; 2007.

29. Schweizer L, Koelsche C, Sahm F, et al. Meningeal hemangiopericytoma and solitary fibrous tumors carry the NAB2-STAT6 fusion and can be diagnosed by nuclear expression of STAT6 protein. Acta Neuropathol 2013;125:651–8.

30. Mosquera JM, Fletcher CD. Expanding the spectrum of malignant progression solitary fibrous tumor – a study of 8 cases with a discrete anaplastic component—is this dedifferentiated SFT? Am J Surg Pathol 2009;33:1314–21.

31. Collini P, Negri T, Barisella M, et al. High-grade sarcomatous overgrowth in solitary fibrous tumor: a clinico-pathological study of 10 cases. Am J Surg Pathol 2012;36:1202–15.

32. Stacchiotti S, Negri T, Palassini E, et al. Sunitinib malate and figitumumab in solitary fibrous tumor: patterns and molecular bases of tumor response. Mol Cancer Ther 2010;9:1286–97.

33. Hajdu M, Singer S, Maki RG, et al. IGF2 over-expression in solitary fibrous tumours is independent of anatomical location and is related to loss of imprinting. J Pathol 2010;221:300–7.

34. Steigen SE, Schaeffer DF, West RB, et al. Expression of insulin-like growth factor 2 in mesenchymal neoplasms. Mod Pathol 2009;22:914–21.
35. Stacchiotti S, Libertini M, Negri T, et al. Response to chemotherapy of solitary fibrous tumor: a retrospective study. Eur J Cancer 2013;49(10):2376–83.
36. Park MS, Patel SR, Ludwig JA, et al. Activity of temozolomide and bevacizumab in the treatment of locally advanced, recurrent, and metastatic hemangiopericytoma and malignant solitary fibrous tumor. Cancer 2011;117:4939–47.
37. Domont J, Massard C, Lassau N, et al. Hemangiopericytoma and antiangiogenic therapy: clinical benefit of antiangiogenic therapy (sorafenib and sunitinib) in relapsed malignant haemangioperyctoma/solitary fibrous tumour. Invest New Drugs 2010;28:199–202.
38. Mulamalla K, Truskinovsky AM, Dudek AZ. Rare case of hemangiopericytoma responds to sunitinib. Transl Res 2008;151:129–33.
39. George S, Merriam P, Maki RG, et al. Multicenter phase II trial of sunitinib in the treatment of non-gastrointestinal stromal tumor sarcomas. J Clin Oncol 2009;27: 3154–60.
40. Stacchiotti S, Negri T, Libertini M, et al. Sunitinib in solitary fibrous tumor. Ann Oncol 2012;23:3171–9.
41. Van der Graaf WT, Blay JY, Chawla SP, et al. Pazopanib for metastatic soft-tissue sarcoma (PALETTE): a randomised, double-blind, placebo-controlled phase 3 trial. Lancet 2012;379:1879–86.
42. Quek R, Wang Q, Morgan JA, et al. Combination mTOR and IGF-1R inhibition: phase I trial of everolimus and figitumumab in patients with advanced sarcomas and other solid tumors. Clin Cancer Res 2011;17:871–9.
43. Sleijfer S, Ray-Coquard I, Papai Z, et al. Pazopanib, a multikinase angiogenesis inhibitor, in patients with relapsed or refractory advanced soft tissue sarcoma: a phase II study from the European Organisation for Research and Treatment of Cancer-Soft Tissue and Bone Sarcoma Group (EORTC study 62043). J Clin Oncol 2009;27:3126–32.
44. Schwartz GK, Tap WD, Qin LX, et al. Cixutumumab and temsirolimus for patients with bone and soft-tissue sarcoma: a multicentre, open-label, phase 2 trial. Lancet Oncol 2013;14:371–82.
45. Hornick JL, Fletcher CD. PEComas: what do we know so far? Histopathology 2006;48:75–82.
46. Crino PB, Nathanson KL, Henske EP. The tuberous sclerosis complex. N Engl J Med 2006;355:1345–56.
47. Wagner AJ, Malinowska-Kolodziej I, Morgan JA, et al. Clinical activity of mTOR inhibition with sirolimus in malignant perivascular epithelioid cell tumors: targeting the pathogenic activation of mTORC1 in tumors. J Clin Oncol 2010;28:835–40.
48. Argani P, Aulmann S, Illei PB, et al. A distinctive subset of PEComas harbors TFE3 gene fusions. Am J Surg Pathol 2010;34:1395–406.
49. Malinowska I, Kwiatkowski DJ, Weiss S, et al. Perivascular epithelioid cell tumors (PEComas) harboring TFE3 gene rearrangements lack the TSC2 alterations characteristic of conventional PEComas: further evidence for a biological distinction. Am J Surg Pathol 2012;36:783–4.
50. Marrari A, Hornick JL, Butrynski JE, et al. Malignant perivascular epithelioid cell tumors (PEComas): a retrospective analysis of 24 patients to define clinical history and response to therapy [abstract 39396]. Presented at the Connective Tissue Oncology Society (CTOS) 16th annual meeting, Chicago, November, 2011.
51. McCormack FX, Inoue Y, Moss J, et al. Efficacy and safety of sirolimus in lymphangioleiomyomatosis. N Engl J Med 2011;364:1595–606.

52. Wolff N, Kabbani W, Bradley T, et al. Sirolimus and temsirolimus for epithelioid angiomyolipoma. J Clin Oncol 2010;28:e65–8.

53. Italiano A, Delcambre C, Hostein I, et al. Treatment with the mTOR inhibitor temsirolimus in patients with malignant PEComas. Ann Oncol 2010;21:1135–7.

54. Shitara K, Yatabe Y, Mizota A, et al. Dramatic tumor response to everolimus for malignant epithelioid angiomyolipoma. Jpn J Clin Oncol 2011;41:814–6.

55. Bissler JJ, McCormack FX, Young LR, et al. Sirolimus for angiomyolipoma in tuberous sclerosis complex or lymphangioleiomyomatosis. N Engl J Med 2008;358:140–51.

56. Krueger DA, Care MM, Holland K, et al. Everolimus for subependymal giant-cell astrocytomas in tuberous sclerosis. N Engl J Med 2010;363:1801–11.

57. Subbiah V, Trent JC, Kurzrock R. Resistance to mammalian target of rapamycin inhibitor therapy in perivascular epithelioid cell tumors. J Clin Oncol 2010;28: e415.

58. Higa F, Uchihara T, Haranaga S, et al. Malignant epithelioid angiomyolipoma in the kidney and liver of a patient with pulmonary lymphangioleiomyomatosis: lack of response to sirolimus. Intern Med 2009;48:1821–5.

59. Stockman DL, Miettinen M, Suster S, et al. Malignant gastrointestinal neuroectodermal tumor: clinicopathologic, immunohistochemical, ultrastructural, and molecular analysis of 16 cases with a reappraisal of clear cell sarcoma-like tumors of the gastrointestinal tract. Am J Surg Pathol 2012;36:857–68.

60. Antonescu CR, Nafa K, Segal NH, et al. EWS-CREB1: a recurrent variant fusion in clear cell sarcoma–association with gastrointestinal location and absence of melanocytic differentiation. Clin Cancer Res 2006;12:5356–62.

61. Romeo S, Dei Tos AP. Soft tissue tumors associated with EWSR1 translocation. Virchows Arch 2010;456:219–34.

62. Limon J, Debiec-Rychter M, Nedoszytko B, et al. Aberrations of chromosome 22 and polysomy of chromosome 8 as non-random changes in clear cell sarcoma. Cancer Genet Cytogenet 1994;72:141–5.

63. Negri T, Brich S, Conca E, et al. Receptor tyrosine kinase pathway analysis sheds light on similarities between clear-cell sarcoma and metastatic melanoma. Genes Chromosomes Cancer 2012;51:111–26.

64. Hocar O, Le Cesne A, Berissi S, et al. Clear cell sarcoma (malignant melanoma) of soft parts: a clinicopathologic study of 52 cases. Dermatol Res Pract 2012; 2012:984096.

65. Jones RL, Constantinidou A, Thway K, et al. Chemotherapy in clear cell sarcoma. Med Oncol 2011;28:859–63.

66. Stacchiotti S, Grosso F, Negri T, et al. Tumor response to sunitinib malate observed in clear-cell sarcoma. Ann Oncol 2010;21:1130–1.

67. Stacchiotti S, Palassini E, Negri T, et al. Sunitinib malate in clear cell sarcoma [abstract 1496P]. Presented at ESMO annual meeting, Prague, September, 2012.

68. Mir O, Boudou-Rouquette P, Larousserie F, et al. Objective response to sorafenib in advanced clear-cell sarcoma. Ann Oncol 2012;23:807–9.

69. Davis IJ, McFadden AW, Zhang Y, et al. Identification of the receptor tyrosine kinase c-met and its ligand, hepatocyte growth factor, as therapeutic targets in clear cell sarcoma. Cancer Res 2010;70:639–45.

70. Rutkowski P, Van Glabbeke M, Rankin CJ, et al. Imatinib mesylate in advanced dermatofibrosarcoma protuberans: pooled analysis of two phase II clinical trials. J Clin Oncol 2010;28:1772–9.

Emerging Therapies for Soft-Tissue Sarcomas

Alice Levard, MD, Louis Tassy, MD, Philippe A. Cassier, MD*

KEYWORDS

- Sarcoma • Tumor • Cancer • Therapy • Drug development

KEY POINTS

- Despite significant progress in our understanding of the biology underlying the clinical heterogeneity of soft-tissue sarcomas (STS), only a few subtypes of sarcoma can currently be treated using rationally selected therapies.
- Inhibition of tumor angiogenesis has proved to be a rational target in STS, but much remains to be done to derive predictive markers.
- Alternative strategies to target angiogenesis are currently under evaluation in clinical trials.
- More work is needed to identify predictive markers not only in sarcomas but also in other solid tumors.
- Future trials should include pretreatment and posttreatment tumor biopsies to allow the identification of predictive factors if the drug is found to be active in a subset of patients, and to enable hypothesis-generating translational research, which will help plan the following generation of studies in STS.

INTRODUCTION

Sarcomas are heterogeneous group of tumors that arise from tissues of mesenchymal origin. As a whole they are rare tumors and account for only 1.5% of cancers, and the classification of the World Health Organization identifies more than 50 different subtypes. Molecular studies have shown these different subtypes to be biologically different, therefore suggesting that sarcomas are in fact a constellation of very rare diseases, some being even rarer than others. From the clinical perspective sarcomas are divided into soft-tissue sarcomas (STS), bone sarcomas, and gastrointestinal stromal tumors (GIST). GISTs and bone sarcomas are discussed elsewhere in this issue.

Disclosures: AL, LT, and PAC's institution have received research funding from Novartis and Roche. PAC is a coordinating investigator for Novartis and Roche sponsored trials. PAC has received travel reimbursment from Novartis, Roche, PharmaMar. PAC has recevied Honoraria from Novartis, Servier, Glaxo Smith Kline, and PharmaMar.
Department of Medical Oncology, Léon Bérard Cancer Center, 28 rue Laennec, Lyon 69008, France
* Corresponding author.
E-mail address: cassierp@hotmail.com

Hematol Oncol Clin N Am 27 (2013) 1063–1078
http://dx.doi.org/10.1016/j.hoc.2013.07.011
0889-8588/13/$ – see front matter © 2013 Elsevier Inc. All rights reserved.

This article addresses only emerging therapies for STS, although there are some areas of overlap between the 3 tumor types in terms of drug development.

STS represent both the largest and most heterogeneous group of tumors among sarcomas. The most common subtypes include liposarcomas and leiomyosarcomas, each representing 20% of STS, but this group also includes rarer subtypes such as synovial sarcoma or even rarer entities such as alveolar soft-part sarcoma (ASPS) or epithelioid sarcoma. Although our knowledge of STS biology has grown considerably over the last few years, such progress has thus far had limited impact on patient management. Management of localized disease relies on complete surgical excision with adequate tumor-free margins followed by radiotherapy. Treatment of advanced disease is based on systemic therapy using doxorubicin, ifosfamide, dacarbazine, and trabectedin used either sequentially or in combination. Gemcitabine has also been shown to have some activity in leiomyosarcoma, either alone or combined with docetaxel or dacarbazine. Pazopanib was recently approved for the treatment of patients with advanced pretreated STS excluding liposarcoma. This review discusses emerging therapies for sarcomas, arbitrarily divided into broad-spectrum approaches for drugs or compounds that have shown clinical activity but for which the precise mode of action remains to be elucidated, and subtype-specific approaches whereby drugs are used to treat some sarcoma subtypes based on current understanding of sarcoma biology (**Fig. 1**).

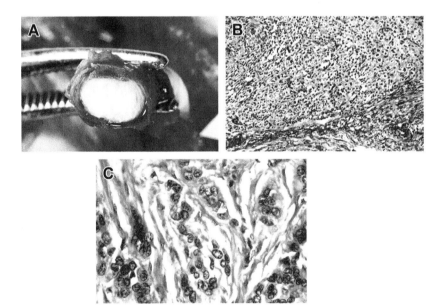

Fig. 1. (*A*) In this patient with an epithelioid sarcoma, the tumor initially arose in the distal portion of the tendon sheath of the extensor pollicis longus. At amputation, as demonstrated in this photograph, the tumor was found to be in the subsynovial space, wrapping around the tendon. (*B*) Photomicrograph of an epithelioid sarcoma shows plump, oval to polyhedral cells that have a dense eosinophilic cytoplasm. The predominant pattern here is epithelial, but in other areas a spindle fibrosarcomatous appearance can be expected (hematoxylin-eosin [H&E], original magnification ×10). (*C*) Higher-power view of nests of epithelioid cells (H&E, original magnification ×40). (*From* Bullough PG. Orthopaedic pathology. St Louis (MO): Mosby; 2010. p. 533–49; with permission.)

BROAD-SPECTRUM APPROACHES
Cytotoxic Agents

Although very few cytotoxic agents remain in the development pipeline of the bigger pharmaceutical companies, several smaller pharmas are still developing "optimized" versions of older cytotoxic or newer cytotoxic agents. Several drugs are currently being developed for the treatment of advanced sarcomas, including eribulin, TH302, and INNO-206. The development of palifosfamide, a new formulation of the active metabolite of ifosfamide, one of the few drugs considered active in STS, was halted in spring 2013 following the interim analysis of a randomized phase III trial (Ziopharm press release, March 26, 2013).

Eribulin mesylate (HALAVEN and formerly E7389) is a synthetic analogue of halichondrin B, which acts as an inhibitor of microtubule dynamics. Schöffski and colleagues[1] treated 128 patients with advanced STS with eribulin mesylate. As did previous European Organization for Research and Treatment of Cancer (EORTC) Soft Tissue and Bone Sarcoma Group studies, this phase II study comprised 4 cohorts: adipocytic sarcoma (n = 37), leiomyosarcoma (n = 40), synovial sarcoma (n = 19), and a cohort of other sarcomas (n = 32). The primary end point was 12-week progression-free survival (PFS) in each cohort (this arbitrary outcome measure is based on the work of Van Glabbeke and colleagues[2] showing that active agents in second line provide a 12-week PFS rate of 40% or more). Fifteen of 32 (47%), 12 of 38 (32%), 4 of 19 (21%), and 5 of 26 (19%) of patients in the adipocytic, leiomyosarcoma, synovial sarcoma, and "other" sarcoma cohorts were progression-free at 12 weeks.[1] Based on these results, a phase III trial comparing eribulin with dacarbazine is currently enrolling patients with liposarcoma and leiomyosarcoma.

TH-302 is a 2-nitroimidazole prodrug of the DNA alkylator, bromo-isophosphoramide mustard. TH-302 is designed to be activated and to release bromo-isophosphoramide mustard under conditions of severe hypoxia. In a phase I/II trial in patients with advanced STS, Ganjoo and colleagues[3] found that TH-302 at 300 mg/m^2 could be safely administered with doxorubicin. In the phase II part of the study, 60 patients with various subtypes of advanced STS were enrolled. The response rate (RR) was 29% (17 of 58 evaluable patients) and the median PFS was 6.7 months, both of which are higher than expected for doxorubicin alone.[3] The Sarcoma Alliance for Research through Collaboration is currently running a phase III trial of doxorubicin alone versus doxorubicin combined with TH-302 in the United States and other parts of the world.

INNO-206, or aldoxorubicin, is a doxorubicin conjugate whereby doxorubicin is attached to an acid-sensitive linker that binds covalently to cysteine-34 in circulating albumin. The proposed mechanism of action is that following intravenous injection, aldoxorubicin binds to albumin, which accumulates in tumor sites where the acidic environment will cleave the linker and release doxorubicin. The main advantage is to allow accumulation of doxorubicin in tumors while preserving normal tissues, with the aim of increasing the therapeutic index of doxorubicin. In a phase I/II trial, the maximum tolerated dose was determined to be 350 mg/m^2. Three of 16 patients (19%) had a partial response (PR) while 10 had stable disease (SD) as their best response.[4] Aldoxorubicin is currently being evaluated in comparison with doxorubicin as first-line chemotherapy in a randomized phase II trial.

Targeting Angiogenesis

As illustrated by the recent approval of pazopanib, inhibition of tumor angiogenesis is a viable therapeutic option in the management of STS. Sunitinib and sorafenib were evaluated in several phase II trials conducted in parallel with the initial pazopanib phase II trial conducted by the EORTC. Although 2 phase II trials failed to demonstrate significant activity for sunitinib,[5,6] in the phase II trial reported by Maki and colleagues,[7] the median PFS and the 3-month progression-free rate with sorafenib were quite similar to those found with pazopanib by the Europeans, but because of different trial designs these results were considered insufficient to declare the compound active as a single agent. Other phase II trials have since been reported and have shown similar results in terms of PFS, although the RR varied from 0% to 15%, likely reflecting disease heterogeneity.[8,9] Sorafenib was also evaluated in the treatment of sarcomas combined with other treatment modalities such as chemotherapy, radiotherapy, and/or surgery. A phase I trial lead by the Grupo Espanol de Investigacion de Sarcomas reported the feasibility of ifosfamide (6 g/m^2 every 3 weeks) combined with sorafenib (400 mg twice a day), and 5 of 12 patients in this study achieved (SD) for 5 months or more. In a phase II trial, D'Adamo and colleagues[10] tested the combination of sorafenib and dacarbazine, and observed a 10% RR and 29% clinical benefit rate (complete response [CR] + PR + SD >18 weeks) in patients with advanced synovial sarcoma and leiomyosarcoma. In this study, 4 of 4 patients with malignant peripheral nerve sheath tumors (MPNST) had progressive disease (PD) as their best response. Overall, these observations suggest that sorafenib has activity in a subset of patients with STS. However, the benefit of combining this agent with chemotherapy remains to be demonstrated. Of note, the pathologic RR seen in preoperative trials combining sorafenib with chemoradiation[11] does not appear to differ much from that observed with chemoradiation alone.[12,13] Likewise, 3 phase Ib trials (2 in Europe and 1 in Australia) are investigating the feasibility of sunitinib combined with radiation, but none of them have as yet reported any results. Aside from evaluation of these tyrosine kinase inhibitors, several studies are currently ongoing, exploring the role of bevacizumab in combination with various chemotherapy regimens as well as radiotherapy. In adult sarcoma patients, Verschraegen and colleagues[14] recently reported the results of a phase Ib trial of bevacizumab in combination with gemcitabine and docetaxel (GD). In this trial, bevacizumab and docetaxel were given at relatively low (and fixed) doses of 5 mg/kg and 50 mg/m^2 every 2 weeks, whereas the dose of gemcitabine was increased from 1000 mg/m^2 (on day 1 every 2 weeks) by 250-mg/m^2 increments. Encouraging efficacy was seen in this study, with an RR of 31.5% (11 of 35 evaluable patients) in presumably treatment-naïve patients. A phase II trial in patients with selected advanced sarcomas (leiomyosarcoma, undifferentiated pleomorphic sarcoma, pleomorphic liposarcoma, rhabdomyosarcoma, and angiosarcoma) previously treated with zero or one previous regimen has completed accrual, while a phase III trial comparing GD with GD without bevacizumab is currently recruiting patients with advanced uterine leiomyosarcomas. Other studies are also currently ongoing in pediatric patients with advanced sarcomas. Of interest, the first phase II trial evaluating bevacizumab in STS combined doxorubicin and bevacizumab. In this study the high rate of grade 2 to 4 cardiac toxicity (6 of 17 patients) contrasted with an RR (12%) that did not seem to be different from that of the single agent doxorubicin.[15] Studies combining bevacizumab and radiotherapy have shown promising results in terms of pathologic response.[16]

Brivanib, a small tyrosine kinase inhibitor targeting vascular endothelial growth factor receptor (VEGFR) and fibroblast growth factor receptor (FGFR) kinases, was assessed in several tumor types in a large, multicohort phase II trial, using an independent randomized discontinuation design in each cohort.[17] Two hundred fifty-one patients with sarcomas were enrolled in this study (leiomyosarcoma, n = 60; liposarcoma, n = 61; angiosarcoma, n = 20; other sarcomas, n = 110).[18] One hundred thirty-three patients and 35 patients came off study for progression or other reasons, respectively, within the first 12 weeks. Seven patients (3%) had a PR and continued on open-label brivanib while 76 patients who had SD at 12 weeks were randomized. Median PFS was 2.6 months for patients in the brivanib arm versus 1.4 months in the placebo arm. This study met its primary end point for patients with FGFR2-positive tumors (median PFS 2.8 vs 1.4 months; hazard ratio = 0.58, P = .08, prespecified α of 0.1).[18]

Other approaches targeting the tumor vasculature are currently being evaluated. One such approach is the development of vascular targeted agents using NGR peptide. NGR-hTNF is human tumor necrosis factor α targeted to the tumor vasculature using NGR peptide. Several studies have shown promising activity of this agent in combination with various chemotherapy regimens, and a phase II trial of NGR-hTNF alone or combined with doxorubicin is currently under way in unselected STS. Similarly, several studies with inhibitors of angiogenesis, either alone (axitinib, angiotensin-(1-7), pomalidomide, tivozanib, MORAb-004) or combined with chemotherapy (cisplatin + AVE8062), are ongoing or have completed accrual and await reporting.

Targeting the PI3K-Akt-mTOR Pathway and IGF1R

Numerous translational and preclinical studies have suggested an important role for the PI3K-Akt-mTOR pathway in sarcomagenesis[19–21] as well as in the prognosis of STS.[22] Of note, aside from PTEN (phosphatase and tensin homologue) loss, genetic events involving the PI3K-Akt-mTOR pathway have been found to be relatively rare in sarcomas. Barretina and colleagues[23] reported PIK3CA mutations in 6 of 207 patients (3%), including 4 of 21 (18%) with myxoid round-cell liposarcoma. These data have provided the rationale for testing the clinical utility of inhibitors of the PI3K-Akt-mTOR pathway in patients with sarcomas. So far only rapalogs (analogue of rapamycin: ridaforolimus, temsirolimus, and sirolimus also known as rapamycin), which are inhibitors of mTORC1 (and not mTORC2), have been tested in clinical trials, and overall the results have been disappointing.

Ridaforolimus (MK8669, deforolimus, or AP23573) was assessed in a phase II study on 212 patients with advanced pretreated STS[2] who were stratified into 4 groups: leiomyosarcoma (n = 57), bone sarcoma (n = 54), liposarcoma (n = 44), and other STS (n = 57). Ridaforolimus was administered as an intravenous infusion, 12.5 mg daily for 5 days every 2 weeks. The primary end point was clinical benefit rate (CBR), defined as CR, PR, or SD for more than 16 weeks. The CBR was 29.5% in patients with liposarcoma, 33.3% in patients with leiomyosarcoma, and 21.2% in the group with other STS. The median PFS was similar in the different cohorts, ranging from 14.3 to 16.1 weeks. No predictive biomarkers have emerged. Based on these results suggesting an essentially cytostatic effect, a randomized, placebo-controlled, phase III study (SUCCEED)[3] evaluating ridaforolimus as maintenance therapy for patients with advanced STS who achieved SD or PR with first-, second-, or third-line chemotherapy was launched. In total, 711 patients were enrolled, 364 in the placebo arm and 347 in the ridaforolimus arm. This trial demonstrated a small but statistically significant benefit for ridaforolimus in terms of PFS (median PFS 17.7 weeks vs 14.6 weeks, $P<.001$), but no impact on overall survival. Moreover, the side effects were not negligible, especially stomatitis, thrombocytopenia, and pneumonitis, which occurred in 9%, 10%, and 3% of ridaforolimus-treated patients versus less than 1% each with placebo. Finally, as in many previous trials, no preselective biomarkers to assess the role of this targeted therapy were required. Merck Sharp & Dohme submitted an application for approval from the Food and Drug Administration, which was rejected.

Temsirolimus, which is approved for the management of patients with clear-cell renal cell carcinoma and mantle cell lymphoma, was evaluated in single-arm phase

II trial that enrolled 41 patients. Despite the choice to perform the study in a first-line advanced disease setting, the RR was low (5%) and the median PFS was short: 2.0 months (95% confidence interval 1.8–3.5).[4]

Activity of sirolimus was assessed in combination with metronomic oral cyclophosphamide in a single-arm, open-label, phase II trial. Forty-nine patients with advanced sarcomas (41 STS, 8 bone sarcomas) were enrolled in this study. Only 1 patient had a PR (RR 2%), and the median PFS and overall survival were 3.4 months and 10 months, respectively.[24]

Richter and colleagues[25] reported preliminary results of a phase II trial of everolimus in sarcomas, GIST, and ASPS. Two of 15 patients (13%) in the sarcoma cohort had SD, and no data were reported for the ASPS cohorts. However, the findings are in line with those of other rapalogs reported previously.

Based on these disappointing results the future of mTOR inhibitors in the management of STS remains uncertain. Great hope was set on combinations with chemotherapeutic agents (gemcitabine) and with other targeted agents (anti–insulin-like growth factor receptor 1 [IGF1R] monoclonal antibodies). However, here again the results reported thus far have been disappointing. Two phase Ib studies combining rapalogs and IGF1R inhibitor suggested interesting activity in sarcomas (either bone or soft tissue, or both). In one of these studies, everolimus 10 mg daily was given orally, combined with intravenous figitumumab every 3 weeks, to 21 patients.[26] One patient with solitary fibrous tumor had a PR and 11 patients remained on study for more than 3 months.[26] In another phase Ib study, Naing and colleagues[27] assessed the safety profile of cixutumumab combined with temsirolimus. In this study, 2 patients with Ewing sarcoma had a CR and 3 other patients had tumor shrinkage of less than 30% per RECIST (Response Evaluation Criterion for Solid Tumors) lasting from 8 to 27 months. The most frequent drug-related adverse events were mucositis, hyperglycemia, hypercholesterolemia, and thrombocytopenia.[27] The most recently reported study is an open-label phase II study of temsirolimus combined with the IGF1R monoclonal antibody cixutumumab (formerly IMC-A12), which was a 3-strata study: IGF1R-positive STS (arm A), IGF1R-positive bone sarcomas (arm B), and IGF1R-negative sarcomas (arm C) (bone and soft tissue). The primary objective was PFS at 12 weeks independently assessed in each cohort using a Simon 2-stage design. Four hundred eighteen patients were screened and 174 enrolled in the study: 57 in arm A, 54 in arm B, and 63 in arm C. The 12-week PFS rates were 32%, 35%, and 42% for cohorts A, B, and C, respectively, and were therefore close to the predefined threshold for activity based on the EORTC criteria.[2] A total of 10 PRs were seen, mostly in patients with bone sarcoma (5 Ewing sarcoma, 3 osteosarcoma, and 1 chondrosarcoma), with only 1 patient with solitary fibrous tumor achieving a PR in the STS arm. Another finding of this study is that the primary chosen biomarker (ie, IGF1R expression) does not seem to predict activity in STS, although it does seem to provide some predictive information in bone sarcomas.[28] Although this study met its primary end point,[28] the future of IGF1R inhibitors in the management of sarcomas is uncertain, as most pharmaceutical companies have stopped the development of such compounds.

Histone Deacetylase Inhibitors

Inhibition of histone deacetylase (HDAC) provides a novel approach for cancer treatment. HDAC deacetylates histones as well as other substrates relevant to cancer therapy, including the chaperone protein HSP90 and tubulins. HDAC inhibitors were shown to have activity in preclinical models of translocation-related sarcomas (synovial sarcoma, Ewing sarcoma).[29–31] The French sarcoma group (GSF/GETO) performed a single-arm phase II trial with panobinostat (formerly LBH589), a pan-HDAC inhibitor, in patients with advanced STS. In this study, 48 patients with advanced pretreated (median 2 lines of prior therapy) STS (liposarcoma, n = 11; leiomyosarcoma, n = 10; MPNST, n = 6; synovial sarcoma, n = 6) were treated with panobinostat given orally on Mondays, Wednesdays, and Fridays. One of the findings of this study was that 40 mg of panobinostat thrice a week was too toxic in this heavily pretreated patient population, and the dose had to be reduced to 20 mg after enrollment of the first 12 patients. From the efficacy standpoint, there were no PRs and only 6 patients (12.5%) were progression-free at 6 months.[32] A study with vorinostat has completed accrual but only pharmacokinetic data from this study have yet been reported.[33] Other studies are currently ongoing combining HDAC inhibitors with doxorubicin (PXD-101 and PCI-24781). Overall, despite very promising preclinical data, clinical results with HDAC inhibitors as single agents have been disappointing, and their development in solid tumors in general remains uncertain.

Hedgehog, Wnt, and Notch Signaling

Notch and Hedgehog (Hh) pathways play major roles in the development of pluricellular organisms. Their oncogenic role has emerged in recent decades.

The Hh pathway involves several actors: the Hh ligand, 2 transmembrane proteins called Patched (PTCH) and Smoothened (SMO), and transcription factors from the GLI family. In the absence of the Hh ligand, PTCH inhibits the activity of SMO. Binding of Hh ligand to PTCH relieves SMO from its inhibition by PTCH. Activated SMO leads to the release of activator forms of GLI, a zinc-finger transcription factor that then regulates the expression of several target genes involved in tumorigenesis.[34] Most of the currently available Hh inhibitors are small-molecule inhibitors of SMO, although some agents currently in preclinical development target Hh ligands.

In humans, Notch signaling is based on 4 Notch receptors (1–4) and 5 ligands (Delta-Like-1, -3, and -4 [DLL-1, DLL-3, and DLL-4] and Jagged-1 and Jagged-2 [JAG1 and JAG2]). Both ligand and receptor are cell-membrane bound in this system. On ligand binding, the intracellular part of Notch (NOTCH-IC) is released and translocates to the nucleus, where it binds to the transcription factor named CSL. Release of NOTCH-IC is in part due to cleavage from the membrane by γ-secretase. Most of the Notch-signaling inhibitors currently in development are actually inhibitors of γ-secretase. Physiologically, Notch signaling is involved in maintenance of an undifferentiated state, cell-fate decision, and induction of terminal differentiation. Notch signaling has been reported to be involved in human tumors both as an oncogene and as a tumor suppressor, suggesting that its transforming potential may be dependent on context and dosage.[35] This proposal seems to be true for sarcomas, as some reports have linked overexpression/activation of Notch signaling to a more aggressive phenotype (increased invasion and motility in rhabdomyosarcoma or proliferation in osteosarcoma)[36,37] while others have shown that Notch signaling is downregulated by the EWS-FLI1 fusion protein in Ewing sarcoma,[38] indicating a putative tumor-suppressing role for Notch in this disease.

Although activity of SMO inhibitors has been disappointing in chondrosarcoma, it is worth noting that the Hh pathway plays an important role in other sarcomas such as rhabdomyosarcoma or osteosarcoma.[39] Furthermore, recent preclinical studies suggest that combination of Hh and Notch pathway inhibitors may be synergistic in some sarcoma subtypes displaying activation of both pathways.[40] A phase I/II trial testing a combination of GDC-0449, an Hh inhibitor, and RO4929097, a γ-secretase inhibitor, was recently reported.[41] In this study, 34 patients with sarcomas of varying histology were treated with fixed doses of GDC0449 and increasing doses of RO4929097. Although no PRs were noted, durable SD (>16 weeks) was seen in 4 patients (12%). Based on these findings, the investigators recommend further clinical development of the combination in sarcomas.[41]

SUBTYPE-SPECIFIC APPROACHES
Targeting Angiogenesis in Vascular Tumors

Vascular tumors represent a heterogeneous group of tumors that either arise from or mimic vascular structures, and usually include angiosarcoma, epithelioid hemangioendothelioma (EHE), and hemagiopericytoma/solitary fibrous tumor (SFT). Targeting angiogenesis in these tumors has been seen as a rational approach because of the presumed vascular origins of these tumors. Several agents have been evaluated in these indications, but the most significant body of literature is found with sorafenib, which was evaluated in a specific trial as well as in several disease-specific cohorts in larger phase II trials. In the phase II trial reported by Maki and colleagues,[7] 37 patients with vascular tumors (angiosarcoma in 34, giant hemangioma in 1, and SFT in 2 cases) were treated with sorafenib. One patient had a CR, 4 had a PR (RR = 14%), and 21 had SD as their best response while the median PFS for this stratum was 3.8 months. Using a similar design the Southwest Oncology Group conducted a phase II trial (SWOG 0505) in 3 subgroups: vascular sarcoma, liposarcoma, and leiomyosarcoma. Because of the statistical design (Simon 2-stage design with a primary end point of RR ≥25%), the study was terminated after the first stage (total N = 37). None of the 8 patients with vascular tumors (5 angiosarcoma and 3 SFT) had a confirmed response. The French sarcoma group conducted a 4-strata phase II trial with sorafenib in patients with tumors of vascular origin (the ANGIONEXT study). In the first cohort, 41 patients with angiosarcoma (26 superficial and 15 visceral angiosarcoma) were treated: the best RR was 14.6% and the 9-month PFS rate (primary end point) was 2.4%, suggesting only minimal activity.[42] Of note, no KnockDown Resistance (KDR)/VEGFR2 mutation was found in any of the 27 patients for whom tumor material was available for analysis. These findings contrast with those of Antonescu and colleagues,[43] who found KDR/VEGFR2 mutations in 4 of 40 angiosarcoma samples, all KDR-mutated samples being from breast angiosarcomas. The reasons for these discrepancies are unknown, but the limited sample size of both studies may be a possible explanation. In a retrospective translational study D'Angelo and colleagues[44] reported Myc and Flt4 amplification in angiosarcoma of the breast responding to antiangiogenic therapy. In a separate cohort of the ANGIONEXT study, 15 patients with SFT and 5 patients with EHE were also treated with sorafenib.[45] In this group, 2 patients with EHE had a PR, and the 6-month and 9-month PFS rates were 38.8% and 33.3%, suggesting activity of sorafenib in these subsets. Results from 2 European retrospective studies suggest that antiangiogenic tyrosine kinase inhibitors have meaningful clinical activity in patients with SFT.[46,47] However, interpretation of these results is difficult, owing to the lack of any historical controls for these rare diseases (**Fig. 2**).

Several case reports have suggested activity of bevacizumab as a single agent in angiosarcoma and EHE. In a recently published phase II trial, 30 patients (23 angiosarcomas, 7 EHE), half of whom had received prior systemic therapy, were treated with bevacizumab (15 mg/kg every 3 weeks). Two of 23 patients with angiosarcoma (9%) and 2 of 7 patients with EHE (29%) achieved a PR. The median PFS was 12.4 weeks, and was longer in the EHE group (9 months, but more indolent disease) than in the

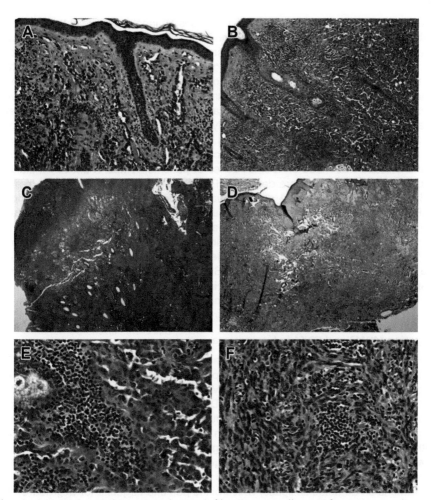

Fig. 2. Cutaneous angiosarcoma is an infiltrative, usually vasoformative, malignant neoplasm of dermis (*A, B*), with superficial ulceration (*C*) and/or mild to moderate lymphocytic inflammatory response (*D–F*) in almost half the cases: vasoformative cutaneous angiosarcoma with a lymphocytic response (*E*) and spindled cutaneous angiosarcoma with a lymphocytic response (*F*). (*From* Abedalthagafi M, Rushing EJ, Auerbach A, et al. Sporadic cutaneous angiosarcomas generally lack hypoxia-inducible factor 1α: a histologic and immunohistochemical study of 45 cases. Ann Diagn Pathol 2010;14(1):15–22; with permission.)

angiosarcoma group (2.8 months). The French sarcoma group (GSF/GETO) is currently conducting a randomized phase II study of paclitaxel with or without bevacizumab in patients with angiosarcoma.

Targeting Angiogenesis in Alveolar Soft-Part Sarcoma

ASPS is a very rare sarcoma (less than 1% of all sarcomas) characterized by a specific t(X;17) translocation, and is part of the family of microphthalmia transcription factor (MITF)-associated tumors, which also comprises clear-cell sarcoma and translocation-associated renal cell carcinoma. In ASPS, the t(X;17) fuses chromosomes 17q25 and Xp11.2, which results in the fusion of the ASPSCR1 and TFE3 genes (the latter being part of the MITF family). ASPS is an indolent but relentless disease with a high rate of metastasis to the lung and bone. The first report suggesting activity of antiangiogenic agents in ASPS was a case report from the MD Anderson Cancer Center regarding a 9-year-old patient with metastatic ASPS who had durable PR after treatment with bevacizumab in combination with interferon-α.[48] Since then, several other case series have shown activity of sunitinib, and a recent study reported activity of cediranib (AZD2171). In the report by Stacchiotti and colleagues,[49] 9 patients were treated with sunitinib 37.5 mg continuously, 5 of whom had a long-lasting PR and 3 SD; only the remaining patient had PD as best response, and the median PFS was 17 months. The first report of activity of cediranib (a VEGFR1–3 selective inhibitor) in this disease was made on a small series of patients treated in phase I/II trials.[50] In this report the investigators described PR or CR in 4 of 7 patients (57%) treated with cediranib 45 mg daily. A phase II trial of cediranib in patients with advanced ASPS was subsequently launched by the National Cancer Institute. In this study Kummar and colleagues[51] treated 46 patients (of whom 43 were evaluable for response) with advanced ASPS with cediranib, 30 mg daily. Twenty-eight patients (61%) had received at least one line of therapy for advanced disease. In this study the RR was 35% (15 of 43) and 26 had SD. The precise reason why these tumors respond to these inhibitors is unknown. However, the activity of these agents may be hypothesized to be mediated by the inhibition of the VEGF/VEGFR pathway, as bevacizumab, which is also active, only targets VEGF.

Targeting MDM2 and CDK4 in Liposarcoma

Amplification of the long arm of chromosome 12 has long been a diagnostic marker for well-differentiated and dedifferentiated liposarcoma (WD/DD-LPS). This amplicon targets, among other genes, MDM2 (HDM2) and CDK4. Amplification of MDM2 is recognized as a diagnostic criterion for WD/DD-LPS (as it appears to be constant in this disease) while CDK4 amplification is found in approximately 90%. Several agents targeting MDM2 and CDK4 are currently in development. Thus far the clinical results with agents targeting MDM2 and CDK4 suggest only minimal single-agent activity. Of interest is that molecular studies have suggested that targeting either of these genetic alterations with short-hairpin RNA leads to reduction in proliferation.[23]

MDM2 is an E3 ubiquitin ligase, which binds p53 and targets it for degradation by the proteasome. Most of the agents currently in development target the MDM2-p53 interaction. Ray-Coquard and colleagues[52] reported a phase 0 pharmacodynamic trial with RG7112, an orally bioavailable inhibitor of MDM2-p53. In this study, following an initial tumor biopsy 20 patients with biopsiable and/or operable, recurrent, WD/DD-LPS were given RG7112, 2500 mg daily for 5 days every 28 days for 1 to 3 cycles before undergoing resection or rebiopsy. This study met its pharmacodynamic end point, demonstrating reactivation of the p53 transcriptional program and induction of apoptosis between the pretreatment and posttreatment biopsy samples. Regarding efficacy, only 1 PR was seen and 14 patients had SD as their best response, although the treatment had limited duration. Other MDM2 inhibitors, including second-generation nutlin-3 analogues, are currently in clinical development, but no results with these agents have yet been reported.

CDK4 is a cyclin-dependent kinase that regulates the G1-S transition in the cell cycle and sits downstream of cyclin D1. Inhibitors currently in development are kinase inhibitors targeting, in most cases, both CDK4 and CDK6, and in some instances have a broader spectrum. Dickson and colleagues[53] reported the results of a phase II trial with the CDK4/6 PD0332991 in patients with CDK4-amplified WD/DD-LPS. Forty-four patients with advanced WD/DD-LPS were screened for CDK4 amplification (by fluorescent in situ hybridization) and Rb expression (by immunohistochemistry). The rationale for the screening of Rb expression is that CDK4 inhibition requires an active Rb to lead to cell-cycle arrest. Forty-two patients were positive for CDK4 amplification, 41 were Rb positive, and 29 patients with pretreated liposarcoma (median 1 line of prior therapy) were enrolled in the therapeutic cohort. The primary end point in this study was 12-week PFS, which was set at a 40% level to declare interest in the drug. In fact the 12-week PFS rate was 70%, and this study was therefore declared positive for its primary end point. The median PFS was 18 weeks (4.1 months), but no responses were reported. A placebo-controlled phase III trial evaluating PD0332991 in patients with advanced liposarcoma is currently in preparation (Philippe A. Cassier, personal communication, 2012).

mTOR Inhibition in Perivascular Epithelioid Cell Tumors

Perivascular epithelioid cell tumors (PEComas) are a very rare subgroup of mesen-chymal tumors that exhibit myo-melanocytic differentiation. These tumors belong to the same family of tumors as lymphangioleiomyomatosis and angiomyolipomas, which can be seen in patients with tuberous sclerosis complex, a disease caused by inactivating mutations of TSC1 or TSC2. TSC1 and TSC2 are upstream inhibitors of mTOR complex 1 (mTORC1), and their inactivation leads to increased activity of mTORC1, thus forming the basis for activity of rapalogs (which only inhibit mTORC1) in this group of diseases.[54] Case reports and small series have highlighted the frequent loss of either TSC1 or TSC2 in sporadic PEComas and angiomyolipomas,[55,56] with subsequent activation of TORC1 downstream signaling.[57] Interesting clinical activity has been seen with rapalogs (sirolimus and temsirolimus) in PEComa.[58–60] However, this has not been universally observed and responses are short lived in some pa-tients.[61,62] An industry-sponsored phase II trial with BEZ235, a dual PI3 kinase/mTORC1/2 inhibitor, is currently open to enrollment.

OTHER APPROACHES

Other studies on STS are currently ongoing, with a variety of agents. Among these, one could cite two phase II studies sponsored by the National Cancer Institute assess-ing alisertib (formerly MLN8237), an aurora kinase A inhibitor, which has shown (modest) antitumor activity in other solid tumors[62,63]: one in patients with advanced STS and the other in patients with advanced uterine sarcomas. Other interesting studies investigate the role of ipilimumab, a CTLA4 (Cytotoxic T-Lymphocyte Antigen 4)-targeting monoclonal antibody, combined with dasatinib. Although STS have not historically been regarded as immunosensitive tumors, the advent of newer immuno-therapies (such as CTLA4, PD-1, PD-L1, and 4-1BB targeting monoclonal antibodies) suggests that immunotherapy may be effective in many different tumor types, including ones previously not identified as immunosensitive. Dasatinib, which has been shown to have activity against sarcoma cell lines in vitro, may in addition serve as an immunomodulator in combination with ipilimumab, as suggested by studies in chronic myelogenous leukemias.

SUMMARY AND PERSPECTIVES

Despite significant progress in our understanding of the biology underlying the clinical heterogeneity of STS, only a few subtypes of sarcomas can currently be treated using rationally selected therapies. Inhibition of tumor angiogenesis has already proved to be a rational target in STS; much, however, remains to be done to derive predictive markers. Alternative strategies to target angiogenesis, either alone or combined with chemotherapy, are currently under evaluation in clinical trials. Some subtypes of sarcomas such as ASPS seem to be sensitive to inhibitors of angiogenesis, but the underlying mechanism remains unclear.

Like tumor angiogenesis, the PI3K-Akt-mTOR pathway is also a very attractive target in solid tumors. Numerous preclinical and translational studies have demonstrated the role of PI3K-Akt-mTOR pathway activation in the prognosis of STS. However, clinical results with first-generation inhibitors of mTOR have been disappointing. Despite these drawbacks, more work is probably needed to identify predictive markers in sarcomas but also in other solid tumors. Indeed, several newer inhibitors of this pathway (PI3K inhibitors, Akt inhibitors, or dual PI3K/mTOR inhibitors) are currently in development, and clear molecular markers are still missing and may significantly differ between agents. Here again, some sarcoma subtypes are clearly more sensitive than others to mTOR inhibitors.

Despite the fact that several studies are still recruiting STS of various histotypes, trials in selected histologies are clearly the way forward in clinical sarcoma research, as exemplified by several recent trials led by large cooperative groups. Cooperation is of paramount importance in enrolling patients with rare tumors and maintaining trial duration as short as possible. Although our understanding of sarcoma biology has improved over the last decade, much remains to be done in terms of therapeutic target identification and validation. Given the significant heterogeneity of these diseases, it is likely that we will not have relevant tumor models for all sarcomas in the coming years. We are therefore bound to lead and design trials that will have only limited preclinical background, if not empiric or opportunity guided. In an effort to derive as many data as possible from these clinical experiences, future trials should include pretreatment and posttreatment tumor biopsies to allow the identification of predictive factors if the drug is found to be active in a subset of patients, but also to enable hypothesis-generating translational research that will help plan the following generation of studies in STS.

REFERENCES

1. Schöffski P, Ray-Coquard IL, Cioffi A, et al. Activity of eribulin mesylate in patients with soft-tissue sarcoma: a phase 2 study in four independent histological subtypes. Lancet Oncol 2011;12:1045–52.
2. Van Glabbeke M, Verweij J, Judson I, et al. Progression-free rate as the principal end-point for phase II trials in soft-tissue sarcomas. Eur J Cancer 2002;38: 543–9.
3. Ganjoo KN, Cranmer LD, Butrynski JE, et al. A phase I study of the safety and pharmacokinetics of the hypoxia-activated prodrug TH-302 in combination with doxorubicin in patients with advanced soft tissue sarcoma. Oncology 2011;80: 50–6.
4. Chawla SP, Chua V, Hendifar A, et al. Phase Ib/II study of INNO-206 (EMCH-doxorubicin) in patients with soft tissue sarcoma. ASCO Meeting Abstracts. 2013.
5. George S, Blay JY, Casali PG, et al. Clinical evaluation of continuous daily dosing of sunitinib malate in patients with advanced gastrointestinal stromal tumour after imatinib failure. Eur J Cancer 2009;45:1959–68.
6. Tariq MS, Agresta S, Vigil CE, et al. Phase II study of sunitinib malate, a multitargeted tyrosine kinase inhibitor in patients with relapsed or refractory soft tissue sarcomas. Focus on three prevalent histologies: leiomyosarcoma, liposarcoma and malignant fibrous histiocytoma. Int J Cancer 2011;129:1963–9.

7. Maki RG, D'Adamo DR, Keohan ML, et al. Phase II study of sorafenib in patients with metastatic or recurrent sarcomas. J Clin Oncol 2009;27:3133–40.
8. Bertuzzi A, Stroppa EM, Secondino S, et al. Efficacy and toxicity of sorafenib monotherapy in patients with advanced soft tissue sarcoma failing anthracycline-based chemotherapy. J Clin Oncol (Meeting Abstracts) 2010;28:10025.
9. Ryan CW, Von Mehren M, Rankin CJ, et al. Phase II intergroup study of sorafenib (S) in advanced soft tissue sarcomas (STS): SWOG 0505. J Clin Oncol (Meeting Abstracts) 2008;26:10532.
10. D'Adamo DR, Keohan ML, Carvajal RD, et al. A phase II trial of sorafenib (S) and dacarbazine (D) in leiomyosarcoma (LMS), synovial sarcoma (SS), and malignant peripheral nerve sheath tumor (MPNST). J Clin Oncol (Meeting Abstracts) 2011;29:10025.
11. Meyer JM, Perlewitz KS, Hayden JB, et al. Phase I study of neoadjuvant chemoradiation (CRT) plus sorafenib (S) for high-risk extremity soft tissue sarcomas (STS). J Clin Oncol (Meeting Abstracts) 2012;30:10011.
12. DeLaney TF, Spiro IJ, Suit HD, et al. Neoadjuvant chemotherapy and radiotherapy for large extremity soft-tissue sarcomas. Int J Radiat Oncol Biol Phys 2003;56:1117–27.
13. Pisters PW, Patel SR, Prieto VG, et al. Phase I trial of preoperative doxorubicin-based concurrent chemoradiation and surgical resection for localized extremity and body wall soft tissue sarcomas. J Clin Oncol 2004;22:3375–80.
14. Verschraegen CF, rias-Pulido H, Lee SJ, et al. Phase IB study of the combination of docetaxel, gemcitabine, and bevacizumab in patients with advanced or recurrent soft tissue sarcoma: the Axtell regimen. Ann Oncol 2012;23:785–90.
15. D'Adamo DR, Anderson SE, Albritton K, et al. Phase II study of doxorubicin and bevacizumab for patients with metastatic soft-tissue sarcomas. J Clin Oncol 2005;23:7135–42.
16. Yoon SS, Duda DG, Karl DL, et al. Phase II study of neoadjuvant bevacizumab and radiotherapy for resectable soft tissue sarcomas. Int J Radiat Oncol Biol Phys 2011;81:1081–90.
17. Ratain MJ, Schwartz GK, Oza AM, et al. Brivanib (BMS-582664) in advanced solid tumors (AST): results of a phase II randomized discontinuation trial (RDT). J Clin Oncol (Meeting Abstracts) 2011;29:3079.
18. Schwartz GK, Maki RG, Ratain MJ, et al. Brivanib (BMS-582664) in advanced soft-tissue sarcoma (STS): biomarker and subset results of a phase II randomized discontinuation trial. J Clin Oncol (Meeting Abstracts) 2011;29:10000.
19. Hernando E, Charytonowicz E, Dudas ME, et al. The AKT-mTOR pathway plays a critical role in the development of leiomyosarcomas. Nat Med 2007;13:748–53.
20. Gutierrez A, Snyder EL, Marino-Enriquez A, et al. Aberrant AKT activation drives well-differentiated liposarcoma. Proc Natl Acad Sci U S A 2011;108:16386–91.
21. Friedrichs N, Trautmann M, Endl E, et al. Phosphatidylinositol-3'-kinase/AKT signaling is essential in synovial sarcoma. Int J Cancer 2011;129:1564–75.
22. Setsu N, Yamamoto H, Kohashi K, et al. The Akt/mammalian target of rapamycin pathway is activated and associated with adverse prognosis in soft tissue leiomyosarcomas. Cancer 2012;118:1637–48.
23. Barretina J, Taylor BS, Banerji S, et al. Subtype-specific genomic alterations define new targets for soft-tissue sarcoma therapy. Nat Genet 2010;42:715–21.
24. Schuetze SM, Zhao L, Chugh R, et al. Results of a phase II study of sirolimus and cyclophosphamide in patients with advanced sarcoma. Eur J Cancer 2012;48:1347–53.

25. Richter S, Pink D, Hohenberger P, et al. Multicenter, triple-arm, single-stage, phase II trial to determine the efficacy and safety of everolimus (RAD001) in patients with refractory bone or soft tissue sarcomas including GIST. J Clin Oncol (Meeting Abstracts) 2010;28:10038.

26. Quek R, Wang Q, Morgan JA, et al. Combination mTOR and IGF-1R inhibition: phase I trial of everolimus and figitumumab in patients with advanced sarcomas and other solid tumors. Clin Cancer Res 2011;17:871–9.

27. Naing A, LoRusso P, Fu S, et al. Insulin growth factor-receptor (IGF-1R) antibody cixutumumab combined with the mTOR inhibitor temsirolimus in patients with refractory Ewing's sarcoma family tumors. Clin Cancer Res 2012;18:2625–31.

28. Schwartz GK, Tap WD, Qin LX, et al. Cixutumumab and temsirolimus for patients with bone and soft-tissue sarcoma: a multicentre, open-label, phase 2 trial. Lancet Oncol 2013;14:371–82.

29. Kutko MC, Glick RD, Butler LM, et al. Histone deacetylase inhibitors induce growth suppression and cell death in human rhabdomyosarcoma in vitro. Clin Cancer Res 2003;9:5749–55.

30. Ito T, Ouchida M, Ito S, et al. SYT, a partner of SYT-SSX oncoprotein in synovial sarcomas, interacts with mSin3A, a component of histone deacetylase complex. Lab Invest 2004;84:1484–90.

31. Sakimura R, Tanaka K, Nakatani F, et al. Antitumor effects of histone deacetylase inhibitor on Ewing's family tumors. Int J Cancer 2005;116:784–92.

32. Cassier PA, Lefranc A, Penel N, et al. Efficacy and safety of panobinostat (LBH-589), a histone-deacetylase inhibitor (HDACi), in patients (pts) with advanced, previously treated soft tissue sarcoma (STS) and sex cord tumors (SCT): a study from the French Sarcoma Group. J Clin Oncol (Meeting Abstracts) 2012;30: 10027.

33. Schmitt T, Andres B, Liu L, et al. Pharmacokinetic analyses of vorinostat in patients with metastatic soft tissue sarcoma. J Clin Oncol (Meeting Abstracts) 2012;30:10041.

34. Ng JM, Curran T. The Hedgehog's tale: developing strategies for targeting cancer. Nat Rev Cancer 2011;11:493–501.

35. Ranganathan P, Weaver KL, Capobianco AJ. Notch signalling in solid tumours: a little bit of everything but not all the time. Nat Rev Cancer 2011;11:338–51.

36. Roma J, Masia A, Reventos J, et al. Notch pathway inhibition significantly reduces rhabdomyosarcoma invasiveness and mobility in vitro. Clin Cancer Res 2011;17:505–13.

37. Tanaka M, Setoguchi T, Hirotsu M, et al. Inhibition of Notch pathway prevents osteosarcoma growth by cell cycle regulation. Br J Cancer 2009;100:1957–65.

38. Ban J, nani-Baiti IM, Kauer M, et al. EWS-FLI1 suppresses NOTCH-activated p53 in Ewing's sarcoma. Cancer Res 2008;68:7100–9.

39. Kelleher FC, Cain JE, Healy JM, et al. Prevailing importance of the hedgehog signaling pathway and the potential for treatment advancement in sarcoma. Pharmacol Ther 2012;136:153–68.

40. Wang CY, Wei Q, Han I, et al. Hedgehog and Notch signaling regulate self-renewal of undifferentiated pleomorphic sarcomas. Cancer Res 2012;72: 1013–22.

41. Gounder MM, Dickson MA, Wu N, et al. A first-in-human, phase Ib combination study to assess safety, pharmacokinetics (PK), and pharmacodynamics (PD) of a hedgehog inhibitor, GDC-0449, with a Notch inhibitor, RO4929097, in patients with advanced sarcoma. J Clin Oncol (Meeting Abstracts) 2012;30: 10004.

42. Ray-Coquard I, Italiano A, Bompas E, et al. Sorafenib for patients with advanced angiosarcoma: a phase II Trial from the French Sarcoma Group (GSF/GETO). Oncologist 2012;17:260–6.

43. Antonescu CR, Yoshida A, Guo T, et al. KDR activating mutations in human angiosarcomas are sensitive to specific kinase inhibitors. Cancer Res 2009; 69:7175–9.

44. D'Angelo SP, Antonescu CR, Keohan ML, et al. Activity of sorafenib in radiation-associated breast angiosarcomas harboring MYC and FLT4 amplifications. J Clin Oncol (Meeting Abstracts) 2012;30:10019.

45. Chevreau C, Le Cesne A, Ray-Coquard I, et al. Phase II study of sorafenib mesylate (So) in patients (pts) with evolutive and advanced epithelioid hemangioendothelioma (EHE) or hemangiopericytoma/solitary fibrous tumor (SFT). J Clin Oncol (Meeting Abstracts) 2012;30:10020.

46. Stacchiotti S, Negri T, Libertini M, et al. Sunitinib malate in solitary fibrous tumor (SFT). Ann Oncol 2012;23:3171–9.

47. Levard A, Derbel O, Meeus P, et al. Outcome of patients with advanced solitary fibrous tumors: the Centre Leon Berard experience. BMC Cancer 2013; 13:109.

48. Azizi AA, Haberler C, Czech T, et al. Vascular-endothelial-growth-factor (VEGF) expression and possible response to angiogenesis inhibitor bevacizumab in metastatic alveolar soft part sarcoma. Lancet Oncol 2006;7:521–3.

49. Stacchiotti S, Negri T, Zaffaroni N, et al. Sunitinib in advanced alveolar soft part sarcoma: evidence of a direct antitumor effect. Ann Oncol 2011;22:1682–90.

50. Gardner K, Judson I, Leahy M, et al. Activity of cediranib, a highly potent and selective VEGF signaling inhibitor, in alveolar soft part sarcoma. J Clin Oncol (Meeting Abstracts) 2009;27:10523.

51. Kummar S, Allen D, Monks A, et al. Cediranib for metastatic alveolar soft part sarcoma. J Clin Oncol 2013;31(18):2296–302.

52. Ray-Coquard I, Blay JY, Italiano A, et al. Effect of the MDM2 antagonist RG7112 on the P53 pathway in patients with MDM2-amplified, well-differentiated or de-differentiated liposarcoma: an exploratory proof-of-mechanism study. Lancet Oncol 2012;13:1133–40.

53. Dickson MA, Tap WD, Keohan ML, et al. Phase II trial of the CDK4 inhibitor PD0332991 in patients with advanced CDK4-amplified well-differentiated or de-differentiated liposarcoma. J Clin Oncol 2013;31(16):2024–8.

54. McCormack FX, Inoue Y, Moss J, et al. Efficacy and safety of sirolimus in lymphangioleiomyomatosis. N Engl J Med 2011;364:1595–606.

55. El-Hashemite N, Zhang H, Henske EP, et al. Mutation in TSC2 and activation of mammalian target of rapamycin signalling pathway in renal angiomyolipoma. Lancet 2003;361:1348–9.

56. Pan CC, Chung MY, Ng KF, et al. Constant allelic alteration on chromosome 16p (TSC2 gene) in perivascular epithelioid cell tumour (PEComa): genetic evidence for the relationship of PEComa with angiomyolipoma. J Pathol 2008;214:387–93.

57. Kenerson H, Folpe AL, Takayama TK, et al. Activation of the mTOR pathway in sporadic angiomyolipomas and other perivascular epithelioid cell neoplasms. Hum Pathol 2007;38:1361–71.

58. Wagner AJ, Malinowska-Kolodziej I, Morgan JA, et al. Clinical activity of mTOR inhibition with sirolimus in malignant perivascular epithelioid cell tumors: targeting the pathogenic activation of mTORC1 in tumors. J Clin Oncol 2010;28: 835–40.

59. Italiano A, Delcambre C, Hostein I, et al. Treatment with the mTOR inhibitor temsirolimus in patients with malignant PEComa. Ann Oncol 2010;21:1135–7.

60. Pedersen JV, Benson C, Tunariu N, et al. A retrospective study from the Royal Marsden Hospital (RMH) of patients with malignant perivascular epithelioid cell tumors (PEComa) receiving treatment with sirolimus (SI) or temsirolimus (TSI). J Clin Oncol (Meeting Abstracts) 2012;30:10038.

61. Subbiah V, Trent JC, Kurzrock R. Resistance to mammalian target of rapamycin inhibitor therapy in perivascular epithelioid cell tumors. J Clin Oncol 2010;28: e415.

62. Macarulla T, Cervantes A, Elez E, et al. Phase I study of the selective Aurora A kinase inhibitor MLN8054 in patients with advanced solid tumors: safety, pharmacokinetics, and pharmacodynamics. Mol Cancer Ther 2010;9:2844–52.

63. Matulonis UA, Sharma S, Ghamande S, et al. Phase II study of MLN8237 (alisertib), an investigational Aurora A kinase inhibitor, in patients with platinum-resistant or -refractory epithelial ovarian, fallopian tube, or primary peritoneal carcinoma. Gynecol Oncol 2012;127:63–9.

Index

Note: Page numbers of article titles are in **boldface** type.

A

Adjuvant therapy, for soft tissue sarcomas of extremities and trunk wall, 925–928
  of GIST, 894–899
    clinical trials, 894–896
    future developments in, 899
    imatinib dose, 897–898
    management of recurrence during, 899
    patient follow-up during and after, 898
    preoperative imatinib, 896–897
    role of tumor mutation analysis, 897
    selection of patients for, 894
Aggressive fibromatosis. *See* Desmoid tumors.
Alveolar soft-part sarcoma, targeted therapies in, 1051–1052
  targeting angiogenesis in, 1071–1072
Angiogenesis, emerging therapies for soft tissue sarcomas targeting, 1065–1067
  targeting of, in alveolar soft-part sarcoma, 1071–1072
  targeting of, vascular tumors, 1070–1071
Angiosarcomas, and other sarcomas of endothelial origin, **975–988**
    angiogenesis *versus* vasculogenesis and growth of endothelial tumors, 977
    causes of, 977–978
    demographics, 976–977
    emerging therapeutic options, 983
    genetic changes in, 978–979
    pathologic abnormality of, 979–980
    primary therapy, 980–981
    scope of diagnoses, 976
    treatment of recurrent disease, 981–983
  localized, treatment for, 923–924
  of the breast, treatment of, 930–931
    primary, 930–931
    secondary, 931
Anthracyclines, for leiomyosarcomas, 962–963
Anti-inflammatory medications, in management of desmoid tumors, 995–996
Antiangiogenic inhibitors, for leiomyosarcoma, 965
Antiapoptosis, in chondrosarcoma therapy, 1035–1036
Aromatase inhibitors, in chondrosarcoma therapy, 1037
Atypical lipomatous tumor, localized, treatment for, 922–923

B

Bisphosphonates, in osteosarcoma treatment, 1029
Bone morphogenetic protein (BMP) signaling, in osteosarcoma therapy, 1024–1028

Hematol Oncol Clin N Am 27 (2013) 1079–1090
http://dx.doi.org/10.1016/S0889-8588(13)00125-1
0889-8588/13/$ – see front matter © 2013 Elsevier Inc. All rights reserved.

hemonc.theclinics.com

United States Postal Service

Statement of Ownership, Management, and Circulation
(All Periodicals Publications Except Requestor Publications)

1. Publication Title	2. Publication Number									3. Filing Date
Hematology/Oncology Clinics of North America	0	0	2	-	4	7	3			9/14/13

4. Issue Frequency	5. Number of Issues Published Annually	6. Annual Subscription Price
Feb, Apr, Jun, Aug, Oct, Dec	6	$367.00

7. Complete Mailing Address of Known Office of Publication *(Not printer) (Street, city, county, state, and ZIP+4®)*

Elsevier Inc.
360 Park Avenue South
New York, NY 10010-1710

Contact Person
Stephen R. Bushing

Telephone *(Include area code)*
215-239-3688

8. Complete Mailing Address of Headquarters or General Business Office of Publisher *(Not printer)*

Elsevier Inc., 360 Park Avenue South, New York, NY 10010-1710

9. Full Names and Complete Mailing Addresses of Publisher, Editor, and Managing Editor *(Do not leave blank)*

Publisher *(Name and complete mailing address)*

Linda Belfus, Elsevier, Inc., 1600 John F. Kennedy Blvd. Suite 1800, Philadelphia, PA 19103-2899

Editor *(Name and complete mailing address)*

Patrick Manley, Elsevier, Inc., 1600 John F. Kennedy Blvd. Suite 1800, Philadelphia, PA 19103-2899

Managing Editor *(Name and complete mailing address)*

Barbara Cohen – Kligerman, Elsevier, Inc., 1600 John F. Kennedy Blvd. Suite 1800, Philadelphia, PA 19103-2899

10. Owner *(Do not leave blank. If the publication is owned by a corporation, give the name and address of the corporation immediately followed by the names and addresses of all stockholders owning or holding 1 percent or more of the total amount of stock. If not owned by a corporation, give the names and addresses of the individual owners. If owned by a partnership or other unincorporated firm, give its name and address as well as those of each individual owner. If the publication is published by a nonprofit organization, give its name and address.)*

Full Name	Complete Mailing Address
Wholly owned subsidiary of	1600 John F. Kennedy Blvd., Ste. 1800
Reed/Elsevier, US holdings	Philadelphia, PA 19103-2899

11. Known Bondholders, Mortgagees, and Other Security Holders Owning or Holding 1 Percent or More of Total Amount of Bonds, Mortgages, or Other Securities. If none, check box → ☐ None

Full Name	Complete Mailing Address
N/A	

12. Tax Status *(For completion by nonprofit organizations authorized to mail at nonprofit rates) (Check one)*
The purpose, function, and nonprofit status of this organization and the exempt status for federal income tax purposes:
☐ Has Not Changed During Preceding 12 Months
☐ Has Changed During Preceding 12 Months *(Publisher must submit explanation of change with this statement)*

PS Form 3526, September 2007 (Page 1 of 3 (Instructions Page 3)) PSN 7530-01-000-9931 PRIVACY NOTICE: See our Privacy policy in www.usps.com

---

13. Publication Title	14. Issue Date for Circulation Data Below
Hematology/Oncology Clinics of North America	June 2013

15. Extent and Nature of Circulation			Average No. Copies Each Issue During Preceding 12 Months	No. Copies of Single Issue Published Nearest to Filing Date
a. Total Number of Copies *(Net press run)*			793	722
b. Paid Circulation (By Mail and Outside the Mail)	(1)	Mailed Outside-County Paid Subscriptions Stated on PS Form 3541. *(Include paid distribution above nominal rate, advertiser's proof copies, and exchange copies)*	294	251
	(2)	Mailed In-County Paid Subscriptions Stated on PS Form 3541 *(Include paid distribution above nominal rate, advertiser's proof copies, and exchange copies)*		
	(3)	Paid Distribution Outside the Mails Including Sales Through Dealers and Carriers, Street Vendors, Counter Sales, and Other Paid Distribution Outside USPS®	202	173
	(4)	Paid Distribution by Other Classes Mailed Through the USPS (e.g. First-Class Mail®)		
c. Total Paid Distribution *(Sum of 15b (1), (2), (3), and (4))*		▶	496	424
d. Free or Nominal Rate Distribution (By Mail and Outside the Mail)	(1)	Free or Nominal Rate Outside-County Copies Included on PS Form 3541	116	113
	(2)	Free or Nominal Rate In-County Copies Included on PS Form 3541		
	(3)	Free or Nominal Rate Copies Mailed at Other Classes Through the USPS (e.g. First-Class Mail)		
	(4)	Free or Nominal Rate Distribution Outside the Mail (Carriers or other means)		
e. Total Free or Nominal Rate Distribution *(Sum of 15d (1), (2), (3) and (4))*		▶	116	113
f. Total Distribution *(Sum of 15c and 15e)*		▶	612	537
g. Copies not Distributed *(See instructions to publishers #4 (page #3))*		▶	181	185
h. Total *(Sum of 15f and g)*		▶	793	722
i. Percent Paid *(15c divided by 15f times 100)*		▶	81.05%	78.96%

16. Publication of Statement of Ownership
☐ If the publication is a general publication, publication of this statement is required. Will be printed in the October 2013 issue of this publication. ☐ Publication not required

17. Signature and Title of Editor, Publisher, Business Manager, or Owner

[signature] Stephen R. Bushing – Inventory/Distribution Coordinator

Date September 14, 2013

I certify that all information furnished on this form is true and complete. I understand that anyone who furnishes false or misleading information on this form or who omits material or information requested on the form may be subject to criminal sanctions (including fines and imprisonment) and/or civil sanctions (including civil penalties).

PS Form 3526, September 2007 (Page 2 of 3)

Moving?

Make sure your subscription moves with you!

To notify us of your new address, find your **Clinics Account Number** (located on your mailing label above your name), and contact customer service at:

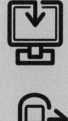

Email: journalscustomerservice-usa@elsevier.com

800-654-2452 (subscribers in the U.S. & Canada)
314-447-8871 (subscribers outside of the U.S. & Canada)

Fax number: 314-447-8029

Elsevier Health Sciences Division
Subscription Customer Service
3251 Riverport Lane
Maryland Heights, MO 63043

*To ensure uninterrupted delivery of your subscription,
please notify us at least 4 weeks in advance of move.

Printed and bound by CPI Group (UK) Ltd, Croydon, CR0 4YY

03/10/2024

01040492-0005